Cardiology and Cardiac Catheterisation

To my wife Margaret

J.B.

To my wife Susan and daughters Elizabeth and Sarah

D.W.M.M.

In memory of Ray Kelly
doctor, colleague, friend

Cardiology And Cardiac Catheterisation

The Essential Guide

Edited by

John Boland
Physiologist and Senior Hospital Scientist, Cardiac Catheterisation Unit,
St Vincent's Hospital, Sydney, Australia

and

David W.M. Muller
Interventional Cardiologist and Director, Cardiac Catheterisation Unit,
St Vincent's Hospital, Sydney, Australia

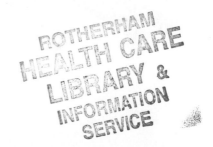

harwood academic publishers
Australia · Canada · France · Germany · India · Japan · Luxembourg
Malaysia · The Netherlands · Russia · Singapore · Switzerland

Amsteldijk 166
1st Floor
1079 LH Amsterdam
The Netherlands

British Library Cataloguing in Publication Data

A catalogue record for this book is available from the British Library.

ISBN 90-5823-131-3

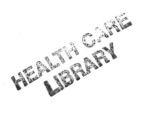

Cover design by Lee McLachlan

Preface

The field of cardiovascular medicine has catapulted forward in the past few years, owing to significant changes in our approach to patients with acute ischemic heart disease, valvular abnormalities, and prevention of serious arrhythmias. Back in the 1980s, cardiology was revolutionized by an aggressive approach to restoring coronary blood flow in acute myocardial infarction. This took several years to become standard practice, but the spirit of more aggressive management has been transmitted to virtually all diagnoses and treatments in cardiology and cardiac surgery. Of note, these changes have only come about as an outgrowth of intensive clinical investigation, with rigorous, large-scale randomised trials and insightful mechanistic studies. The buzz word of 'evidence-based medicine' has been a cornerstone for accepting many of the newer and more active strategies.

It is hard to find a reference source that captures the latest developments in a comprehensive way. But this book carefully edited by John Boland and David Muller is a superb contribution to our field. This monograph covers core clinical areas such as the electrocardiogram, pressure wave forms, physiological monitoring. Building on this theme, there is heavy emphasis on the physiologic approach to the patient, with chapters on cardiac output and shunts, determination of oxygen status, use of pressure–volume loops for assessing left ventricular function, and two chapters dedicated to interpreting pressure waveforms. With fundamental reviews of atherosclerosis, coagulation, and cardiovascular pharmacology, all of the latest therapies are reviewed including anticoagulants, new anti-platelet agents, and reperfusion therapy. Not just the pharmacology is reviewed, but also device therapies including stenting, vascular closure devices, catheter-based reperfusion of acute myocardial infarction, endovascular therapy of the carotid and peripheral vasculature, approach to valvular diseases, and the potential for angiogenesis and gene therapy. Some particularly useful and hard to find chapters are included on radiation safety, nursing considerations, infection control, haemodynamic monitoring in transplant patients, and evidence-based cardiac catheterisation.

In aggregate, this book is a unique monograph which covers many vital aspects of cardiovascular medicine and surgery in a thorough, refreshing, and highly pragmatic fashion. It will undoubtedly be well received by the cardiology physician, trainee, and nurse community. John Boland and David Muller, together with their superb expert contributors, deserve kudos for their fine work.

Eric J. Topol, MD
Chairman, Department of Cardiology
Cleveland Clinic Foundation
Cleveland, OH, USA

Contents

Foreword

Cardiac catheterisation began in 1929 when Werner Forsmann exposed a vein in his left arm, introduced a ureteric catheter under local anaesthetic, walked to the x-ray department and advanced it under fluoroscopic guidance into the right atrium. This was lost in the world literature until a Frenchman A. F. Cournard and an American D. W. Richards in 1941 used the technique to measure cardiac output and pulmonary artery pressures. In 1947 Lewis Dexter and his colleagues used cardiac catheterisation to study and diagnose congenital heart disease.

In Australia, catheterisation of the right heart began in two Sydney hospitals, at Royal Prince Alfred Hospital in 1947 and at St Vincent's Hospital in 1954. At St Vincent's Hospital, the studies were carried out in a small room in the x-ray department under fluoroscopic guidance. There was no image intensification and no check or control of radiation safety. Pressures were recorded using cumbersome equipment that often took an hour or more to calibrate, and pressure waveforms were recorded using either direct writing pens or photographic equipment. There were no display screens or computers. Catheters were re-used and were sterilised by boiling in water. It was not unusual for the patient to experience rigors after the procedure as a result of pyrogens within the catheter. In the first year 104 cases were performed.

The senior doctors had learned the techniques in Great Britain and America, but were largely self-taught. They instructed assisting nurses and later junior medical, scientific and technical staff. Collective knowledge and expertise were passed down by word and example. There was no course and no textbook to introduce the newcomer to the mysteries of cardiac output, the Fick principle, or the changes in waveform in the different cardiac chambers.

In 1957, catheterisation via the left brachial artery began, and Dr Geoff Benness performed the first coronary areteriogram in Australia at St Vincent's Hospital in 1962. Harry Windsor performed the first human heart transplant in Australia in 1968, which established St Vincent's Hospital as Sydney's cardiac biopsy centre for the next decade. Staff at St Vincent's performed Australia's first intracoronary thrombolysis in 1979 and Australia's first coronary angioplasty in 1980. Since then St Vincent's has played a prominent role in interventional cardiology by leading the way in applying new interventional techniques and hosting interventional demonstration courses.

This progress in interventional cardiology has been made possible by dramatic advances in instrumentation and technology. Image intensification, display screens, computers, sophisticated catheters and percutaneous techniques have revolutionised the cardiac catheterisation laboratory, where several disciplines interact in a very sophisticated environment to provide quality patient care. Despite these advances, until now there has been no textbook to which the newcomer could turn for appropriate information.

John Boland and David Muller have now filled this void by editing a valuable contribution covering all aspects of the techniques and problems encountered in both the cardiac diagnostic and research laboratories. Their co-authors are experienced cardiologists and scientists from Australia and overseas.

I hope that this excellent monograph will be widely read and prove of great help to the many medical, nursing and health professional support staff without whom modern procedural cardiology would not be possible.

Emeritus Professor John B. Hickie, AO

Acknowledgements

A publication of this scope would not have been possible without the dedicated involvement of many individuals.

In particular, we would like to express our appreciation to our corporate sponsors for their confidence and support, and to the many companies that provided material for inclusion in this text. We are also grateful to all our contributors for their collaboration in this production, and for editorial assistance. In this respect we are much indebted to Dr Albert Ambroglio, Dr Carl Holbeck, Professor Kanji Inoue, Dr Joyce Low, Dr Preston Mason, Dr Julie Mundy, Sr Sally Newport and Dr Marcia Zucker for their helpful guidance in reviewing parts of this book.

We are especially grateful to Julie Murray of Medici Graphics for her artistic contributions in preparing the illustrations, mostly as original artwork, also to Bill Cheung for photographic reproductions, and to Harwood Academic Publishers for their unstinting professionalism in producing the finished publication.

To the many staff at St Vincent's Hospital, and all others whose assistance in numerous ways facilitated this work, our heartfelt thanks for their confidence and support over a demanding but particularly satisfying period.

This production is proudly sponsored by:

Boston Scientific Corporation Pty Ltd, 4A Lord Street, Botany, NSW, 2019

Eli Lilly Australia Pty Ltd, 112 Wharf Road, West Ryde, NSW, 2114

GE/Marquette Medical Systems Australia Pty Ltd, Forest Corporate Centre, Suite 3, 17 Rodborough Road, Frenchs Forest, NSW, 2086

Medical Applications Pty Ltd, 56 Buffalo Road, Gladesville, NSW, 2111

Medtel Australia Pty Ltd, 5 Orion Road, Lane Cove, NSW, 2066

Medtronic Pty Ltd, Unit 4/446 Victoria Road, Gladesville, NSW, 2111

St Jude Medical Australia Pty Ltd, 10b/10 Mallett Street, Camperdown, NSW, 2050

Contributors

Arnold, Ruth MBBS, FRACP, Cardiac Transplant Unit, St Vincent's Hospital, Sydney, NSW, Australia, 2010

Baron, David MBBS, FRACP, FCCP, Interventional Cardiologist, Department of Cardiology, St Vincent's Hospital, Sydney, NSW, Australia, 2010.

Boland, John BSc, MSc (Pathology), Physiologist, Senior Hospital Scientist, Cardiac Catheterisation Unit, St Vincent's Hospital, Sydney, NSW, Australia, 2010

Brouwer, S. RN, Ba HSc (Nursing), Dip H Sc, Nurse Unit Manager, Cardiac Catheterisation Laboratory, St Vincent's Hospital, Sydney, NSW, Australia, 2010

Campbell, Claudia N. BS, MS (Microbiol) Marketing Manager, Clinical and Regulatory Affairs, International Technidyne Corporation, 8 Olsen Avenue, Edison NJ 08820, USA

Campbell, Terence J. MD, PhD, FRACP, FACC, Professor of Medicine, St Vincent's Hospital and The University of New South Wales, Sydney, NSW, Australia, 2033

Carroll, Gerard MBBS (Hons), FRACP, Consultant Cardiologist, Director Cardiac Catheterisation Unit, Calvary Hospital, Wagga Wagga, NSW, Australia, 2650

Chew, Derek MBBS, Department of Cardiology, Austin & Repatriation Medical Center, Heidelberg, Victoria, Australia, 3084.

Colombo, Antonio MD, Director, Cardiac Catheterisation Laboratory, Columbus Hospital, Milan, Italy; Director of Investigational Angioplasty, Lenox Hill Hospital, New York, USA

Cross, Peter PhD CPhys MInstP MAAPM MACPSEM, Radiological Physicist, Department of Radiation Oncology, St Vincent's Hospital, Sydney, NSW, Australia.

Faddy, Steven B. App.Sc (Biomedical Sc), AICTA, MAIMS, Physiologist, Scientific Officer, Cardiac Catheterisation Unit, St Vincent's Hospital, Sydney, NSW, Australia, 2010

Feneley, Michael P. MD, FRACP, FACC, Associate Professor of Medicine, Director of Cardiology, St Vincent's Hospital, Sydney, NSW, Australia, 2010

Gavaghan, Tom MBBS, FRACP, Consultant Cardiologist, Sydney Adventist Hospital, 185 Fox Valley Road, Wahroonga, NSW, Australia, 2076

Greenfield, Jerry MBBS (Hons), BSc (Med), Senior Endocrinology Registrar, St Vincent's Hospital, Sydney, NSW, Australia, 2010

Hadjipetrou, Peter MBBS, FRACP, Interventional Cardiologist, St Andrew's Hospital Heart Institute, Brisbane, QLD, Australia, 4004

Harkness, Jock MBBS, DCP (LON), FRCPA, FASM, Director of Microbiology, St Vincent's Hospital, Sydney, NSW, Australia, 2010

Hayward, Christoper S. BmedSc, MD, FRACP, Cardiologist, Department of Cardiac Medicine, National Heart and Lung Institute, Imperial College, London, United Kingdom

Horrigan, Mark MBBS, FRACP, Deputy Director of Cardiology, Department of Cardiology, Austin & Repatriation Medical Centre, Heidelberg, Victoria, Australia, 3084.

Isner, Jeffrey M. MD, FACC, Chief, Vascular Medicine, Chief, Cardiovascular Research, Professor of Medicine and Pathology, Tuft's University School of Medicine, St Elizabeth's Medical Center, Boston, MA, USA

Juul, Marcus BSc, Physiologist, Scientific Officer, Thoracic Medicine Department (Lung Function Unit), Bryan Dwyer Department of Anaesthetics, St Vincent's Hospital, Sydney, NSW, Australia, 2010

Kelly, Raymond P. MD FRACP FACC, Cardiologist, Associate Professor of Medicine, Department of Cardiology, St Vincent's Hospital, Sydney, NSW, Australia, 2010

Kelly, Steven ADDR, Dip App Sc, B Med Sc, MIR, Product Manager, Medical Applications Pty Ltd, 56 Buffalo Road, Gladesville, NSW, Australia, 2111.

Keogh, Anne MBBS, MD, FRACP, Cardiologist, Associate Professor of Medicine, Senior Lecturer in Medicine, Cardiac Transplant Unit, St Vincent's Hospital, Sydney, NSW, Australia, 2010

Koo, Kim L. RN, CM, CCNC, Dip N Mgt, Nurse Unit Manager, Cardiac Catheterisation Laboratory, St Vincent's Hospital, Sydney, NSW, Australia, 2010

Kuchar, Dennis L. MB, BS (Hons), MD, FRACP, FACC, Interventional Cardiologist, Director, Coronary Care Unit, St Vincent's Hospital, Sydney, NSW, Australia, 2010

Lee, Chris Applications Specialist, GE Marquette Medical Systems Aust Pty Ltd, Forest Corporate Centre Suite 3, Rodborough Road, Frenchs Forest, NSW, Australia, 2086.

Lemmon, Jennifer RN, B Nurs, ICC, Infection Control Clinical Nurse Consultant, St Vincent's Hospital, Sydney, NSW, Australia, 2010

Losordo, Douglas W. MD, FACC, Associate Professor, Divisions of Cardiology and Cardiovascular Research, St Elizabeth's Medical Center, Tuft's University School of Medicine, Boston, MA, USA

Lowe, Harry C. MB, BCh, FRACP, Cardiologist and Postgraduate Scholar, Centre for Thrombosis and Vascular Research, University of New South Wales, Sydney, NSW, Australia, 2006

Macdonald Peter MBBS, PhD, FRACP, Cardiologist, Associate Professor of Medicine, Cardiac Transplant Unit, St Vincent's Hospital, Sydney, NSW, Australia, 2010

Maree, Aran MB, MRCPI, Cardiologist, Cardiac Catheterisation Unit, St Vincent's Hospital, Sydney, NSW, Australia, 2010.

Mumford, Drew MBBS (Hons), BSc (Med), Senior Cardiology Registrar, St Vincent's Hospital, Sydney, NSW, Australia, 2010

Muller, David W.M. MD, FRACP, FACC, Associate Professor of Medicine, Director, Cardiac Catheterisation Laboratories, St Vincent's Hospital, Sydney, NSW, Australia, 2010.

Nankivell, Brian J. MD (Syd), BSc, MSc (Pharmacology), PhD, MRCP (UK), FRACP, Consultant Physician and Nephrologist, Department of Medicine, University of Sydney, Westmead Hospital, NSW, Australia, 2145

Nicholson, Anthony BVSc, PhD, Dip ACVA, Senior Hospital Scientist, Bryan Dwyer Department of Anaesthetics, St Vincent's Hospital, Sydney, NSW, Australia, 2010.

Oldfield, Geoffrey S. MBBS, FRACP, Consultant Cardiologist, John Hunter Hospital, Newcastle, NSW, Australia, 2300; Director CCU, Catheterisation & Angioplasty Laboratory, Lake Macquarie Hospital, Newcastle, NSW, Australia, 2290

Roy, Paul MBBS, FRACP, FACC, FSCA, FRCP, Interventional Cardiologist, Department of Cardiology, St Vincent's Hospital, Sydney, NSW, Australia, 2010.

Sammel, Neville MB BCh, FRACP, FACC, DDU, Cardiologist, St Vincent's Hospital, Sydney, NSW, Australia, 2010.

Thorburn, Charles W. MA, FRCP, FRACP, Cardiologist, Department of Cardiology, St Vincent's Hospital, Sydney, NSW, Australia, 2010

Vale, Peter R MD, FRACP, Cardiologist and Vascular Physician, Divisions of Vascular Medicine and Cardiovascular Research, St Elizabeth's Medical Center, Tuft's University School of Medicine, Boston, MA, USA

Wilson, Michael K. BSc (Med), MBBS, FRACS (General and Cardiothoracic Surgery), Cardiothoracic and Transplant Surgeon, St Vincent's Hospital, Sydney, NSW, Australia, 2010

Winlaw, David S. MB BS(Hons), MD, FRACS, Fellow in Cardiothoracic Surgery, St Vincent's Hospital, Sydney, NSW, Australia, 2010.

Zucker, Marcia L. BSc (Biol), MA (Biochem) PhD (Molecular Biology), Director of Clinical Research, Clinical and Regulatory Affairs, International Technidyne Corporation, 8 Olsen Avenue, Edison NJ 08820, USA

Chapter 1

The Cardiac Imaging System

Digital Cardiac Angiography

Steven Kelly

History

In November 1895, whilst experimenting with a cathode ray tube, Wilhelm Conrad Roentgen, a physicist at the University of Wurtzburg in Germany, saw a weak flickering greenish light on a piece of cardboard coated with a fluorescent chemical preparation. Roentgen later verified that the cathode ray tube was the source of invisible rays with an unexpected power of penetration.

A month later the first image of human anatomy, the hand of Roentgen's wife, was obtained using an exposure time of some 30 minutes. He told his wife; 'I am doing something that will cause people to say "Roentgen has gone mad"'. Whether this quote can be actually attributed to Roentgen or not, the statement well describes the furor following the presentation of his paper, *A New Type of Rays*.

Today, just over 100 years later, the ability to see into the living body without the need for surgical invasion is perhaps the most historically significant advance in medical diagnostics, having far-reaching implications for medical therapy, specifically in the area of cardiovascular disease.

In 1929 Werner Forssmann introduced a catheter into his own right atrium via the antecubital vein. His intention was to develop a method of rapid delivery for medications. In the same year the first x-ray tube featuring a rotating anode disc was released.

Over the next 30 years, cardiac catheterisation developed from a method by which cardiac physiology could be studied experimentally, to an established clinical investigational technique used in the diagnosis of congenital and valvular heart disease. In 1959 cardiac catheterisation became the preferred method for the investigation of coronary artery disease.

Advances in radiological and cardiac imaging techniques over the same period included development of the mechanical cassette changer, the AOT film changer, the image intensifier (1952) and acceptance of 35 mm cine film to capture rapid sequence x-ray images. These developments formed a technical framework on which early imaging systems in the cardiac laboratory were based. In the 1960s television provided an interactive means of obtaining clinical information from an x-ray source.

Cardiologists of the early 1970s, in collaboration with various imaging companies, helped to develop the first dedicated cardiac stand and generator, using 35 mm cine film as the recording medium. The first dedicated cardiac stands of this period were based on a parallelogram or U-arm using conventional x-ray generators and featured the image intensifier above the patient.

In 1976 the Optimus Modular 200 x-ray generator and Polydiagnost C (parallelogram based) gantry were introduced. The combination of this generator and gantry formed the backbone of many cardiac centres worldwide for the next 20 years. This generator, with its tetrode switching of high-tension voltages, was the first to incorporate the 'measuring shot' technique, eliminating the need to predetermine the exposure parameters of voltage, current and time.

Advances in cardiac surgery during the 1970s led to coronary artery bypass surgery becoming a viable clinical option for patients suffering coronary artery disease. During this period, significant technological refinements in both surgery and cardiac catheterisation techniques created a need for an increased diagnostic yield from cardiac imaging, resulting in the first digital cardiac imaging systems in late 1985.

The enormous demand placed on imaging equipment by routine diagnostic procedures, and more so by prolonged interventional procedures, saw further technical advances in imaging equipment in early 1989, and again an advance specifically tailored to the needs of cardiac imaging. The Maximus Rotalix Ceramic (MRC) x-ray tube featured a continuously rotating anode with liquid metal lubricated spiral groove bearing technology. This x-ray tube provided a mechanism by which the enormous heat loadings produced by cardiac procedures could be effectively dissipated and, just as importantly, provided a significant reduction in radiation dose.

Since the initial use of 35 mm cine film as a recording medium, several alternatives have been used, all essentially for cost-saving purposes. These alternatives documented the procedure in an analogue format, of poorer quality than the images obtained digitally at the time of the examination. In early 1995 this problem was overcome by digital archive systems and compact disc technology.

Table 1.1. Major events in the development of cardiac imaging equipment.

1895	Discovery of x-rays
1896	Use of x-rays for medical diagnosis
1906	First contrast-filled image of the renal system
1929	First heart catheterisation by Forssmann on himself
1929	Development of an x-ray tube with a rotating anode disc
1945	Visualisation of the coronary arteries
1946	Automatic x-ray exposures with IONTOMAT
1952	X-ray image intensifiers
1953	Cut-film changer with 6 exposures/sec for angiography
1970s	Commercial deliveries of the first dedicated cardiac catheterisation systems (mainly to the USA)
1985	The first Digital Cardiac Imaging (DCI) system
1989	Maximus Rotalix Ceramic (MRC) x-ray tubes. The first x-ray tube to contain a continuously rotating anode and liquid metal lubricated spiral groove bearing technology
1990	1024 x 1024 imaging matrix
1991	The first fully integrated (fibre optic) system network
1992	Archiving of cardiac images to compact disc as per the ACC/NEMA DICOM standard
1993	Integrated second generation digital Charge Coupled Device (CCD)-based imaging chain
1998	The first cardiac digital network for distribution of cardiac catheterisation studies within the hospital.

Current technology

A modern cardiac laboratory is no longer an x-ray imaging system based on or modified from angiography equipment used in radiology. Today's cardiac laboratory consists of:

1. X-ray generator capable of pulsed fluoroscopy at rates equal to minimum acquisition rates of 12.5 frames per second (fps) and allowing digital acquisition at rates up to 50 fps. An achievable current of 1000 milliamperes (mA) at 100 kilovolts (kV) is essential.
2. X-ray tube incorporating a continuously rotating anode and utilising liquid metal lubricated spiral groove bearing technology and an oil heat exchanger.
3. Image intensifier (ii) combined with either a video camera or a digital output Charged Coupled Device (CCD) camera.
4. Monitor(s).
5. An analogue to digital (A/D) converter.
6. Digital storage device.
7. Archive device +/- review station.
8. Networking capabilities for multi-laboratory/multi-center archive and review.

Specifications and instrumentation

Typical cardiac catheterisation imaging equipment is shown in Fig. 1.1.

Where does it all begin?

X-rays are produced within an x-ray tube when electrons from the cathode filament bombard and interact with a rotating disc of metal, the anode. The anode and cathode are mounted a short distance apart. A high voltage is applied between the anode (positive terminal) and the source of electrons, the cathode filament (negative terminal). A high voltage is required to accelerate electrons from the cathode filament and is obtained from a transformer which converts mains voltages to the voltages required for diagnostic imag-

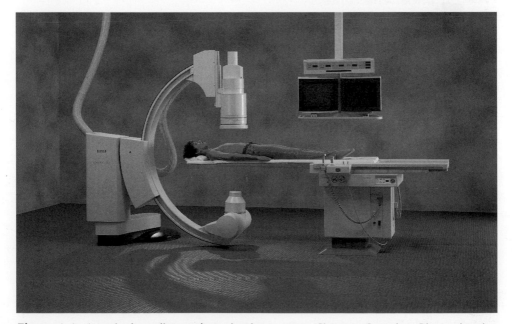

Figure 1.1. A typical cardiac catheterisation system (Siemens Coroskop Plus), showing position of patient on examination table, X-ray tube and image intensifier.

ing, 40 kilovolts to 130 kilovolts (kV). This transformer and other components form the basis of the x-ray generator. Bombardment of electrons on the heavy metal of the anode results in generation of x-rays. The anode contains a high proportion of a heavy metal such as molybdenum or tungsten, as heavy metals maximise generation of x-ray energy.

X-ray generators used in cardiac imaging are microprocessor-controlled and contain medium- to high-frequency converters. The kilowatt (kW) is the unit used to describe the power output of x-ray generators. For cardiac imaging up to 100 kW of power are required.

What is image quality?

The clinical information obtained in cardiac imaging is a function of spatial resolution and the dynamic contrast range displayed. Image contrast is affected by high voltage. A high kV results in increased penetration and consequently in reduced image contrast. Due to the inherent properties of the iodine-based contrast medium used in cardiac imaging, subtle differences in image contrast are most evident when images are acquired at 70 kV. The high-frequency generators used in cardiac imaging require high output power to provide images to occur around this 70 kV value.

Because cardiac structures move during acquisition, a short generator switching time ('exposure time') is required, this value being fixed at approximately 8 milliseconds (ms). To then be able to acquire images without motion artifact and at voltages best suited to iodine-based contrast (70kV), the x-ray generator must operate at currents of at least 500–600 mA, and typically at values up to 1000 mA. This is required to maximise contrast resolution.

The high-voltage supply from the x-ray tube accelerates electrons from the cathode. If this voltage varies over time, the x-ray output will change during an exposure, thus influencing image quality. Modern x-ray generators are therefore designed to have very low variation in the higher voltages. The control unit of a generator controls tube current and exposure time, controls anode rotation and has other additional functions.

'The bit under the table'

The x-ray tube is contained within a metal housing lined with lead shielding. The tube housing provides the mechanical connection between the x-ray tube and the rest of the x-ray system and is filled with oil in order to conduct heat away from the x-ray tube. X-rays are emitted through an opening in the metal housing. The tube is provided with a window made of a very light material such as beryllium or thin glass to permit unrestricted outflow of x-rays in the chosen direction.

A collimator (a mechanism to attenuate, or focus, or restrict a beam of energy into a narrow field or column) is mounted on the x-ray tube housing. The collimator limits the x-ray beam to the minimum area needed for the diagnostic procedure. This protects patient and operator from unnecessary radiation and improves image quality by reducing the amount of scattered radiation. An iris diaphragm located within the collimator produces a circular field of irradiation focused onto the image intensifier. The collimator also contains two pairs of lead shutters that can be adjusted to limit the beam area through a rectangular field. A semi-transparent wedge-shaped filter is incorporated within the collimator to overcome attenuation differences between different anatomical areas. The ability to position this filter and also the collimator shutters under Last Image Hold (LIH) conditions (i.e. without need for fluoroscopy) has recently been implemented in some cardiac imaging systems. This can lead to significantly reduced radiation doses to both patient and operators.

The rotating anode of the x-ray tube is coupled to the static part of the tube by liquid metal lubricated spiral groove bearings that have replaced ball bearings in the anode support construction. Unlike conventional x-ray tubes, the anode in x-ray tubes of dedicated cardiac imaging equipment rotates continuously. This produces an instantaneous response from the x-ray tube when fluoroscopy or digital x-ray images are required. Added benefits of this technology include silent operation and an extended x-ray tube lifetime due to 'wear-free' operation.

When electrons strike the anode target disc, approximately 1% of the total energy generated is converted into actual x-ray. The other 99% of the electron beam energy generates heat. In conventional x-ray tubes this excess heat is stored in the anode, then transmitted outwards from the anode through the tube envelope by heat radiation and convection. Only a small amount of heat is transmitted by point heat conduction due to the limited area provided by conventional x-ray tubes equipped with ball bearing construction. Direct cooling of the anode disc has solved the frustrating problem of long waiting times previously experienced in cardiac imaging while the x-ray tube cooled. Spiral groove bearing construction provides the mechanism by which approximately 50% of excess heat generated from within the x-ray tube may be transferred via conduction, compared with the 1% transferred by conventional x-ray tubes.

The cathode contains one or more filaments that are heated by the filament current in order to release electrons. The cathode cup is shaped to focus the electrons onto a specific point on the anode known as the focal spot. When a high voltage is applied between the anode and cathode, electrons flow with increasing velocity towards the anode. The filament current determines the quantity of electrons emitted at a given voltage and thus the amount of x-rays produced by the x-ray tube. The total flow of electrons is the tube current. This quantity is expressed in milliamperes (mA). Most x-ray tubes are equipped with two filaments, producing two focal spots of different sizes.

The x-ray tube load is defined as the amount of energy absorbed by the tube during an exposure and is expressed in kilowatt-seconds or kilojoules. This measure is a function of tube current, exposure time and voltage. Electrons hitting other parts of the x-ray tube rather than the focal spot also produce x-rays. These are referred to as extra-focal or off-focus radiation; they affect the contrast resolution of the image and can be reduced by appropriate collimation.

Images from a big light bulb?

The place at which the x-ray-derived image is formed is the image intensifier tube. The image intensifier was developed to replace the fluorescent screen seen in earlier x-ray imaging systems. It provides a far brighter image for continuous viewing at a much lower dose and is available in a range of sizes for different clinical applications. A 23 cm (9") image intensifier with further field sizes of 18 cm (7") and 13 cm (5") for magnified viewing are typical for cardiac imaging. A recent trend to provide imaging systems capable of both cardiac and systemic angiography has seen the successful application of larger 30 cm (12") image intensifiers.

The image intensifier converts each impinging x-ray photon into several light photons. One x-ray photon of high energy releases many light photons and, in accordance with the principle of the conservation of energy, the released light photons will have a lower energy. Adjacent to the input phosphor is the photo cathode. This converts the photons of visible light into a cloud of low-energy electrons. High-voltage electrodes accelerate the low-energy electrons towards the output screen. The output screen, composed of a caesium iodine phosphor, converts the high-energy electrons into a bright visible image. Each impinging x-ray photon is converted into several photons of visible light, being much brighter than initially on the input phosphor as a result of electron acceleration and the small size of the output screen compared with the input screen. The gain of the intensifier is often expressed as the conversion factor Gx, which is the amount of light emitted per incoming photon.

The visible light image produced by the image intensifier is further processed by the television system, which converts the visible light image into an electronic or video signal. The image distributor incorporates a light sensor that measures the total amount of light during the exposure and a photodiode for automatic dose rate control. The television camera is designed specifically for cardiac angiographic applications with appropriate sensitivity, lag and contrast dynamic range.

Whatever happened to cine film?

Digital imaging offers enhanced image quality and new diagnostic and analytical possibilities. A digital cardiac image is composed of 512 x 512 or 1024 x 1024 picture elements (pixels).

Quantitative analysis of coronary vessel profile and densitometric flow, as well as ventricular functionality, can be derived from the digital image data. A digital image consists of a set of numbers that can be displayed by assigning a grey level to each number. The maximum number of different grey levels that can be distinguished by the human eye is about 64. Assigning the full range of numbers to the total number of grey levels provides a display of the total brightness range in the image. However, it is also possible to assign a smaller range of numbers to the total number of grey levels, in which case an average level and a smaller window width are used so that numbers outside this window are displayed in white or black. This technique is used for optimum display of a smaller attenuation range such as that in cardiac imaging.

What do we do with these digital images?

Recent developments in computer technology (cost and performance) have now made it viable to store digital images directly onto a large-capacity computer network. Images are stored in the long term (5–7 years) on a juke box system onto Magneto Optical Discs (MODs), and short term (1 month) on a RAID system on the main computer server. A network of Windows N.T.™ based workstations provides on-line access to cardiac angiographic examinations from various locations within the hospital (e.g. cardiology, theatres, coronary care).

Future directions

Cardiac catheterisation laboratories of the next decade will evolve through developments in (i) digital recording media, (ii) replacement of the conventional imaging chain, and (iii) radiation dose management.

Digital recording media

Development of on-line digital archive and review networks in larger centers will incorporate networks containing not only cardiac images, but also data from other diagnostic modalities. Along with physicians' reports, total patient management will be possible within the entire hospital environment and between associated departments and institutions.

The ability to archive dynamic cardiac images to compact disc (CD) has been steadily accepted as the most economical, most accessible, and most functional alternative available. Despite the finite resolution of cine film, costs associated with its use have become prohibitive and its functionality is limited to archive and review. Alternative formats include laser disc and SVHS tapes. These formats, however, document data in an analogue format, degrading the original data, and have also become expensive by comparison with compact discs. Image quality of the digital cardiac laboratory can now be efficiently transferred onto a medium that records the original digital data.

Use of compact disc technology has enhanced departmental productivity and allowed data exchange between sites. The ability to transfer cardiac images via CD into a Windows environment has enabled the same applications and functionality previously associated with the personal computer (PC) workstation to apply to cardiac examinations, such that CD archives on PC-based workstations now provide a platform on which mini-network systems can be organised and extended into the office. It is also possible to use software applications such as Powerpoint and Word for reviewing, reporting, research and staff or patient education.

Over the next few years advances in CD technology will permit use of higher capacity compact discs. This may lead to changes in the ACC/NEMA DICOM standard and to the number of procedures that may be archived to a single CD. These changes may become more appropriate if Digital Versatile Disc (DVD) technology is applied to digital archiving. In late 1997 Philips Electronics launched Digital Versatile Disc in Australia. Designed initially for the home cinema market, DVD provides digital recording and state-of-the-art data compression technology to record vast amounts of information (e.g. an entire movie) onto a single 12 cm disc. DVD, which resembles the compact disc, may permit recording multiple patient studies onto a single disc. The application of DVD as an archive medium will improve the cost effectiveness of digital archiving as hardware associated with DVD recording becomes more available, and when the medium itself becomes more affordable. The ability to archive the cardiac examination onto a medium in which the original digital information is stored could be one of the most significant advances in cardiac imaging in recent times.

Direct digital imaging (replacement of the image intensifier)

The most significant technological advance to occur over the next few years will involve replacement of the conventional imaging chain (image intensifier, TV camera/CCD camera and A/D convertor) by a cesium iodide scintillator in combination with photosensors having an active amorphous silicon (a-Si) read-out matrix. This development will be the most significant advance in both cardiac and radiological x-ray imaging since Roentgen's initial experiments with the cathode ray tube. The application of silicon solid-state detectors will complete the transition of conventional x-ray technology to the digital age. Implementation of this detector technology will have application and ramifications for dynamic cardiac imaging, but will impact more significantly in conventional radiology.

Over the past 20 years a number of different methods have evolved to capture radiographic images digitally. The first advance involved the x-ray image being transferred to a storage phosphor as an analogue signal and then being converted into a digital data file at the 'reader'. The storage phosphor was contained within a 'plate' and handled similarly to a conventional x-ray film/cassette. It reacted linearly and demonstrated a high dynamic range.

More recent advances used the optical coupling of Charged Coupled Devices (CCDs), but were limited by the analogue information provided from the interaction of x-irradiation on the image intensifier. The first generation CCD had the major disadvantage of extreme optical reduction caused by the relatively small CCD surface area available. Second generation CCDs have overcome this problem somewhat due to significant increases in the surface area now available from these devices.

Use of amorphous selenium to convert x-irradiation directly into an electrical charge that is then either electrostatically sampled or read with a matrix of active switching devices had limited application as a result of the low signal-to-noise ratio experienced during fluoroscopy.

Using cesium iodide/a-Si solid state detectors has overcome some earlier problems and has shown promise in overcoming certain problems associated with specific applications, namely low-dose fluoroscopy. A substantial component of the development in this area has resulted from a research and development consortium organised between Philips Medical System, Siemens Medical Engineering Group and Thompson Electroniques. The combined focus of this cooperation has resulted in the clinical evaluation of bi-plane cardiac systems featuring conventional imaging chains in one plane being directly compared against the cesium iodide/a-Si system in the other plane. Currently a lower then acceptable signal-to-noise ratio for fluoroscopy has delayed adaptation of this technology to cardiac applications, especially as the increase in interventional procedures has made quality fluoroscopy increasingly important at the lowest possible level of radiation.

A possible outcome of solid-state detectors in cardiac imaging may be the re-design of the cardiac gantry once the weight of the image intensifier/TV camera has been replaced by these lighter image receptors. Gantries will operate more quickly, occupy less space and be capable of more complex projections.

Radiation dose management

Patient and operator radiation exposure has previously been considered an unavoidable procedural and occupational risk. Radiation dose management can now be realised. Currently available technologies such as x-ray tubes equipped with spiral groove bearings, and the associated benefits of x-ray spectral beam filtration, combined with integrated radiation dose reports, real-time dose read-out and accumulated dose warnings have caused significant changes in occupational exposure.

The radiation dose-saving benefits derived from spiral groove bearing x-ray tubes is a consequence of the enormous heat dissipation properties of these devices and the ability of these x-ray tubes to function under the extra stress of additional copper and aluminum filtration. The resultant reductions in radiation dose are essential considerations in today's climate of occupational health and safety. Patient or staff litigation as a consequence of not providing the safest possible work and clinical environment remains a major concern.

Clinical case studies continue to be presented demonstrating radiation injuries as a result of cardiac procedures. Procedures such as angioplasty and electrophysiological studies have resulted in numerous and perhaps avoidable cases of patient trauma. As a result, cardiologists and laboratory staff are becoming more aware of the need to reduce radiation exposure. The radiation dose within the cardiac laboratory may now be managed and, by utilising appropriate systems, reduced to acceptable levels.

The immediate future

X-ray imaging equipment used for cardiac investigation and intervention will change significantly over the next decade as a result of the convergence of all x-ray modalities, and as an adaptation of complementary technologies. Current imaging technologies of associated modalities such as magnetic resonance angiography (MRA), computerised tomographic angiography (CTA) and 3-dimensional angiography may see a further convergence, this time of the clinical diagnostic applications applied to cardiac imaging, irrespective of modality. A similar diagnostic result may one day be achievable from quite differing modalities using separate imaging sources (magnetic field, x-irradiation, ultrasound), with the modality of choice dependent on the requirements of therapeutic intervention and the level of invasiveness deemed acceptable.

Chapter 2

The Physiological Monitoring System

Chris Lee

The cardiac catheterisation laboratory

A modern cardiac catheterisation laboratory demands the highest quality in equipment design and performance, a specification that computerised instrumentation systems are well placed to meet. This is particularly true of the system responsible for monitoring cardiac and haemodynamic physiology, with the specific requirements for accuracy, safety and reliability inherent in invasive cardiovascular investigations.

System requirements

Any physiological monitoring system must include provision for the haemodynamic measurement system, which plays a primary role in detecting alterations in patient status and quantifying haemodynamic measurements. There are unique requirements in areas such as equipment mounting, cabling and display screens. Also, there are specific regulations regarding power reticulation and earth leakage. It is recommended that an emergency power supply be installed, particularly if the haemodynamic system is used as a vital signs monitor.

Physiologic and haemodynamic presentation

Physiological signals are presented on large, high-resolution displays for the physician and system operator, enabling all parameters to be easily observed and monitored by staff. Displayed on the operator screen are various control windows and menus permitting system functions to be accessed. Controls are also available via the keyboard and protocol-based command sequences. These protocols are similar to short programs which, when executed, perform a series of functions that would otherwise require many specific operator actions and may be customised for many specific procedure types (Table 2.1). As a result, computerised instrumentation has revolutionised patient monitoring and data analysis in the catheter laboratory.

Physiological signals such as pressure waveforms are sampled by the haemodynamic system, and signal analysis algorithms are automatically applied to obtain the required data. A simple example is the electronic identification of systole, diastole and mean for the arterial pressure waveform, or analysis for the 'a' wave, 'v' wave and mean values of a venous or pulmonary artery wedge pressure. Similar signal analysis is used for physiological determinates such as thermal dilution cardiac output, non-invasive blood pressure and

Table 2.1. Example of a Right and Left Heart case protocol written for the GE Marquette Mac-Lab.

RIGHT & LEFT HEART

Patient arrives	(1ART,2VEN,GRAT9,phs1,nxt)
	(1g200,2g40,s25,1I,2II,3AVF,4E-,crun,lon)
Patient is a Child	(PED)
Patient is an Adult	(ADULT)
Log staff	(staff)
Zero both pressures	(z1,z2,sb2)
***** RIGHT SIDE 'P2' *****	
RA insert	(sb2,g40,2RA)
Measure RA	(mRA)
RV advance	(2RV)
Measure RV	(mRV)
PA advance	(2PA)
Measure PA	(mPA)
PCWedge advance	(2PCW)
Measure PCWedge	(mPCW)
Transpulm.grad.'PCW' [START]	(WP,2PCW,cPCW)
Unwedge catheter now.	
Transpulm.grad.'PA' [STOP]	(2PA,cPA,WOFF)
Pullback PA-RV	(2PA,PBPARV)
Pullback RV-RA	(2RV,PBRVRA)
Cardiac output	(co)

.

*** LEFT CORONARY INJECTIONS ***
*** RIGHT CORONARY INJECTIONS ***

***** LEFT SIDE *** 'P1' ***	200 mmHg Set
Ao measure	(sb1,1g200,1Ao,mAo)
LV measure & LVEDP	(1LV,cLV,s50,1g40,nxt)
	(cLV,s25,1g200)
V-GRAM performed	(phs2)
LV measure & LVEDP	(1LV,cLV,s50,1g40,nxt)
	(cLV,s25,1g200)
LVEDP & PCWSimultaneous	(g40,s50,nxt)
for mitral valve.	(1LV,2PCW,nxt)
	(DCVLM,s25,1g200)
LV to Ao pullback	(sb1,1LV,PBLVAO)
Review measurements	(ALT_L)
End of case.'Print report'	(fr)
Review measurements	(ALT_L)
End of case.'Print reports'	(fr)

---

intracardiac electrograms. In addition, if specific groups of measurements are made during a procedure then certain derived parameters are automatically calculated and are made available immediately. This effectively eliminates laborious techniques such as hand planimetry to measure mitral valve gradients, along with tedious measurement of values such as diastolic filling times or systolic ejection times. The immediate availability of calculated determinates such as vascular resistance or valve area is invaluable during an interventional study.

Pressure measurement

Accuracy and stability are imperatives in all physiological measurement systems. Although transducers are now available pre-calibrated, it is important for all pressure channels used in the system to have identical gain settings and to be calibrated to the known static calibration pressure of a mercury column. This is because pressure values are often compared simultaneously between chambers and/or vessels and such comparative measurements must be proven accurate.

Older transducers (e.g. Gould, Statham) require regular sterilisation, maintenance and calibration. Modern transducers are available as sterile, disposable, pre-calibrated single-use units. Depending on individual infection control practices, they may be either 'fixed' to

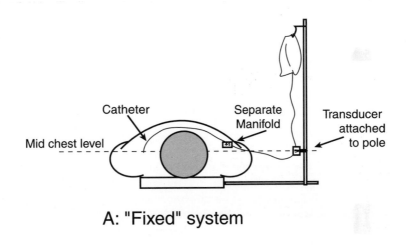

A: "Fixed" system

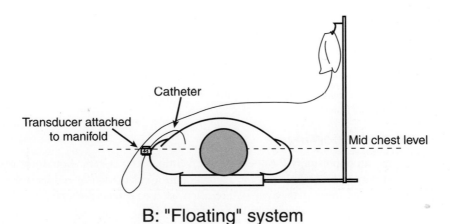

B: "Floating" system

Figure 2.1. *Difference between a transducer system attached to a pole at mid-chest level ('fixed') and one attached to a moveable manifold ('floating').*

a bedside pole (permitting re-use) at mid-chest level, or attached directly to a manifold ('floating') (Fig. 2.1). Some manifolds incorporate a built-in transducer. In either case, all transducers must be balanced ('zeroed') to atmospheric pressure at mid-chest level immediately prior to use to avoid false high or low pressure signal bias. Balancing compensates for the effect of atmospheric pressure (760 mmHg at sea level), making atmospheric pressure equivalent to zero mmHg in relation to internal body measurements. Mid-chest level is normally taken as half the height of the patient's chest from the table top, along the mid-axillary line.

With a 'fixed' transducer independent of a manifold, pressures are accurate irrespective of manifold level. With a 'floating' transducer attached to a manifold, the manifold unit must be positioned at mid-chest level whenever a pressure is measured, otherwise hydrostatic pressure exerted by the column of fluid in the flush line may affect readings. Raising a transducer 1.34 cm above mid-chest level induces an artifactual drop of 1 mmHg in recorded pressure; conversely, lowering the transducer 1.34 cm raises recorded pressure by 1 mmHg. Such differences may become critical in evaluating right heart pressures and valve gradients.

Although not usual practice, the zero port may be extended by a length of tubing from the transducer body. In such cases the transducer may be offset from mid-chest level provided the zero port itself remains at this level throughout the procedure. This is because with this set-up modern pressure amplifier systems can compensate for small amounts of transducer offset.

Equipment design and performance

Most haemodynamic systems are modular in design, permitting a high degree of versatility in application (Fig. 2.2). Multi-parameter data acquisition modules with ward monitor compatibility make the patient interface simple and highly flexible, allowing parameters such as electrocardiogram, pulse oxymetry, respiration, non-invasive blood pressure and thermal dilution cardiac output to be directly available. All physiological information is usually recorded in real time onto the system hard drive and may be recalled at any time during the case for review. Controls of a haemodynamic system must permit detailed access to all functions and there must be provision for institutional details, display setup, automatic data logging, hardware settings and a means of back-up.

It is often desirable to divide physiological data into time blocks in an effort to compare changing physiological states. This may perhaps permit a baseline set of haemodynamic data to be taken for comparison with a later set of data taken as a result of a valve dilatation procedure or administration of a drug. With entry of blood oxymetry values intracardiac shunts can be calculated (Qp/Qs), and if a cardiac output is measured or an estimated Fick cardiac output made, then these are presented as relative pulmonary and systemic blood flows.

Data log and reporting

There is always an opportunity for operator intervention, as a system should not permit any measured data to be included in the record or in a calculation of results unless the operator has verified those data. Systems are often used as a record-keeping facility enabling information such as oxygen saturation from blood samples, clinical procedures, staff, supplies, drugs, contrast media and complications to be entered during the study and logged into a configured case report. The cardiac catheterisation study data and config-

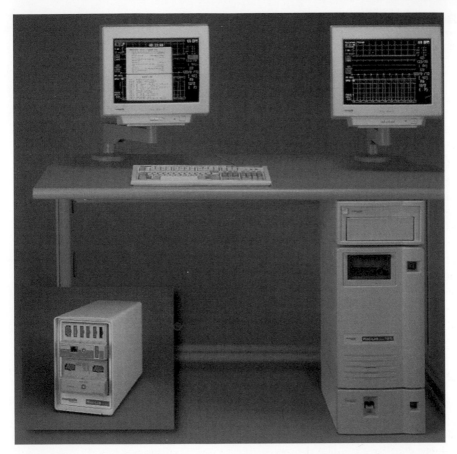

Figure 2.2. *GE Marquette Mac-Lab EX5000 haemodynamic recording system. TRAM signal acquisition unit inset.*

ured report may be printed on the integrated recorder or placed on floppy disk for post-case editing if required. Also, it may be possible for information to be sent via local area network to a clinical review station where the cardiac catheterisation report, including all measurements, calculations and procedural information, can be stored for inclusion in the global patient record. This information record may be used for laboratory audits or even inventory control.

Summary

The modern cardiac catheterisation laboratory in a busy unit has a need for rapid patient turnover. To facilitate this the haemodynamic system must have a well designed user interface with clear and logical controls, thus reducing the amount of operator time required to obtain the required information. The system must be accurate and safe for the operator and patient. At the conclusion of the study all physiological and calculated information should be presented, along with records of supplies or case complications in a clear and precise report format suitable for inclusion into the patient record.

Further reading

1. GE Marquette Medical Systems MAC-Lab cardiac catheterization system operators manual PN 416299-001, 1993.
2. Kern MJ. *The Cardiac Catheterisation Handbook*, 3rd ed. St Louis: Mosby, 1999.

Chapter 3

Laboratory Coagulation and Antiplatelet Assays

Marcia L. Zucker and Claudia Campbell

B edside coagulation systems provide a critical link in the successful management of invasive procedures. Quality of care is improved when clinicians have immediate diagnostic information upon which to base anticoagulation and transfusion management decisions.[1] Whole blood coagulation analysers have become the systems of choice for routine point-of-care management of haemostasis in various clinical settings. One system, the Hemochron® analyser, provides two independent technologies: the standard test tube-based whole blood coagulation analysers and a novel semi-automated microcoagulation system.

Both technologies offer the three most commonly requested coagulation assays, the Activated Clotting Time (ACT), Prothrombin Time (PT) and the Activated Partial Thromboplastin Time (APTT). These tests are utilised in a wide variety of clinical settings as haemostasis screening tools and for monitoring anticoagulant therapy. In addition, the test tube based systems offer Thrombin Time (TT) and fibrinogen assays to monitor residual heparin and fibrin(ogen)opathies as well as a selection of dosing systems for heparin and protamine dose determinations (Table 3.1). Use of the dosing assays has been shown to reduce transfusion requirements and blood product usage in patients undergoing cardiopulmonary bypass.[2,3]

Test tube-based whole blood coagulation assays are performed by introducing into the test tube a whole blood sample (fresh or citrated, 0.4 to 2.0 cc, depending on the test), and vigorously agitating from end to end 10 times. The tube is then inserted into the instrument. Mechanical detection of a fibrin clot in the blood sample automatically terminates the test, causing a digital timer to display the coagulation time in seconds. Tracking of test results by patient and operator is easily accomplished using onboard data management features in the Response instrument.

Microcoagulation systems offer a menu of point-of-care coagulation tests less influenced by operator technique, by using a mechanical endpoint clotting mechanism in which clot formation occurs within a disposable test cuvette. Following introduction of the whole blood sample (one drop of fresh whole blood) the instrument precisely measures a 15 µL sample and automatically moves it into the test channel within the cuvette. The remainder of the blood sample, not needed for testing, is automatically drawn into the waste channel of the cuvette. Sample/reagent mixing and test initiation are also performed automatically, requiring no operator interaction. After mixing with the reagent, the sample is moved back and forth within the test channel and observed photo-optically for a decrease in movement of the blood sample due to clot formation in the channel.

Table 3.1. Summary of various coagulation assays available with the Hemochron 401, 801, Response, Jr., Jr. II and Signature coagulation analysers.

Coagulation test		Tube or cuvette	Instrument	Most frequent applications
Activated clotting times	ACT (celite)	Black top tube	401/801/Response	Bypass/ PTCA[a]/ CATH[b]/ CCU[c]
	ACT (kaolin)	Gold top tube	401/801/Response	Bypass/ PTCA
	ACT+	Gold print cuvette	Jr/ JrII /Signature	Bypass/ PTCA
	ACT-LR	Green print cuvette	Jr/ JrII /Signature	CATH/ CCU/ Dialysis/ ECMO[d]/ haemofiltration
	ACT (glass)	Clear top tube	401/801/Response	Dialysis/ ECMO/ haemofiltration
Activated partial thrombo-plastin times	APTT	Blue top tube	401/801/Response	ICU[e]/ CCU/ ECMO
	APTT	Blue print cuvette	JrII /Signature	ICU/ CCU/ ECMO/ dialysis
	APTT (citrated)	Light grey top tube	401/801/Response	ICU/ CCU
Prothrombin times	PT	Purple top tube	401/801/Response	ICU/ CCU
	PT	Cranberry print cuvette	Jr/ JrII	ICU/ CCU/ OAC[f]
	PT (citrated)	Light purple top tube	401/801/Response	ICU/ CCU
	PT (citrated)	Light blue label cuvette	JrII	ICU/ CCU
Thrombin-based tests	TT	Rose top tube	401/801/Response	ICU/ CCU
	HNTT	Brown top tube	401/801/Response	ICU/ CCU
	HiTT	Turquoise top tube	401/801/Response	Bypass
	Fibrinogen	Light brown top tube	401/801/Response	ICU/ CCU/ Radiology
Dosing assays	HRT480	Lime green top tube	401/801/Response	Bypass
	PRT200	Peach top tube	401/801/Response	Bypass
	PRT400	Red top tube	401/801/Response	Bypass
	PDA-O	Orange top tube	401/801/Response	Bypass/ CCU/ ICU

[a]PTCA = percutaneous transluminal angioplasty; [b]CATH = cardiac catheterisation suite; [c]CCU = cardiac care unit; [d]ECMO = extracorporeal membrane oxygenation; [e]ICU = intensive care unit; [f]OAC = outpatient anticoagulation clinic.

Test tube types are identified by colour-coded caps, cuvettes by colour-coded labels. Refer to text for specific nature of each test (ACT = activated clotting time, APTT = activated partial thromboplastin time, PT = prothrombin time, TT = thrombin time, HiTT = high-dose thrombin time, HNTT = heparin neutralised thrombin time, HRT = heparin response test, PRT = Protamine response test, PDA-O = protamine dose assay-orange).

Clinical applications

Coronary angiography, angioplasty and stenting

Optimal target ACT clotting times for percutaneous transluminal coronary angioplasty (PTCA)[4] and diagnostic angiography[5] still remain somewhat dependent on the clinical site. However, it is generally agreed that using the ACT to monitor heparin dosage, rather than relying on empirical dosing regimens, can assist the clinician in achieving proper anticoagulation and potentially reduce ischaemic complications.[6] During PTCA, stenting and vascular angioplasty, moderate to high doses of heparin are given to patients to avoid thrombotic complications associated with invasive procedures. Intra-procedural monitoring in these arenas generally requires that the ACT remain above a target time of 300 seconds,[7,8] particularly in view of the incidence of ischaemic complications during PTCA, such as abrupt closure and the high rate of restenosis.[9] The Celite® (diatomaceous earth)-activated ACT (FTCA510) has been the standard by which many of these target ACT times were determined. The Hemochron Jr. offers two different ACT tests which may be used in this application. The ACT-LR is a Celite-based ACT that has been optimised to monitor low to moderate heparin levels (ACT < 400 seconds) and is not suitable where the ACT exceeds 400 seconds. For most interventional cardiology procedures, this is the system of choice. For institutions requiring clotting time values in the 400 to 450 second range, the ACT+, a kaolin/silica-based ACT, has been optimized for monitoring moderate to high levels of heparin (ACT ranges > 300 seconds).

Platelet inhibitors

Platelet glycoprotein IIb/IIIa receptors participate in the process of platelet aggregation and presumably play an important role in the occurrence of ischaemic complications during or after PTCA. The new glycoprotein IIb/IIIa inhibitor pharmaceuticals, such as ReoPro® (abciximab, Eli Lilly & Co.), have been shown to reduce ischaemic events and post-procedural thrombosis.[10] However, heparin dosages and ACT target times must be evaluated in conjunction with these drugs due to the potential for increased bleeding complications.[11] Specifically, in clinical trials of ReoPro, it was demonstrated that use of low-dose, weight-adjusted heparin in conjunction with ReoPro resulted in fewer bleeding complications than when a standard dose heparin protocol was employed.[12] It is controversial whether the Celite ACT is elevated in the presence of ReoPro. Irrespective of this, the recommended target time of 250 seconds for anticoagulation of ReoPro-treated patients was determined using the celite ACT, therefore these targets are accurate when celite-based ACTs are used. As more platelet-inhibiting agents such as Aggrastat® (tirofiban, Merck & Co.) and Integrelin® (eptifibatide, COR Therapeutics) become available, it is important that the effect of these agents upon the ACT be carefully evaluated.

Antifibrinolytic agents

The test traditionally used to monitor high doses of heparin used during surgery requiring cardiopulmonary bypass (CPB) is the Celite ACT. An ACT time of 480 seconds[13] has been widely accepted as indicative of adequate heparinisation. The Celite ACT has been the standard of care in this setting for more than 25 years. Alternative ACT tests, including kaolin ACT[14] and the ACT+ have been increasingly used since the advent of aprotinin (Trasylol®, DuPont) treatment to reduce post-operative blood loss.[15] The kaolin ACT has been shown to be unaffected by moderate levels of aprotinin,[16] and the ACT+ is not influenced by aprotinin at any level examined.[17] It must be noted that both the kaolin-activated ACT and the ACT+ have been shown to result in clotting times that differ from

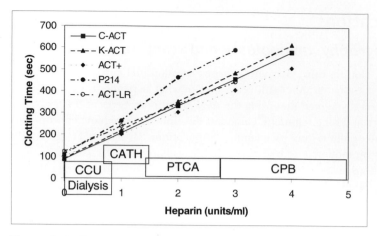

Figure 3.1. *Heparin dose response of Hemochron ACT assays showing the effect of heparin dosage on blood clotting time as measured by 5 different assay types. Heparin dosage and the corresponding target clotting times for various clinical situations are indicated by boxes along the horizontal axis.*
C = Celite, K = kaolin, ACT = activated clotting time, CCU = coronary care unit, CATH = cardiac catheterization, PTCA = coronary angioplasty, CPB = cardio-pulmonary bypass.

the standard Celite system (Fig. 3.1). The kaolin test runs 5–10% longer than the Celite, while the ACT+ can run as much as 10–15% lower than the standard.[16,17] An alternative to ACT testing in CPB, with or without aprotinin treatment, is the High Dose Thrombin Time (HiTT).[18] This assay utilises a thrombin-based reagent and is highly correlated with laboratory anti-IIa heparin activity.[19]

Heparin neutralisation

The use of individualised heparin and protamine dosing systems has been shown to significantly reduce postoperative blood loss and post- and intraoperative transfusion requirements.[2,20] In primary operation patients, this reduction was shown to be comparable to that achieved through aprotinin usage.[2] The Heparin Response Test (HRT) for heparin dosing and the Protamine Response Test (PRT) for protamine dosing are run in parallel with standard Celite ACT tests to allow an accurate prediction of a specific patient's dosing needs. The use of the HRT/PRT system has led to conspicuous cost savings over the use of empirical dosing regimens.[21]

Postoperatively, heparin neutralisation must be confirmed to preclude excessive blood loss during patient recovery. Two test systems are available for this purpose. The first, the Protamine Dose Assay-Orange (PDA-O) is similar to the PRT in that it is a protamine titration assay based on the Celite ACT.[22] The TT/HNTT system (Thrombin Time/Heparin Neutralised Thrombin Time) can also be used for this application. The TT is exquisitely sensitive to very low levels of heparin, while the HNTT is insensitive to heparin levels up to 1.5 units per ml. In the presence of low-level (residual) heparin, the TT will be elevated while the HNTT is normal. However, if the fibrinogen level of the patient's blood is low, both the TT and HNTT will be elevated.[22,23]

Heparin rebound

The mechanism of heparin rebound is still undetermined. One theory is that excess heparin resides in the vascular bed and is released back into circulation upon re-warming of the patient.[24] Studies have demonstrated that the paired TT/HNTT tests showed a better correlation to heparin concentration measurement by a laboratory anti-Xa assay than the laboratory TT,[24] or the ACT or APTT tests.[23] Thus, the TT/HNTT test combination can be used by the clinician to diagnose heparin rebound and can differentiate this condition from fibrinogen depletion.[24]

Critical care

Post-catheterisation decisions as to when to remove the femoral sheath can be expedited using the ACT or the APTT. By using rapid bedside tests to monitor patients for sheath removal, the clinician can potentially remove the sheath earlier without compromising patient outcome. In general, sheath removal should be deferred until the ACT is < 170 secs. The Celite ACT and the APTT on the Hemochron, as well as the APTT and the ACT-LR on the Hemochron Jr. have all been used for this application.

The United States Department of Health recommends performing APTT and PT tests to determine whether the patient has a clotting factor deficiency before administering fresh frozen plasma.[25] When such tests are performed using point-of-care systems at the patient's bedside, significant reductions in usage of blood products to treat microvascular bleeding can be realised.[1]

Warfarin

Outpatient management of warfarin therapy is a rapidly expanding segment of anticoagulation management. The use of point-of-care PT/INR testing allows the optimisation of clinic resources, removes the delay inherent in communicating results from the laboratory to the clinician and the additional delay as the result is finally communicated to the patient. Additionally, monitoring PT/INR using a fingerstick sample is less traumatic to the patient than venipuncture. This can lead to improved compliance in monitoring regimens.

Platelet aggregation assays

The processes leading to platelet aggregation and secretion are discussed in detail in Chapter 10. Simply, platelets respond to the action of agonists such as ADP, collagen, thrombin and adrenaline. This results in a change in the conformation of the membrane glycoprotein IIb/IIIa, exposing binding sites for soluble plasma proteins such as fibrinogen and von Willebrand factor (vWF) and allowing cross-linking of adjacent activated platelets into aggregates.

Platelet aggregation assays use a modified spectrophotometer (aggregometer) that measures changes in light transmission as individual platelets form aggregates. The rate or extent of change in light transmission is used as a measure of platelet aggregation. Whole blood is diluted 9:1 with sodium citrate. Platelet-rich plasma is obtained by centrifuging at 250g for 10 minutes,[26] 1600g for 3 minutes[26] or 150g for 30 minutes.[27] Platelet-rich plasma should be kept at ambient temperature and it is also favourable to maintain the pH around 7.7.[26] Plastic[27,28] or siliconised glass[27] tubes and syringes should be used for blood collection and handling of platelet-rich plasma.

Platelet aggregation is sensitive to drug effects and it is recommended that patients withhold all medications for at least one week prior to the test. In particular, aspirin and aspirin-containing medications,[26-28] non-steroidal anti-inflammatory drugs[26,28] and antihistamines[27,28] should be avoided. Alcohol, cocaine, tricyclic antidepressants and dipyridamole may also reduce platelet aggregation.[28]

After addition of the agonist (except adrenaline) there is an initial fall in light transmittance as platelets change from discoid shape to spherical. An increase in transmittance follows as aggregates form. There are two phases of aggregation, resulting in two waves on the light transmittance trace. Primary aggregation is due to agonist stimulation. This phase is reversible and is not associated with platelet secretion. Secondary aggregation is due to the irreversible formation of large aggregates in response to platelet secretion. If the concentration of agonist is high, the first and second waves may merge into one on the transmittance trace.

Common agonists

ADP The aggregation response of ADP (adenosine diphosphate) is concentration dependent. The second phase of aggregation requires synthesis of thromboxane A_2 and is inhibited by cyclooxygenase inhibitors such as aspirin.

Adrenaline Platelet stimulation by adrenaline is not preceded by change in platelet shape. The second phase is also dependent on thromboxane A_2 synthesis. Adrenaline solution should be freshly prepared and kept in the dark.

Thrombin Addition of thrombin produces a fibrin clot which obscures analysis of platelet aggregation. Washed or gel-filtered platelets may be used to remove exogenous fibrinogen.

Collagen There is an initial lag period as collagen polymerises into fibrils small enough to activate platelets.

Arachadonic acid This test is used to assess the action of platelet cyclooxygenase.

Ristocetin This antibiotic initiates platelet aggregation and secretion through von Willebrand factor binding to GPIb/IX allowing fibrinogen to bind to GPIIb/IIIa.

Other Platelet aggregation assays may also be performed in the presence of serotonin, aggregated gamma globulin, bovine factor VIII, antiplatelet antibodies, calcium ionophore, prostaglandin endoperoxide analogue and polysine.

Normal ranges should be established by each laboratory. Studies have shown that ADP, adrenaline, collagen, arachadonic acid and ristocetin usually achieve 60–90% platelet aggregation in normal patients.[28]

References

1.   Despotis GJ, Santoro SA, Spitnagel KM *et al.* Prospective evaluation and clinical utility of on-site monitoring of coagulation in patients undergoing cardiac operation. *J Thorac Cardiovasc Surg* 1994; **107**:271-79.
2.   Jobes DR, Aitken GL, Shaffer GW. Increased accuracy and precision of heparin and protamine dosing reduces blood loss and transfusion requirements in patients undergoing primary cardiac operations. *J Thorac Cardiovasc Surg* 1995; **110**:36-45.
3.   Fitch JCK, Geary KLB, Mirto GP *et al.*. Individualized versus empiric dosing of heparin and protamine during cardiac surgery: impact on postoperative bleeding and transfusions. In preparation.
4.   Vacek JL, Bellinger RL and Phelix J. 1988. Heparin bolus during cardiac catheterization. *Amer J Cardiol* 1988; **62**:1314-17.
5.   Hansell H. ACT levels for interventional procedures. *Cath Lab Digest* 1996; **4**:4-5.
6.   Voyce SJ, Weiner BH and Becker RC. ACT monitoring: Current applications in the angioplasty suite. *Cardio News* 1993; Feb:69-73.
7.   Ogilby JD, Kopelman HA, Klein LW and Agarwal JB. 1989. Adequate heparinization during PTCA: Assessment using activated clotting times. *Cath Cardiol Diag* 1989; **18**:206-09.
8.   Brack MJ, Hubner PJB, Gershlick AH. Anticoagulation after intracoronary stent insertion. *Br Heart J* 1994; **72**:294-96.

9.   Ellis SO. Elective coronary angioplasty: technique and complications. In: Topol E (ed). *Textbook of interventional cardiology*. Philadelphia: WB Saunders 1990, pp.199-222.

10.   The EPIC Investigators. Use of a monoclonal antibody directed against the platelet glycoprotein IIb/IIIa receptor in high-risk coronary angioplasty. *N Eng J Med* 1994; **330**:956-61.

11.   Lincoff AM. Heparin and control of bleeding complications during platelet glycoprotein IIb/IIIa receptor antagonist therapy during percutaneous coronary revascularization. *J Inv Cardiol* 1996; **8**:15B-20B.

12.   Lincoff A, Teheng J, Bass T *et al*. A multicentre, randomised, double-blind pilot trial of standard versus low dose weight-adjusted heparin in patients treated with the platelet GP IIb/IIIa receptor antibody c7E3 during percutaneous coronary angioplasty. *J Am Coll Cardiol* 1995; **25**:80-81A.

13.   Bull BS, Korpman RA, Huse WM, Briggs BD. Heparin therapy during extracorporeal circulation: 1. Problems inherent in existing protocols. *J. Thorac Cardiovasc Surg* 1975; **62**:674-84.

14.   Wang JS, Lin CY, Hung WT, Karp RB. Monitoring of heparin-induced anticoagulation with kaolin-activated clotting time in cardiac surgical patients treated with aprotinin. *Anesthesiology* 1992; **77**:1080-84.

15.   Murkin JM, Lux JL, Shannon NA *et al*. Aprotinin significantly decreases bleeding and transfusion requirements in patients receiving aspirin and undergoing cardiac operations. *J Thorac Cardiovasc Surg* 1994; **107**:554-61.

16.   Zucker ML, Walker C, Jobes DR, LaDuca FM. Comparison of celite and kaolin based heparin and protamine dosing assays during cardiac surgery: The in vitro effect of aprotinin. *J Extracorp Tech* 1995; **27**:201-07.

17.   Hemochron Jr. ACT+ package insert. International Technidyne Corporation.

18.   Huyzen RJ, Harder MP, Gallandat-Huet RCG *et al*. Alternative perioperative anticoagulation monitoring during cardiopulmonary bypass in aprotinin-treated patients. *J Cardiothorac Vasc Anesth* 1994; **8**:153-56.

19.   Murkin JM, Shannon NA, Turner A. Aprotinin interferes with measures of anticoagulation when using ACT but not when using HITT. *Proc Soc Cardiovasc Anesthes* 1992:175.

20.   Delaria GA, Tyner JJ, Hayes CL, Armstrong BW. Heparin-protamine mismatch. A controllable factor in bleeding after open heart surgery. *Arch Surg* 1994; **129**:945-51.

21.   Jobes DR, Etzioni DA, Stepsis LH, *et al*. Cost effective management of heparin/protamine in cardiopulmonary bypass: Analysis by type of surgery. *Anesthesiology* 1996; **85**:3A.

22.   LaDuca FM, Zucker ML, Walker CE. Assessing heparin neutralization following cardiac surgery: qualitative (thrombin time) versus quantitative (protamine titration) methods. *Perfusion* 1999; **14**:181-7.

23.   Wang JS, Lin CY, Pan C *et al*. Comparative sensitivity of bedside coagulation tests for residual heparin in CABG patients. *Anesthesiology* 1994; **81**:A85.

24.   Wang JS, Lin CY, Albertucci M *et al*. Identification of heparin rebound by measurement of whole-blood thrombin time in CABG patients. *Anesthesiology* 1992; **77**:A144.

25.   Transfusion Alert 1989. Indications for the use of red blood cells, platelets and fresh frozen plasma. NIH Publication 1989; No. 89:297a. US Department of Health and Human Services.

26.   Bennett JS. Platelet aggregation. In: Beutler E, Lichtman MA, Coller BS, Kipps TJ. (eds). *Williams Haematology* (5th ed). New York: McGraw Hill 1995, pp L114-17.

27.   Maile JB. *Laboratory medicine hematology* (6th ed). St. Louis: Mosby 1982 (Appendix: Methods)

28.   Brown BA. *Hematology: Principles and procedures* (5th ed). Philadelphia: Lea and Febiger 1988, pp 259-62.

Chapter 4

Non-invasive Physiological Monitoring

Anthony Nicholson

Pressure monitoring

Accurate measurement of blood pressure is an essential component of cardiac catheterisation. For systemic arterial pressure measurements, this is routinely achieved by one of three indirect methods: sphygmomanometry, oscillometry, digital tonometry (Penaz's continuous method), or by invasive catheterisation (see Chapter 8). Advantages of non-invasive techniques include their relative simplicity, ease of application, ready acceptance by patients, speed of response and reliability. As a consequence of such advances, non-invasive physiological monitoring is being utilised in a wide variety of situations, one of which is to support catheter readings during coronary angiography.

Oscillometry

Oscillometry is the most widely used non-invasive technique for arterial blood pressure measurement. The principle of this technique involves occlusion of a peripheral artery by a cuff that is inflated then deflated in a step-wise fashion to allow detection of oscillations caused by pulsatile blood flow. The cuff has two hoses: one is for cuff inflation and defla-tion, the other for measurement of the pulsatile oscillations by a solid-state pressure trans-ducer.[1]

When first applied to a patient the cuff is inflated to a pressure of about 160 mmHg, or else inflated to a pressure about 30 to 40 mmHg greater than the previously measured systolic pressure. The cuff is then repeatedly deflated in steps of about 7 mmHg until the pressure transducer within the device is able to detect pressure wave oscillations transmit-ted along the tubing. After each deflation, pressure within the cuff is kept constant to allow detection of these oscillations. Each two consecutive oscillations are compared, and these pairs are averaged with the value stored. The cuff is then deflated and further paired com-parisons of oscillation amplitude are made. The point at which there is a sudden and marked increase in oscillation amplitude is considered the systolic blood pressure; diastolic pressure is the point at which the amplitude falls away suddenly. The mean pressure is taken as the point of maximal averaged amplitude.[1]

The best-known oscillometric device is the Dinamap (Critikon Inc.). Dinamap is an acronym for 'Device for Indirect Non-invasive Automatic Mean Arterial Pressure'. More recent models have more sophisticated algorithms for pressure determination as well as for artifact rejection. Many studies have compared the reliability and accuracy of this device with direct pressure measurements. Reliability is the consistency of multiple results from one individual over time, whereas accuracy is the similarity between results from the device and those obtained simultaneously by direct arterial measurement. The accuracy of the Dinamap is < 5 ± 8 mmHg when compared with direct central arterial measurements.[1] Consequently, the Dinamap, or a similar device, is used as the sole blood pressure monitoring device during general anaesthesia, as well as with other less invasive procedures. These devices are also capable of displaying the pulse rate measured during each pressure determination.

For accurate measurements the cuff should be the correct size; cuff width should be 40% of the limb circumference.[2] If this is not possible it is preferable that the cuff be oversized rather than undersized: with undersized cuffs, measurements tend to be too high whilst with oversized cuffs, measurements may still be reasonably accurate or at worst marginally low. The cuff should have all air expelled before being wrapped snugly around the limb. The most commonly used limb is the upper arm, although measurements are possible from the forearm and the ankle. Ideally the cuff is placed at the same level as the heart, to avoid discrepancies due to hydrostatic pressure.

Penaz's continuous method

In this technique a small inflatable cuff is placed around a finger. The cuff contains an infrared photoplethysmograph that measures volume changes of the finger due to pulsatile blood flow in the digital arteries.[3] There is a feedback loop to control cuff inflation based on the volume measurement, such that the cuff is inflated to the point where the volume in the artery is kept constant (i.e. it is volume clamped). The result is that transmural pressure across the artery wall is zero and cuff pressure is equal to intra-arterial pressure.[3] The servocontrol system responds to the continuous plethysmographic finger volume measurement so that resulting pressure measurements are also continuous.

The output display for this device is a continuous waveform that resembles that from an intra-arterial catheter placed into the radial artery. Consequently, the display includes not only systolic, diastolic and mean blood pressures but also the pulse rate.

To obtain the most accurate measurements, initial readings are calibrated against results for a Dinamap pressure determination at the same time; but even without this the results are still clinically reliable. As a result of pulse wave distortion associated with the peripheral arterial system, the measured systolic pressure is usually a few mmHg higher than that measured directly in more central arteries.[3] Although not as common as the Dinamap or other oscillometric devices, this method is also reliable and accurate when applied properly. Commercially available devices are marketed as either 'Finapres' or 'Portapres'.

Pulse oximetry

Pulse oximetry has been described as 'arguably the greatest advance in patient monitoring since electrocardiography'.[4] This technique relies on changes in transmission of light through tissue due to pulsatile blood flow to determine the oxygen saturation of haemoglobin.

Two basic principles underlie pulse oximetry. The first is the differing absorbance of red light by oxygenated haemoglobin (oxyHb) and deoxygenated (reduced) haemoglobin (deoxyHb) (the term deoxygenated is now preferred over reduced). The other principle is the change in volume of tissues with pulsatile blood flow. Two light-emitting diodes (LEDs) emit either red (approximately 660 nm wavelength) or infra-red (940 nm) light in pulses of about 400 per second. A photodetector on the other side of the tissue, usually a finger, senses the two lights and also ambient light intensity. A microprocessor calculates the ratio (R) of the absorbances at the two wavelengths at the two tissue blood volumes. The R value obtained is then compared to a table of empirical results obtained from CO-oximetry on whole blood from healthy volunteers to estimate the haemoglobin saturation.[5-7]

Pulse oximetry is able to determine the **arterial haemoglobin oxygen saturation** [SO_2(aB), previously known as functional saturation] of oxyHb present as a percentage of total (functional) haemoglobin detected by these two wavelengths of light:

$$SO_2(aB) = \frac{xyHb}{oxyHb + deoxyHb}$$

whereas the **fractional haemoglobin oxygen saturation** [FO_2Hb(aB), previously known as fractional saturation] also takes into consideration the amount of carboxyhaemoglobin (COHb) and methaemoglobin (metHb) which are non-functional in that they cannot carry oxygen for delivery to the periphery (the IFCC/IUPAC system of nomenclature is used throughout this text):

$$FO_2(aB) = \frac{oxyHb}{oxyHb + deoxyHb + COHb + metHb}$$

Pulse oximetry is also an indicator of the adequacy of peripheral perfusion, and so indirectly reflects cardiovascular function. This is because the pulse oximeter requires a detectable arterial pulse in order to determine saturation.[7] Many pulse oximeters provide a visual display indicating the strength of the pulsatile signal detected. When this display is a continuous waveform it is known as a plethysmograph. The plethysmograph reflects the quality of the pulse detected by the oximeter, and indicates the likely accuracy of the displayed saturation. Many pulse oximeters also have an audible tone (beep) for each pulse wave detected. The pitch of this tone usually increases with decreasing arterial saturation, to act as an audible trend monitor and allow a degree of remote monitoring. Most pulse oximeters display pulse rate as well as arterial saturation and the concordance between the oximeter pulse rate and another method of rate determination (e.g. ECG) is another indicator of the probable accuracy of the pulse oximeter reading.

It is generally accepted that one should aim to maintain arterial saturation above 90%, as this represents an arterial partial pressure of oxygen of 60 mmHg, the turning point of the oxygen-haemoglobin dissociation curve. With arterial oxygen tension below this point there is rapid decline in haemoglobin saturation and increasing risk of organ damage. In healthy individuals at sea level haemoglobin saturation is around 95%, whilst with increasing altitude it decreases to around 92% at 5000 feet and about 88% at 10 000 feet.[5]

Various probes have been designed for use on different parts of the body, with the finger probe being the one most frequently used. Finger probes may also be used on toes, whilst there are also specific probes for the ear lobe, bridge of the nose, and flexible adhesive probes particularly for use in neonates and infants.[5]

Pulse oximeters have been determined to be extremely accurate, with excellent correlation to CO-oximetry in the range of 70 to 100% saturation but are far less reliable at saturations below 70%. Since a saturation of 70% or less is generally indicative of a critical situation, corrective measures together with alternative measurement techniques should be employed if this situation arises.

References

1.   Ramsey M III. Blood pressure monitoring: Automated oscillometric devices. *J Clin Monit* 1991; **7**:56-67.

2.   Vender JS, Gilbert HC. Monitoring the Anesthetized Patient. In: Barash PC, Cullen BF, Stoelting RK (eds). *Clinical Anesthesia,* 3rd ed. Philadelphia: Lippincott-Raven 1997, pp.621-41.

3.   Schmidt T, Jain A. Continuous assessment of finger blood pressure and other haemodynamic and behavioral variables in everyday life. In: Fahrenberg J, Myrtek M (eds). *Ambulatory assessment. computer-assisted psychological and psychophysiological methods in monitoring and field studies.* Seattle: Hogrefe and Huber 1996, pp.1-20. Accessed at: http//www.uni-koeln.de/phil-fak/psych/diagnostik/PUBL/FaTSText on 23/02/99.

4.   Hanning CD, Alexander-Williams JM. Pulse oximetry: a practical review. *Br Med J* 1995; **311**:367-70.

5.   Dorsch JA, Dorsch SE. Pulse Oximetry. In: Dorsch JA, Dorsch SE (eds). *Understanding anesthesia equipment: Construction, care and complications,* 3rd ed. Baltimore: Williams & Wilkins 1994, pp.657-85.

6.   Grace RF. Pulse Oximetry: Gold standard or false sense of security? *Med J Aust* 1994; **160**:638-44.

7.   Schnapp LM, Cohen NH. Pulse oximetry: uses and abuses. *Chest* 1990; **98**:1244-50.

Chapter 5

Determination of Oxygen Status in Human Blood

Marcus Juul

D etermination of oxygen status in human blood is essential in evaluating the severity of conditions that produce oxygen depletion, which ultimately leads to
abnormalities in cellular oxygen metabolism, and results in organ and whole body
functional abnormalities.[1] The ability to measure all the components of oxygen status,
combined with a knowledge of their interaction and variabilities allows for greater scope
in patient management and provides important information on the integrity of the cardiopulmonary system.

Approximately 80% of total oxygen consumption occurs within mitochondria by
oxidative phosphorylation. Oxygen combines with electrons to produce free energy, which
in turn is used to pump H^+ from within the mitochondrion to the cytoplasm against an
electrochemical gradient. The H^+ then diffuses back along its gradient, releasing free energy that is used to produce adenosine triphosphate (ATP) from adenosine diphosphate
(ADP). ATP provides energy for most biological processes. A moderate to severe reduction in oxygen supply causes an increase in the rate of glycolysis (ATP production from
cytoplasmic anaerobic fermentation) in order to maintain cellular energy supply.[1] However glycolysis, unlike oxidative phosphorylation, does not provide sustained energy supply
because the lactate product of glycolysis leads to acidosis, which compromises optimal
cellular function. The remaining 20% of oxygen consumption occurs in subcellular or-
ganelles that are involved in biosynthetic, biodegradative and detoxification oxidations.
Some of the enzymes reacting with oxygen in these processes are sensitive to only moderate decreases in oxygen supply as a result of their low oxygen affinity (e.g. metabolic processes
involved in neurotransmitter production), unlike mitochondrial enzyme activity, which
has a high oxygen affinity.[1] Measurement and maintenance of oxygen status is therefore
essential if biochemical disorders resulting from poor oxygen supply are to be minimised.

Oxygen status of blood is defined by the following parameters: oxygen concentration (content) $ctO_2(B)$, oxygen saturation $SO_2(B)$, oxygen tension $pO_2(B)$ and haemoglobin
concentration $ctHb(B)$. (The IFCC/IUPAC system of nomenclature is used throughout
this text. 'B' means 'in blood').

Oxygen concentration refers to the total amount of oxygen contained within a unit
volume of blood and is commonly expressed as mmol/l, Vol% or mls oxygen per dl of
whole blood. Oxygen is carried in blood in two states:

Dissolved oxygen in blood. The amount of dissolved oxygen in blood depends
upon the $pO_2(B)$ (it also varies slightly with ctHb) and is 0.003 ml/dl blood/mmHg $pO_2(B)$
(concentration solubility coefficient for oxygen in blood, called α).[2,3]

Oxygen bound to haemoglobin, of which oxygen saturation $[SO_2(B)]$ is the percentage that oxygen-bound haemoglobin constitutes of the total haemoglobin capable of carrying oxygen.[4,5] Oxygen bound to haemoglobin constitutes approximately 99% of the oxygen content of blood. Ideally, when fully saturated with oxygen, each gram of normal haemoglobin holds 1.39 ml of oxygen. However, due to the presence of dyshaemoglobins (haemoglobin derivatives incapable of reversibly binding with oxygen molecules) the *in vivo* value for fully saturated haemoglobin is 1.36 ml of oxygen/gm haemoglobin.

Oxyhaemoglobin dissociation curve

The association between $pO_2(B)$ and oxygen saturation is governed by the shape of the oxyhaemoglobin dissociation curve (Fig. 5.1). This curve shows how oxygen tension $[pO_2(B)]$(abscissa) affects the reaction between oxygen and haemoglobin saturation, $SO_2(B)$ (ordinate). The S-shaped curve is due to the haemoglobin molecule having four oxygen binding sub-units each of which binds one oxygen molecule sequentially in four steps. The affinity for haemoglobin is increased as oxygen binds to haemoglobin (i.e. each successive sub-unit combination with oxygen facilitates the next sub-unit combination with oxygen). Conversely, each oxygen dissociation from a sub-unit facilitates further dissociations. This accounts for the steepness of the middle portion of the curve when the haemoglobin is partially saturated. However, at either limit of the curve, the propensity of oxygen to either associate or disassociate from haemoglobin decreases when the sub-units are almost saturated or desaturated with oxygen. This accounts for the curve being flatter at its limits.[4]

The steepness of the middle portion of the curve facilitates oxygen unloading to the tissues because a small decrease in $pO_2(B)$ results in significant dissociation of oxygen from haemoglobin, providing more oxygen for use by tissues. Unloading of oxygen is dependent on factors that can alter the shape and position of the curve on the abscissa. These factors are $pH(B)$, $pCO_2(B)$, blood temperature, 2,3-diphosphoglycerate (2,3-DPG), anaemia and various substances causing formation of dyshaemoglobins. These shifts in the oxyhaemoglobin dissociation curve can be represented by the value p50, which repre-

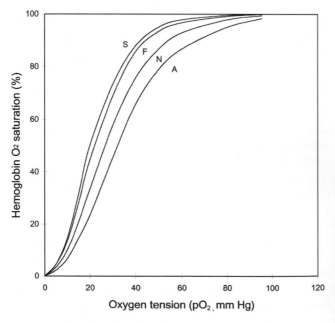

Figure 5.1.Oxyhaemoglobin dissociation curves, showing the relationship between haemoglobin oxygen saturation and oxygen tension in human blood from a smoker (S), foetus (F), normal adult (N, average of male and female) and an anaemic patient (A).

sents the $pO_2(B)$ at which half of all availableO_2 binding sites are occupied and thus represents the haemoglobin-oxygen affinity.[4]

When peripheral factors such as vascular disease, anaemia, heavy exercise and cardiac output are the main limitations to oxygen transport, the p50 increases to facilitate
oxygen unloading (the curve shifts to the right). When the limitation to oxygen transport is
due to poor oxygen diffusion in the lungs, the p50 decreases to reduce oxygen unloading
(the curve shifts to the left). Chemoreceptor control of ventilation, allosteric control of p50
and the diffusing capacities of the lungs and tissues regulate loading and unloading so that
the resultant p50 provides the best level of oxygen transport for all conditions.[6]

The Bohr effect describes the influence that $pH(B)$ and $pCO_2(B)$ have on the
oxyhaemoglobin dissociation curve. It occurs because deoxyhaemoglobin is a weaker acid
than oxyhaemoglobin. In tissue, deoxyhaemoglobin accepts hydrogen ions (produced by
dissociation of carbonic acid which in turn is produced from the reaction between water
and carbon dioxide) under low $pO_2(B)$/high $pCO_2(B)$ conditions. This decreases haemoglobin affinity for oxygen. In the lung, the high $pO_2(B)$/low $pCO_2(B)$ causes oxygen to
combine with haemoglobin. This releases hydrogen ions to combine with carbonic acid to
form bicarbonate, which liberates carbon dioxide and water. The high $pH(B)$ (low acidity/
low $pCO_2(B)$) increases haemoglobin affinity for oxygen.[4]

2,3-DPG is an important regulator of oxygen release by haemoglobin in adults.[4] It
is a product of anaerobic glycolysis in erythrocytes and causes a decrease in haemoglobin
affinity for oxygen. Anaemia triggers an adaptive mechanism causing a decrease in haemoglobin affinity for oxygen. This results from an increase in the 2,3-DPG levels in erythrocytes
during chronic anaemia.[7]

Haemoglobin

The haemoglobin complex has four iron-containing haem groups, i.e. four haemoglobin
monomer molecules. The haemoglobin molecule has four symmetrically arranged pyrroles with a ferrous iron (Fe^{2+}) at its centre and is also combined with the protein globin[8,4]
The globin molecule has four polypeptide chains. Normal adult haemoglobin (HbA) has
two alpha and two beta chains. The alpha polypeptide chains have 141 amino acids and
the beta chains have 146 amino acids. Foetal haemoglobin (HbF), with two alpha chains
and two gamma chains, has a greater affinity for oxygen than does adult haemoglobin,
foetal $pO_2(B)$ being lower than adult $pO_2(B)$ (4). The greater affinity is due to poor binding
of 2,3-DPG by the gamma chains.[2]

The iron is bound to each of the pyrroles and to one of the four polypeptides and
allows for reversible Hb-O_2 combinations. Oxygen or carbon monoxide can bind with the
sixth binding site on the ferrous iron.[4]. One molecule of Fe^{2+} can combine with one molecule of oxygen.[8] By changing the relationship of the polypeptide chains to each other, the
haemoglobin molecule assumes either a relaxed state that favours oxygen binding or a
tense state that decreases oxygen binding. This is achieved by breaking or forming salt-
bridges between the polypeptide chains. The two beta chains lie closer to each other when
oxygen is bound to haemoglobin. This alters oxygen affinity.[2]

The most frequently occurring haemoglobins are:

Deoxygenated (Reduced) haemoglobin (HHb). This is unassociated with oxygen and is bound to H^+ (the term 'deoxygenated' is recommended over 'reduced', as in a
chemical sense no reduction has taken place).

Oxyhaemoglobin (O_2Hb) is the haemoglobin (monomer) molecule with one oxygen molecule reversibly bound to the ferrous ion.

Carbaminohaemoglobin ($HHbCO_2$). This bond causes structural changes in the haemoglobin molecule, decreasing its affinity for oxygen. The haemoglobin-carbon dioxide bond does not occur on the same location on the haemoglobin molecule as the haemoglobin-oxygen covalent bond.[9] Carbon dioxide is not attached to the haem, but to the amino groups.[8]

Dyshaemoglobins (DysHb) are normal haemoglobins that have temporarily or permanently lost the ability at physiological pO_2 to reversibly bind with oxygen. Dyshaemoglobins should be distinguished from **abnormal haemoglobins,** which have genetically determined alterations in the globin moiety. Only a few of these haemoglobins have significantly different oxygen affinity.[10] Abnormal haemoglobins can be produced rarely by alterations of the structure in the haem groups or more commonly by genetic substitution of a single incompatible amino acid for a normal amino acid in an alpha or beta chain.[2]

Common dyshaemoglobins are:

Methaemoglobin (MetHb), sometimes referred to as hemiglobin (Hi), is not useful for carrying oxygen and is normally present in the blood in amounts that are typically below the detection capacity of commercial multiwavelength haemoximeters. Methaemoglobin can be formed by the action of oxidants. This can result from the action of certain substances such as local anaesthetics, cyano compounds, nitrates and nitrites or even via the action of the superoxide anion (O_2^-) that dissociates from the iron instead of O_2, leaving the iron in the ferric state (auto-oxidation). In the ferric state the haem iron does not bind to oxygen. Methaemoglobinaemia can occur via excess formation of methaemoglobin (endogenous or exogenous), limited reduction capacity of methaemoglobin to haemoglobin by erythrocytes from genetic deficiency of the methaemoglobin reductase enzyme, or the increased tendency of the haemoglobin iron to oxidation (found in rare haemoglobinopathies). In some instances oxidants can inhibit metabolic pathways such as oxidative phosphorylation by diffusing into tissues. This inhibits oxygen utilization.[10,11]

Carboxyhaemoglobin (COHb) occurs normally in amounts of less than 3% in non-smokers living in an urban environment. The increase in haemoglobin-oxygen affinity with carboxyhaemoglobin arises from the influence of the single carbon monoxide molecule in the haemoglobin tetramer on the oxygen binding by the other haem groups. As with methaemoglobin, there is a decrease in oxygen capacity with a resultant increase in haemoglobin-oxygen affinity and thus a shift in the oxyhaemoglobin curve to the left. The affinity of carbon monoxide for haemoglobin is approximately 200 times that of oxygen. As well as displacing oxygen, carbon monoxide can enter the cell and inhibit oxidative phosphorylation. The combined effects of carbon monoxide can cause tissue hypoxia, acidosis and central nervous system depression.[10,11] Other haemoglobin derivatives such as Sulfhaemoglobin (SHb), carboxysulfhaemoglobin (SHbCO) and Cyanmethaemoglobin (HiCNHb) are not usually found in significant amounts and account for less than 1% of total haemoglobin.[11]

Determinants of oxygen status

Currently, for determination of blood gas status, the most commonly used blood gas instruments measure pH, pCO_2 and pO_2. These instruments are used in conjunction with a haemoximeter which calculates total haemoglobin concentration (ctHb), measures oxygen saturation, and, with many, the percentage carboxyhaemoglobin (%COHb) [carboxyhaemoglobin fraction(FCOHb) expressed as a percentage] and percentage methaemoglobin (%MetHb)[methaemoglobin fraction(FMetHb) expressed as a percentage] of the total haemoglobin concentration. This arrangement allows derivation of bicarbonate concentration, base excess, oxygen content, concentration of active haemoglobin and the haemoglobin-oxygen affinity determined by p50.[12]

The single most important parameter in the arterial oxygen status is **oxygen content**. The most important component of oxygen content is the **total haemoglobin concentration,** as haemoglobin controls oxygen transport via the **oxyhaemoglobin dissociation curve** (Fig. 5.1).

In the path from alveoli to tissue cells:

The pO_2(aB)(oxygen tension of arterial blood) is a measure of diffusion of oxygen into blood from the lungs but gives no indication of oxygen content.[13] However, pO_2(aB) is a more sensitive diagnostic indicator of respiratory status than oxygen content. This is because the oxyhaemoglobin dissociation curve is flat at normal physiological pO_2(aB) above 70 mmHg. If a patient's pO_2(aB) falls from 90 mmHg to 70 mmHg the proportionate fall of pO_2(aB) will be significant (>20%). The proportionate fall of oxygen content will be insignificant (typically 3–4% for a normal ctHb level).

Oxygen content, cardiac output and/or organ perfusion together determine delivery of oxygen to tissues, where:

DO_2 (oxygen delivery to the tissues) = oxygen content x cardiac output, or,

DO_2 (oxygen delivery to an organ) = oxygen content x organ perfusion.[13]

Tissue end-capillary oxygen tension [pO_2(cB)](oxygen tension of capillary blood) reflects tissue oxygen supply under normal conditions. However since cardiac output and pO_2(cB) are more difficult to measure, oxygen availability is based on arterial blood [oxyhaemoglobin affinity (p50)] alone. Therefore oxygen content and particularly the oxygen content curve [the graphical relationship between oxygen content (ordinate) and pO_2(B) (abscissa)] are predictors of pO_2(cB). In order for oxygen content to be normal, the pO_2(aB), SO_2(aB) and total haemoglobin concentration must be normal.[13] Maintaining a normal pO_2(cB) is crucial because it is the vital parameter in oxygen supply to tissues and is dependent on perfusion parameters, the distribution of capillaries, pO_2(aB) and blood transport properties.[14]

Oxyhaemoglobin dissociation vs oxygen content curves

In order to understand these curves it is important to understand the difference between oxygen saturation and oxygen concentration of blood. **Oxygen saturation of haemoglobin** [SO_2(B)] is the oxyhaemoglobin fraction of active haemoglobin expressed as a percentage, i.e. $SO_2 = nO_2Hb/(nHHb + nO_2Hb)$ where n refers to the amount of substance of the relevant component. It can also be expressed as $SO_2 = cO_2Hb/(cHb + cO_2Hb)$ where c refers to substance concentration of the relevant component. Concentration of active (effective) haemoglobin is defined by ceHb = ctHb - cCOHb - cMetHb - cSHb - cXHb(concentration of unidentified inactive haemoglobin). Oxygen concentration(content) in blood is defined by ctO_2(B) = cO_2Hb(B) + cO_2(B) (concentration of dissolved oxygen in blood).[3]

Oxygen saturation is a derivative that reflects the pO_2(B) via their relationship in the oxyhaemoglobin dissociation curve. Fractional oxygen saturation of haemoglobin (FO_2Hb) is a derivative calculated by haemoximeters capable of measuring the percentage dyshaemoglobins and on its own is not a useful measurement. This is because a decrease in fractional oxygen saturation could be due to several reasons, e.g. a fall in pO_2(B) and/or an increase in dyshaemoglobins, or a decrease in Hb-O_2 affinity.[5] If the plot of oxygen content ctO_2(B) versus oxygen tension pO_2(B) is displayed as the oxygen content curve

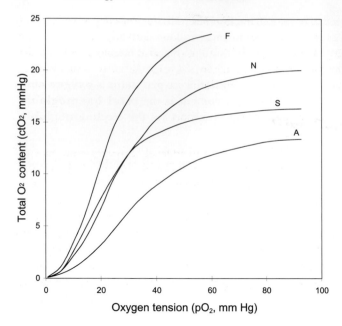

Figure 5.2. *Relationship between the oxygen concentration (content) and oxygen tension in human blood from a foetus (F), normal adult (N, average for male and female), smoker (S) and an anaemic patient (A).*

(Fig. 5.2), the effects of all factors influencing oxygen availability can be seen more clearly than the oxyhaemoglobin dissociation curve. The oxygen content curve for foetal blood shows a greater rise in oxygen content as $pO_2(B)$ increases compared to normal adult blood, and anaemic blood shows a smaller rise in oxygen content as $pO_2(B)$ rises compared to normal adult blood.

The oxyhaemoglobin dissociation curve does not show the effect that changes in haemoglobin concentration have on oxygen carrying capacity. It is therefore limited to illustrating only the differences between haemoglobin-oxygen affinities and not the effects from variations in the amount of haemoglobin available for oxygen transport, as illustrated by the oxygen content curve. The oxygen content curve illustrates and quantifies the ability of blood to release oxygen under different conditions.

New parameters

Apart from the commonly measured and derived parameters already mentioned, new oxygen parameters have been proposed to determine oxygen availability. These are not universally accepted but may provide clinical information for early prophylactic maintenance of oxygen status in critically ill patients, without pulmonary artery catheterisation. These parameters are:

Oxygen Extraction Tension (px). This is the oxygen tension in arterial blood after extraction of 2.3 mmol of oxygen per litre of blood (5.1 ml O_2/dl blood) at constant $pH(B)$ and $pCO_2(B)$. The normal arterio-venous difference in oxygen concentration is 2.3 mmol/l. A px value at or above the normal mixed venous $pO_2(B)$ [$pO_2(vB)$] thus indicates that the arterial blood is capable of releasing the normal amount of oxygen at or above the normal mixed venous oxygen tension. Px includes the effects of all parameters influencing $ctO_2(B)$. It therefore represents the maximum information on oxygen and is available from one arterial sample.[12]

Extractable Oxygen Concentration of Arterial Blood (Cx). This is the concentration of oxygen that can be extracted from arterial blood at a $pO_2(aB)$ of 38 mmHg.

It approximates $pO_2(vB)$ (e.g. a Cx below 1.8 mmol/l suggests cardiac output would need to increase to provide sufficient oxygen to the tissues).[12]

Oxygen Compensation Factor (Qx). This is the standard arterio-venous oxygen content difference (2.3 mmol/l) divided by Cx. Therefore it is the factor by which cardiac output should rise to maintain a $pO_2(vB)$ of 38 mmHg.[12]

Mixed venous oxygen saturation

The standard concepts based on oxygen delivery and a fixed level of oxygen extraction do not account for differences in metabolic oxygen requirements. It has been shown that oxygen delivery to tissues can be increased, resulting in significant increases in oxygen consumption until oxygen demands are met and oxygen consumption no longer increases. For critically ill patients whose oxygen demands are different, assessment of this endpoint would be useful.[15] These patients have a higher dependency of oxygen consumption on oxygen delivery levels that would under normal circumstances be considered adequate.[14] **Mixed venous oxygen saturation** [SO2(vB)] is a component in this determination. Increased oxygen demands are usually met by increased oxygen supply. This is achieved by increasing cardiac output so that mixed venous oxygen saturation is maintained to provide a reserve of oxygen.

Continuous mixed venous oxygen saturation measurements can be made using invasive fibreoptic probes.[13] Measurements are based on reflectance of specific light intensities from blood back to the probes. However, if changes in oxygen consumption are confined to a single organ, the mixed venous oxygen saturation does not change significantly and therefore the benefit of measuring it under these circumstances is questionable.[13] Mixed venous oxygen saturation does provide the ability to determine the matching of tissue oxygen delivery and oxygen consumption as well as the point at which oxygen consumption becomes dependent on tissue oxygen delivery. Mixed venous oxygen saturation monitoring indicates when changes in $PO_2(aB)$ result from changes in mixed venous oxygen saturation and not intrapulmonary shunting. It also provides the means to calculate cardiac output, oxygen consumption and intrapulmonary shunts and is an indicator of significant problems in overall oxygenation rather than single component problems because the latter are normally compensated for by changes in other related components.[16] A normal arterial oxygen saturation means that if the cardiac output is also normal then oxygen supply to the microvascular bed is normal, whilst analysis of mixed venous oxygen saturation indicates whether oxygen is actually delivered to the tissues. The determination of oxygen affinity of blood provides an even greater ability to ensure that supplied oxygen is properly delivered to tissues, and this involves determination of a complete oxyhaemoglobin dissociation curve using the p50, pH(B) and $pCO_2(B)$.[10]

Haemoximetry (CO-oximetry)

The most commonly used instruments for measuring the most important parameters in oxygen content [ctHb(B) and $SO_2(B)$] are the haemoximeters® (CO-oximeters). Their efficiency is gauged by their ability to measure accurately different derivatives of haemoglobin.

The haemoglobin percentages and oxygen saturations measured by haemoximeters use the same principles. They use a colour photometry method for measuring total haemoglobin [ctHb(B)] and concentrations of certain haemoglobin derivatives. Light intensities at specific wavelength channels are measured. The intensities are converted to absorbances from which the concentrations of derivatives are based. From this, the various fractions of haemoglobin are derived. The light intensities are the raw input data used in the algorithms for the instrument. Absorbance 'A' at wavelength λ is defined by:

A = log (I_0/I_s), where I_0 = measured reference light intensity with a clear cuvette sample (i.e. water), I_s = measured intensity with the blood cuvette sample. Subsequent calculations of saturations are based on the Lambert-Beers Law: $Ay^\lambda = E\ y^\lambda \times Cy^\lambda \times L$, where E = proportionality constant (termed molar absorptivity, or the molar extinction coefficient of the particular derivative compound), A = absorbance, L = light path (thickness of cuvette), y = compound derivative, λ= wavelength, C = molar concentration of the compound derivative.[17, 18] Thus, the calculation involves measuring the absorbance of both an unknown sample containing haemoglobin and a sample containing a known amount of haemoglobin and, with algebraic rearrangement, calculating the amount of unknown haemoglobin.[19]

Measurement of percentage oxygenated haemoglobin and percentage deoxygenated haemoglobin requires measurement of the total absorbance at only two wavelengths, e.g. the OSM2 (Radiometer Copenhagen) using 506.5 and 600.0 nm.[17] Measurement of other derivatives requires that the total absorbance must be measured at each of several wavelengths so that the minimum number of total absorbance measurements must equal the number of substances being measured,[19] i.e. in order to obtain solutions for n unknowns, there must be n independent equations. Therefore to measure deoxygenated, carboxy, oxy and methaemoglobins, a haemoximeter must use at least 4 wavelengths of light to produce 4 absorbance equations. The set of equations is called a determined matrix. Additional wavelengths can account for sulfhaemoglobin, interfering effects of foetal haemoglobin, and effects of such factors as thermal changes, turbidity and dyes such as bilirubin and methylene blue. Systems adopting extra wavelengths are referred to as 'overdetermined'. These 'extra' wavelengths, however, do not refer to those needed to compensate for bilirubin etc. but refer to systems with more wavelengths than light-absorbing components in the sample.[11,19]

The direct photometric measurement of concentration of haemoglobin derivatives requires discrete, narrow bands of light so that the small differences of light absorbed by the derivatives can be differentiated. Photometric measurement of the derivatives relies on the specific light absorption characteristics of each haemoglobin derivative at the selected wavelengths (which in turn requires the concentrations of each entity in reference materials to be known by the manufacturer).[19]

Haemoximeter accuracy is determined by the availability of pure reference materials and the accuracy to which the extinction co-efficients (light absorption characteristics) are known for each component and each of the selected wavelengths. When the fractional amounts of haemoglobin derivatives are low, the haemoximeters may not be ideal for differentiating between subjects and populations that have small differences between them, i.e. < 2–2.5%. This is because haemoximeters are designed to measure haemoglobin fractions over a broad analytical range. An additional problem occurs because dyshaemoglobins are such a small portion of the whole that any small variability in the background chromophores can result in large but not clinically significant differences between those dyshaemoglobin quantities. Abnormal haemoglobins can also produce altered absorbance characteristics. Wavelength selection can minimize sensitivity to interfering substances such as bilirubin and turbidity.[19] Interfering compounds absorb light in the same wavelength range as the derivative being measured.[18]

Measurement methods are standard for all haemoximeters. There are two types of light sources used by these instruments. The OSM3 (Radiometer Copenhagen) is an example of one where a white or incandescent light source such as tungsten (maintained at constant intensity) illuminates the haemolyzed sample (haemolyzed to eliminate light scat-\tering caused by red blood cells). Ultraviolet and infrared blocking filters eliminate high and low wavelength light. The visible light passes through the sample, after which it passes through a diffraction grating where the spectrum is separated into individual wavelengths that pass to the photodiodes. The light that some haemoximeters use is referred to as spectral. They use a lamp, neon or thallium hollow-cathode (maintained at constant intensity) that produce multiple precise narrow-band-pass wavelengths called 'lines'. These lines have fixed wavelengths, with the bandwidths being sufficiently narrow that differences to the actual bandwidth characteristics of the entire optical path are insignificant. The spectral lines are selected for analysis by blocking undesired light bands with interference filters. Each wavelength requires a separate filter. The light then passes through the sample and is collected by a single photodiode. The disadvantages of this system are that the wavelengths available may not be optimal for determination of a certain derivative and may allow other absorbing materials apart from haemoglobin derivatives to be measured. Both systems use the reference light intensity measured from water in the cuvette and compare it to the detected light (from the sample) at the photodiode. Absorption can thus be determined.[19]

With the advent of discrete multiwavelength spectrophotometers such as the CO-oximeter 2500 and 270 (Ciba-Corning) using 7 wavelengths, OSM3 (6 wavelengths) and the IL482 (Instrument Laboratories), direct measurement of percentage methaemoglobin, percentage carboxyhaemoglobin and more accurate oxygen saturation readings are possible.[20] Even multiwavelength analysers can be affected by dyshaemoglobins. Percentage of sulfhaemoglobin in blood rarely exceeds 1%; but if a sample were to contain as much as 10% sulfhaemoglobin, it has been reported that the OSM3 (discrete wavelength hemoximeter) will measure percentage of methaemoglobin as being 3.5% less than actual and the percentage carboxyhaemoglobin as being 2.5% higher than actual. However, the OSM3 will display a warning that the percentage sulfhaemoglobin is high.[21] Sulfhaemoglobin has different absorption spectra from deoxyhaemoglobin and has a low oxygen affinity. It is capable of reversibly binding with oxygen although the Sulf-Hb bond is irreversible and its p50 is more than two orders of magnitude (i.e. >100 times) greater than that of normal haemoglobin.[10] Similarly, foetal haemoglobin, which can constitute as much as 90% of the total haemoglobin in newborns, can affect discrete wavelength haemoximeters. A foetal haemoglobin level of 80% in a fully oxygenated sample can cause an error of up to 4% in the SO_2 determination[18] unless compensated for.

The ABL 725 (Radiometer Copenhagen) is an example of a new generation of instruments using full spectrum (visual range), which makes it an overdetermined system. It has a concave holographic grating and employs 128 photodiodes constituting a self-scanning integrated photodiode array. It is capable of measuring a continuous absorption spectrum with a wavelength range of 478–672 nm in 128 channels. It has a spectral resolution of 1.5 nm and a bandwidth of 2 nm. The discrete wavelengths offered by traditional haemoximeters only allow measurement of the spectra for deoxygenated, oxy, carboxy, met and sulf haemoglobins and intralipid, whereas the multiwavelength instruments using the continuous spectrum allow measurement of spectra from conjugated and unconjugated bilirubin and oxy-foetal haemoglobin (O_2HbF).[18]

Oxygen tension (pO_2)

The remaining component of oxygen concentration, $pO_2(B)$, is commonly measured using a Clark electrochemical cell. A platinum cathode is maintained at a negative potential relative to a silver/silver chloride reference electrode (anode), both immersed in electrolyte solution (potassium chloride). Oxygen is reduced at the platinum cathode producing a current proportional to the $pO_2(B)$.[22]

Apart from the *in vitro* methods, intravascular methods have been developed using optical sensors. Light of certain wavelengths illuminates a sample chamber containing dye on a fibreoptic probe. The amount of incident light absorbed by the dye depends on the amount of analyte or, by another method, the intensity of re-emitted radiation at modified wavelengths is determined by the amount of analyte. These instruments can be affected by thrombosis, reduced blood flow and vessel wall effect, i.e. measurement of tissue gas exchange if forced against the vessel wall.[22] Biosensor electrodes using enzymes, antibodies and nucleic acids have been used for *in vivo* blood gas monitoring.[14] Transcutaneous monitoring using heated Clark electrodes placed on the skin are used widely in neonatology for $pO_2(B)$ measurements. Their accuracy is dependent on adequate skin circulation. Another non-invasive method of (oxygen only) blood gas analysis is pulse oximetry (see Chapter 5). However this method presumes, as do the two wavelength haemoximeters, that only oxygenated and deoxygenated haemoglobin are present in the blood.[14]

Assessment of cardiac, pulmonary and circulatory function is enhanced by knowledge of the blood oxygen status, e.g. oxygen saturation analysis from multiple sites allows intracardiac shunts to be localised and quantified. The evolution of instruments capable of accurately measuring the necessary paramaters has been invaluable in clarifying our understanding of the determinants of blood pathophysiology.

References

1. Robin ED. Tissue O_2 Utilization. In: Loeppky, Riedesel (eds). *Oxygen transport to human tissues*. Amsterdam: Elsevier Biomedical 1982, pp.179-86.
2. Ganong WF. *Review of medical physiology*. Sydney: Prentice-Hall 1991, pp.616-19.
3. Wimberley PD, Siggaard-Anderson O *et al.* Haemoglobin oxygen saturation and related quantities: Definitions, symbols and clinical use. *Scand J Clin Lab Invest* 1990; **50**:455-59.
4. Levitzky MG. *Pulmonary physiology*, 3rd ed. New York: McGraw-Hill 1991, pp.137-48.
5. Oeseburg B. Definition, notation and reporting of oxygen quantities in blood. *Blood Gas News* 1995; **4**(1):3-6.
6. Hsai CW. Respiratory function of hemoglobin. *New England Journal of Medicine* 1998; **338**(4):239-47.
7. Zschiedrich H . Therapeutic threshold values for chronic alterations in hemoglobin concentration. In: Zander R, Mertzlufft F(eds). *The oxygen status of arterial blood*. Basel: Karger 1991, pp.174-83.
8. Ross G (ed.). *Essentials of.* Chicago, Year Book Medical Publishers 1979 pp.280-7.
9. Reeder G. *The biochemistry and physiology of hemoglobin*. American Society of Extra-Corporeal Technology Inc, Reston, 1986.
10. Zijlstra WG, Maas AHJ, Moran RF. Definition, significance and measurement of quantities pertaining to the oxygen carrying properties of human blood. *Scand J Clin Lab Invest* 1996; **56**(Suppl.) 224:27-45.
11. Moran RF. Application of hemoglobin derivatives in STAT analysis. *Blood Gas News* 1999; **8**(1):4-11.
12. Siggaard-Anderssen O Wimberley PD, Fogh-Andersen N, Gothgen IH .Arterial oxygen status determined with routine pH/blood gas equipment and multi-wavelength hemoximetry; reference values, precision and accuracy. *Scand J Clin Lab Invest* 1990; **50**(Suppl.) 203:57-66.
13. Zander R. The oxygen status of arterial human blood. In: Zander R, Mertzlufft F, (eds) *The oxygen status of arterial blood*. Basel: Karger 1991, pp.1-13.
14. Waldau T. Blood Gases-measurement and interpretation of results. *Blood Gas News* 1995; **4**(1):7-12.

15. Shapiro BA. Assessment of oxygenation. Today and tomorrow. *Scand J Lab Invest* 1990; **50**(Suppl.) 203:197-202.

16. Ahrens T, Rutherford K. *Essentials of oxygenation.* Boston: Jones & Bartlett 1993, pp.96-7.

17. *OSM2 Hemoximeter user's handbook.* Radiometer Copenhagen, Edition P 1988, pp.65-70.

18. Singer P. Suppression of fetal hemoglobin and bilirubin on oximetry measurement. *Blood Gas News* 1999; **8**(1):12-17.

19. Brunelle J, Degtiarov A, Moran R, Race L. Simultaneous measurement of total hemoglobin and its derivatives in blood using CO-oximeters: Analytical principles; their application in selecting analytical wavelengths and reference methods; a comparison of the results of the choices made. *Scand J Clin Lab Invest* 1996; **56** (Suppl.) 224:47-69.

20. Mertzlufft F. Determination of arterial O_2 saturation: Oxymetry. In: Zander R, Mertzlufft F, (eds). *The oxygen status of arterial blood.* Basel: Karger 1991, pp 89-97.

21. Wu C, Kenny A. A case of sulfhemoglobinemia and emergency measurement of sulfhemoglobin with an OSM3 CO-oximeter. *Clin Chem* 1997; **43**(1):162-6.

22. Mahutte CK. On line arterial blood gas analysis with optodes: Current status. *Clin Biochem* 1998; **31**(3):119-30.

Chapter 6

Radiation Safety in the Cardiac Catheterisation Laboratory

Operator and Patient Exposure Minimisation

Peter Cross

The interventional diagnostic radiology room, and in particular the cardiac catheterisation laboratory, present a unique environment containing several kinds of hazards. One major concern is that of radiation exposure, both to staff and patient. Whereas patients are more likely to experience skin injury from a prolonged examination, staff members may accumulate radiation exposure in a daily work environment that can extend over several years. The risk to both groups can be reduced by an understanding of the physics of radiation, and by practising the safety procedures described in this chapter.

Penetrating radiations are an essential feature of current medical radiodiagnostic practice. These radiations are called ionising radiation because they can ionise and excite molecules in the body, and damage living tissue. Precautions must therefore be taken when working with ionising radiation. For safety considerations, exposure to radiation is classified as:

- **Occupational:** That which is incurred at work by radiation workers such as radiologists, medical fluoroscopists, scientists, technologists and radiographers.
- **Medical:** That which is incurred by individuals as part of their own medical diagnosis or treatment.
- **Public:** That which encompasses all exposures other than occupational and medical. The greatest component in this category is that due to natural or environmental sources.

Ionising radiation is quantified in different ways according to the physical effect measured:

Exposure is a measure of the quantity of ionisation per unit mass of air. The unit of exposure is Coulomb per kilogram ($C\ kg^{-1}$). The unit used until recently was the Roentgen (R), but the sievert (Sv) is the unit now used for radiation protection purposes.

Absorbed dose is a measure of the amount of **energy** imparted to matter per unit mass of irradiated material. The unit of absorbed dose is joule per kilogram ($J\ kg^{-1}$), with the special name gray (Gy). One Gy is equal to 100 rads in the old units.

Equivalent dose (H_T) is a quantity introduced for radiation protection purposes. It relates to harmful effects that may be caused to an organ or tissue by exposure to different types and energies of radiation, each type being given a weighting factor according to its ionising characteristics. The unit of equivalent dose is the same as that for absorbed dose, $J\ kg^{-1}$, with the special name sievert (Sv). Equivalent dose is a descriptor for a specified organ or tissue, and for diagnostic medical radiations the radiation weighting factor is assumed to be unity.

Effective dose (E) is a weighted sum of equivalent doses of all organs and tissues of the body. Different sensitivities of the various organs are described by a tissue-specific weighting factor. The unit of effective dose is also J kg^{-1}, or sievert (Sv).

The majority of average annual radiation dose to the population is from natural sources of radiation. In Australia the environmental effective dose is of the order of 2 mSv (2 x 10^{-3} Sv) annually. A significant component of this effective dose comes from food and drink. There is a substantial amount of natural radioactivity in the human body. It has to contend with about 40 million disintegrations per hour, which corresponds to an activity of 10 kBq (or 0.3 mmCi in the old units). The Becquerel is the unit used to measure radiation protection (1 Bq equals 1 J/kg).

In Australia the National Health and Medical Research Council[1] and state authorities set **dose limits**. These dose limits are consistent with international recommendations[2] for radiation doses that occupationally exposed persons and members of the public can receive. It is not intended that these limits be an allowable level, but rather that the dose should always be kept As Low As Reasonably Achievable (the ALARA principle) and within the limits tabulated below.

Exposure	Occupational	Public
Whole body (effective dose)	20 mSv per year (averaged over 5 consecutive years)	1 mSv per year
Lens of the eye	150 mSv	15 mSv
Skin	500 mSv	15 mSv
Hands and feet	500 mSv	—

Obviously, doses to patients are higher. There are no regulatory limits on the cumulative amount of radiation that a patient may receive from diagnostic or interventional medical procedures.

Radiation levels in the catheterisation laboratory, because of the requirement of extended exposure, are the highest encountered during any commonly performed diagnostic radiological study. It is important therefore that laboratory personnel be aware of these radiation dose levels and methods of their reduction, consistent with obtaining images of adequate diagnostic quality.[3]

Radiation exposure effects are grouped as follows:

• **Stochastic effects**, where there is a probability of an effect at any dose, the probability increasing with dose. In the absence of accurate data at very low doses and at low dose rate, it is assumed that there is zero probability of an effect only at zero dose.
• **Deterministic effects**, where there is no effect until a threshold is reached, beyond which the severity of the effect increases.
• **Hereditary effects**, where subsequent generations are affected.

The purpose of radiation protection is to prevent deterministic effects and to limit stochastic effects to acceptable levels. The major stochastic effects are carcinogenesis and leukaemogenesis, while examples of deterministic effects are cataract formation and skin erythema. The latency period for stochastic effects to become apparent is usually many years, whereas deterministic effects may manifest themselves in only a few days.

Radiation safety measures for the operator and assistants

Radiation exposure to staff in the fluoroscopy room is mostly from radiation scatter from the patient. The primary beam is attenuated and absorbed by the patient and the image receptor (intensifier).

The protection methods used to reduce personnel exposure are to:

Minimise **time**
Maximise **distance**
Maximise **shielding**

Time

As time spent in a radiation field increases, the radiation dose received also increases, so the beam-on time should be kept to an absolute minimum. Exposure may be regulated either at the control panel or at the table-side by the foot pedal. Keeping fluoroscopic beam-on time and the number of image acquisitions for a procedure to a minimum will prevent unnecessary radiation dose to the operator, attending personnel and the patient.

Distance

As distance from a radiation source increases, radiation exposure decreases very rapidly. Doubling the distance between a person and the source reduces exposure by one fourth (1/4), according to the **inverse square law,** the rule that relates distance with dose reduction. It is good practice for personnel to keep as much distance between themselves and the radiation source as is reasonably possible, especially during acquisition as acquisition runs require higher radiation setting factors and generate higher dosages.

Shielding

Lead and concrete are the most commonly used materials for shielding against x-rays. The walls of x-ray rooms are usually lined with laminated lead panels to reduce exposure to areas on the other side of the wall. Viewing areas are additionally protected with transparent lead acrylic windows. The lead equivalence of panels and windows should be 0.5 mm Pb, which will shield protected areas and give approximately 90% reduction of the scattered radiation. Portable or hanging transparent lead acrylic shields can give typically an 85% dose reduction. All personnel who are not positioned behind a radiation barrier must wear a protective lead apron and thyroid collars during the procedure. Aprons and collars must have a shielding value of not less than 0.3 mm lead equivalent at 150kVp. They should be properly stored on a hanger when not in use and handled with care, since the protective lining can be damaged and may compromise their shielding characteristics. Leaded eyewear, fitted with side panels to reduce penetration of lateral scatter, provides an extra measure of protection.

Staff who regularly perform, or who assist in, fluoroscopic procedures are required to wear a personal radiation monitoring device (film or thermoluminescent card holder). For an estimate of effective dose (E), two monitors should be worn. One should be worn underneath a protective lead apron at chest or waist level (measurement H_1). The second should be worn at the neck outside a thyroid collar (measurement H_2). An estimate for E is given by a weighted sum of H_1 and H_2.[4] For example, for fluoroscopy at 90 kVp with an undertable x-ray tube and the fluoroscopist/assistant wearing an apron and collar of 0.5 mm Pb equivalent, an estimate of effective dose (E) is given by:

$$E = 0.5H_1 + 0.025H_2$$

The monitors should be clearly distinguished as to where they are worn to avoid confusion on their readings. Results should be regularly interpreted and reviewed to verify that work practices are adequate.

Radiation safety measures for the patient

The medical value of fluoroscopic x-rays is well recognised, but not so is the potential danger in their use, the assumption being that the benefit to the patient outweighs any radiation risk. It is important that measures are introduced to reduce the likelihood and severity of deterministic effects in fluoroscopically guided interventional procedures that may result in high patient dose.

Skin injuries attributable to x-rays from fluoroscopy have recently been reported.[5] A dramatic but rare example was reported in 1995[6] in which a male patient underwent coronary angiography, coronary angioplasty and a second angiography due to complications all on the same day. It was estimated that the fluoroscopic exposure time exceeded 120 minutes and the skin dose exceeded 20 Gy. Erythema was noticed about one month after the procedure. Skin breakdown continued over the following months with progressive necrosis. The patient eventually required a skin grafting procedure. This case is described in detail, along with others, on the US Food and Drug Administration's Internet site.[6]

Again, in keeping with international standards, in Australia the National Health and Medical Research Council and State Authorities have set output dose rate limits for fluoroscopy units. For continuous or pulsed fluoroscopy, the maximum allowable dose rate in air at the surface of the patient (table surface) is 50 mGy/min without automatic exposure control, and 100 mGy/min with exposure control. However, for fluoroscopy with cine or digital image acquisition, there is no regulation or standard specifying a limit for the dose per frame (image), either at the input to the image intensifier or to the patient surface. In order to evaluate radiation doses received by patients, radiation dose rates should be known for the specific fluoroscopy system and for each mode of operation used during the various procedure types. Ideally, these dose rates should be derived from measurements performed by a radiological physicist at the particular facility.

With this information clinicians involved in interventional procedures can be aware of what length of screening time and number of cine runs, or similar, would lead to a skin dose in the beam exceeding an action level of, say, 1 to 2 Gy, which would correspond to an early (few hours) transient erythema.

As an example, consider the skin dose from a typical procedure. The x-ray output would be about 170 μGy/mAs at 75 cm with 3 mm Al beam filtration, and a typical skin focus distance of 70 cm.

For screening, the technique factors could be 90 kVp, 2 mA for 15 minutes. The skin entrance absorbed dose is then:

$$170 \times (75/70)^2 \times 2 \times 15 \times 60 = 350 \text{ mGy}$$

This corresponds to a dose rate of 23.3 mGy/min; thus it would take approximately 43 minutes of screening on the primary field to reach an entrance dose of 1 Gy.

For image acquisition (cine) the technique factors could be 90 kVp, 100 mA, 3 ms pulse width, and 50 frames/second. The single frame entrance absorbed dose is:

$$170 \times (75/70)^2 \times 100 \times 0.003 = 58.6 \text{ μGy}$$

Assuming 6 cine runs of 7 seconds each, the total number of frames will be 6 x 7 x 50 = 2100, and the total cine absorbed dose is 58.6 x 2.1 mGy = 123.1 mGy.

The total skin absorbed dose from 43 minutes of screening and 6 cine runs would then be 1.123 Gy.

Calculations such as these should be documented for all the protocols used in the cardiac catheterisation laboratory.

In addition, radiological technique factors should be recorded in the patient's notes so that an estimate can be made of the skin absorbed dose if so required. Thus, for screening record the kVp, mA and total screening time, and for cine record the kVp, mA, pulse width, frame rate, and number of cine runs. For both modes of operation a listing of multiple views should be made so that an estimate can be made of the dose to the common region of irradiated skin. The use of a transmission ionisation chamber fitted into an x-ray tube head, post-collimation, can be the most reliable dose measurement technique for dynamic radiological examinations such as fluoroscopy where the projection directions and technique factors are continually varying. The quantity measured is the dose area product (DAP). The maximum skin entrance dose can be deduced from the DAP if field size and x-ray focus skin distance are known.[7]

Discussion on patient exposure dose tends to focus on the absorbed dose of entrance skin directly in the path of the radiation beam that can lead to deterministic effects. Concern is sometimes expressed, both by patients and staff, about the dose to internal organs not in the path of the direct beam, and the possible associated stochastic health effects. This dose to internal organs arises from radiation scatter within the patient, and to a much lesser extent from scatter from the image intensifier close to the patient's surface. Equivalent organ doses and the effective dose to the patient can be calculated for each angiographic projection from the measured skin entrance dose.[8] The total radiation risk to patients consists mainly of risk of lung cancer, as the lungs, being mostly in the direct beam, receive a relatively high dose[9] compared with the female gonad dose (two orders of magnitude less) and with the male gonads, which receive virtually no dose. Female patients of reproductive age may be reassured by placing a lead apron on their pelvic region under the drapes. This will contribute to a 'feel good' factor but will have little effect in reducing the actual radiation dosage received.

Recommendations for safe fluoroscopy practice

Factors that determine radiation dose and dose rate to the patient (and to personnel) during fluoroscopy/fluorography are as follows:

1. Size of the patient

As the beam is positioned over thicker areas of a patient, the penetrability of x-rays decreases. To maintain image quality the kVp and/or mA are controlled either automatically or manually. How this is done will determine the amount of increase in dose rate with increasing patient size.

Dose rates will be greater and dose will accumulate faster in larger patients.

2. Tube current

Entrance dose rates are in direct proportion to tube current.

Keep the tube current as low as possible.

3. Tube kilovoltage (kVp)

Higher kVp is generally required with the larger patient for increased beam penetration (image brightness) but this is accompanied by a lowering of image contrast and increase in x-ray production, the latter being proportional to $(kVp)^2$. From the patient viewpoint, a higher kVp beam is advantageous since it contains less of the softer or low-energy x-rays that contribute to a higher skin dose but not to image formation. Reducing tube current will lower x-ray production but will not affect penetration. It is preferable to operate with a higher kVp and low mA than with a low kVp and a high mA.

Keep the kVp as high as possible to achieve a compromise between image quality and low patient dose.

4. Proximity of x-ray tube to the patient

It is important in all procedures to maintain the x-ray source at maximum distance from the patient's surface (as for personnel). This distance may be limited by the design of the unit, and arising from this it should be remembered that in lateral and oblique projections entrance dose rates at the patient's skin can be much higher than those measured in the PA (or AP) view.

Keep the x-ray tube at maximal distance from the patient.

5. Proximity of image intensifier (ii) to the patient

When the ii is close to the patient, image quality can improve because distortion of anatomy and image blur decrease. Also, the intensity of x-rays required to produce a sufficiently bright image decreases, resulting in a better image with lower patient dose.

Keep the image intensifier as close to the patient as possible.

6. Image magnification

Entrance dose rate at the patient's skin is related to the magnification (ii field size) selected. To a good approximation, dose rates scale inversely with the area of the ii field size. Thus, compared with an 18 cm (7") diameter field, a 13 cm (5") field will require double the dose, and a 23 cm (9") field will require half the dose.

Do not over-use the magnification (small field) mode of operation.

7. X-ray field collimation

Collimators can be manually adjusted to reduce or enlarge the size of the x-ray field. Collimating to the area of interest reduces scatter radiation and so improves image quality. Reducing the field size also reduces the volume of patient tissue being irradiated and decreases the dose to personnel, since less room scatter is generated. Over-collimation, however, can also cut off the area of interest and may lead to repeat screening, thus doubling the original dosage.

Always use tight collimation (when appropriate).

8. Beam-on time

Minimising fluoroscopic beam-on time and the number of image acquisitions for a procedure will prevent unnecessary radiation dose to the patient, fluoroscopist and other personnel. Do not screen when the live image on the TV monitor is not being used. Use the last-image hold after the beam is turned off for continual visualisation.

Keep beam-on time to an absolute minimum.

9. Wedge filter

Wedge filters are used to 'harden' the x-ray beam. They cut out lower energy x-rays, leaving higher energy rays, thereby softening the skin dose. Filters also reduce the need for repeat angiographic runs (acquisitions) that may arise from image 'flaring'.

Use wedge filter.

In summary, it is most important that the potential for approaching or exceeding the threshold for skin injury be recognised and that procedures for avoidance be implemented. Fluoroscopists and radiographers must always adopt procedures that minimise the dose to their patients and to themselves.[10,11]

References

1. National Health and Medical Research Council recommendations and national standard for limiting exposure to ionising radiation. Radiation Health Series 1995, No. 39.
2. ICRP 60. Recommendations of the International Commission on Radiological Protection. Oxford: Pergamon Press, 1991.
3. Johnson LW, Moore RJ, Balter S. Review of radiation safety in the cardiac catheterisation laboratory. *Cathet Cardiovasc Diagn* 1992; **25**:186-94.
4. Rosenstein M. Practical approaches to dosimetry for the patient and staff for fluoroscopic procedures. In: *Proceedings of the 9th Conference of the International Radiation Protection Association.* Vienna 1996; **1**:219-26.
5. Vano E, Larranz L, Sastre JM, *et al.* Dosimetric and radiation protection considerations based on some cases of patient skin injuries in interventional cardiology. *Br J Radiol* 1998; **71**:510-16.
6. Shope, TB. Radiation-induced Skin injuries from fluoroscopy. Center for Devices and Radiological Health, Food and Drug Administration, MD 20857,USA. Internet Site http://www.fda.gov/cdrh/rsnaii.html.
7. Betsou S, Efstathopuolos EP, Katritsis, D, *et al.* Patient radiation doses during cardiac catheterisation procedures. *Br J Radiol* 1998; **71**:634-39.
8. Stern HD, Rosenstein M, Renaud L, Zanki M. Handbook of selected tissue doses for fluoroscopic and cineangiographic examination of the coronary arteries. CDRH (FDA), US Dept Health and Human Services, September 1995.
9. Karpinen T, Parviainen T, Servomaa A. Radiation risk and exposure of radiologists and patients during coronary angiography and percutaneous transluminal angioplasty (PTCA). *Radiation Protection Dosimetry* 1995; **57**, Nos.1-4, 481-5.
10. Faulkner K. Radiation protection in interventional radiology. *Br J Radiol* 1997; **70**:325-6.
11. Vano E, Gonzales L, Guibelalde E, *et al.* Radiation exposure to medical staff in interventional and cardiac radiology. *Br J Radiol* 1998; **71**:954-60.

Chapter 7

Infection Control Procedures

Jennifer Lemmon and Jock Harkness

Infection control has become one of the most important issues facing many clinical disciplines in the last 15 to 20 years, resulting mainly from the emergence of blood-borne viruses such as hepatitis B and C and the human immunodeficiency virus. The field of cardiac catheterisation is no exception and many questions have been raised about the development of a rational approach to infection control precautions while maintaining methods of best practice.

Of particular relevance is the enormous cost of equipment and the reportedly low incidence of infection among patients who have undergone this procedure. Nevertheless, due to the invasive nature of cardiac catheterisation there is an associated risk of infection to the patient, along with the risk of occupational exposure of health care workers (HCWs) to blood or body substances. This section discusses infection control measures required to reduce the risk of disease transmission to both patients and HCWs when cardiac catheterisation is performed.

Patient preparation

One of the most important areas of preparation is the patient's skin at the site of catheter insertion. Correct preparation of the puncture site is required to reduce the number of potentially infectious microorganisms on the patient's skin. If clipping or shaving of the skin site is required, this should be done just before commencing the procedure. The skin site should be washed with a skin disinfectant and prepared using an antimicrobial agent, working from the centre of the intended puncture site to the perimeter.[1] Careful cleansing of the wound site, following aseptic techniques, decreases the risk of bacterial infections caused by organisms such as staphylococcal species.[2]

Equipment sterility

A sterile field must be maintained at all times when performing cardiac catheterisation. Following skin preparation, sterile drapes are used to surround the prepared area in order to prevent contamination from adjacent unprepared areas.[3] This sterile field extends to the catheter table and parts of the machines used for the procedure.

All instruments inserted into a patient must be sterile. Many institutions have re-used cardiac catheters in order to contain the escalating cost of these items. As catheter manufacturers now market their products as disposable single-use items, re-use of this equipment is not recommended and should be discontinued. The risk of contamination from viable pathogens surviving the sterilisation process by remaining within crystalline blood cells is a disturbing scenario that precludes re-use of such items. Several studies, however, have shown no increase in the infection rates of patients who had a re-used catheter inserted, provided that the catheter had been cleaned and sterilised correctly.[4-7]

Pre-packaging

Pre-packaged kits containing disposable catheterisation instruments have increased in popularity in recent years. As use of single-use disposable items is a proven barrier to contamination and spread of infection, they are recommended in cardiac catheterisation.

Disposable transducers can also be included in standard diagnostic catheter kits, but it is up to individual laboratories to decide whether to re-use such equipment.

Standard precautions

The term 'universal precautions' was adopted in Australia to mean that all blood and body substances were considered to be potentially infectious regardless of the patient's infectious status or the perceived risk. In addition, use of gloves was considered a suitable alternative to hand washing.[8] This broad approach was subsequently considered confusing and likely to cause a false sense of security in its application.

As a result, the National Health and Medical Research Council and Australian National Council on AIDS working party on infection control recommended in 1996 the adoption of the alternative 'standard precautions' for treatment and care of all patients. 'Standard precautions' applies to all patients regardless of their perceived infectious status, and pertains to the handling of blood, all other body fluids, non-intact skin or mucous membranes, secretions and excretions (excluding sweat), regardless of whether they contain visible blood.[8]

In late 1999, the term 'standard precautions' was endorsed throughout most organisations applying the major features of universal precautions, blood and body fluid precautions and body substance isolation. As with the National Health and Medical Research Council guidelines, 'standard precautions' apply to all patients receiving care, regardless of their diagnosis or presumed infection status.[9]

Hand washing and hand care

Hand washing is the single most important practice in preventing spread of infection and should occur routinely before significant contact with any patient and after all activities that may have caused contamination of the hands. HCWs involved in cardiac catheterisation must use a surgical hand-wash technique.

A surgical hand wash involves the use of a suitable anti-microbial skin cleanser for thoroughly washing hands, fingernails and forearms to remove dirt and transient bacteria. Five minutes is the recommended minimum period for the first surgical hand wash for the day, while subsequent washes should be three minutes. Hands should be dried thoroughly with a sterile towel prior to donning sterile gloves. Care must be taken not to touch non-sterile items.[3,8]

Suitable hand creams should be used to prevent irritation or sensitivity from repeated hand washing and glove use. HCWs who have cuts or abrasions on their hands should cover them with water-resistant occlusive dressings.

Protective measures

Laslett *et al.* reported that there was no significant increase in infection rates after cardiac catheterisation, whether or not a HCW wore a cap and mask.[10] While this study was useful in determining that the risk of infection to patients is insignificant whether or not a cap and mask are worn, it did not consider the risk to HCWs of accidental exposure to patients' blood or body substances. The authors have also noted that few physicians perform catheterisation without wearing at least a mask, owing to awareness of the risk of exposure to blood.

As HCWs are at risk of exposure to patients' blood or body substances, protective eyewear and a mask or faceshield should be worn along with gloves and gowns for added protection.

Sharps

To prevent potential exposure to blood-borne diseases, sharps must be handled with extreme care at all times. The person who generates the sharp must be responsible for its immediate disposal following use into a clearly labelled puncture-resistant container.[8] Sharps must not be passed by hand between HCWs. A kidney dish or other container must be provided to permit passing to another operator.[8] If a sharp is to be re-used it must be placed in a labelled puncture-resistant container for reprocessing, which must be performed in a way that minimises risk of injury.

Spills

Any blood or body substance spill should be cleaned up immediately. Wearing gloves and other appropriate protective apparel, the HCW should use disposable paper towelling to remove all the spill, then a neutral detergent should be used for cleaning. Contaminated towelling should be placed in a contaminated-waste bag.[8]

Clinical waste

Waste segregation should occur at the point of generation. This means that all disposable waste contaminated with patients' blood or body substances must be disposed of into the appropriate yellow contaminated-waste bags. Non-contaminated disposable waste should be disposed of with general waste. Waste disposal must follow national guidelines or codes of practice and comply with local regulations.[8]

It is ultimately up to the individual operator to implement all appropriate infection control guidelines. In team-oriented environments such as the catheter laboratory, only suitable staff training, supervision and strict adherence to safety requirements will maintain satisfactory standards and ensure the lowest possible infection rate.

References

1. Larson E. APIC guidelines for infection control practice. Guideline for use of topical antimicrobial agents. *Am J Infect Contl* 1988; **16**:253.
2. Grossman W, Bain D. *Cardiac catheterisation angiography and interventions*, 4th ed. Philadelphia: Lea and Febiger 1991, pp37-38.
3. Bennett JV, Brachman PS. *Hospital infections*, 3rd ed. Boston: Little, Brown 1992.
4. Frank U, Herz L, Daschner FD. Infection risk of cardiac catheterisation and arterial angiography with single and multiple use disposable catheters. *Clin Cardiol* 1988; **11**:785-87.

5.   Dunnigan A, Roberts C, McNamara M *et al.* Success of re-use of cardiac electrode catheters. *Am J Cardiol* 1987; **60**:807-10.

6.   O'Donoghue S, Platia EV. Reuse of pacing catheters: A survey of safety and efficacy. *PACE* 1988; **11:**1279-80.

7.   Avitall B, Khan M, Krum D *et al.* Repeated use of ablation catheters: A prospective study. *J Am Coll Cardiol* 1993; **22**(5):1367-72.

8.   National Health and Medical Research Council. *Infection control in the health care setting.* Canberra: Australian Government Publishing Service 1996.

9.   NSW Health Department. *Infection control policy* Circular 99/87. Sydney: NSW Health Department, 1999.

10.   Laslett LJ, Sabin A. Wearing of caps and masks not necessary during cardiac catheterisation. *Cathet Cardiovasc Diagn* 1989; **17**:158-60.

Chapter 8

Pressure Waveforms in the Cardiac Cycle

John Boland

D ynamic blood pressure is the propulsive force generated in the cardiovascular system by ventricular contraction. These rhythmic contractions are responsible for pulsatile blood flow in arteries, which is dissipated into constant low-pressure flow in the capillary circulation. Cardiac catheterisation records pressure from the intracardiac chambers and great vessels by means of catheters inserted directly into arteries or veins, each chamber or vessel having its own distinctive pulse pattern. The pulsatile nature of dynamic blood flow means blood pressure is recorded as a continuous rhythmic waveform, with repeated peaks and troughs that correspond to reported values of systole and diastole respectively. Mean blood pressure is calculated electronically as the integral of the pressure waveform, or the average area under the curve.

Pressure measurement

As the human or mammalian heart is a four-chambered pump with dual circuits to pulmonary and systemic circulations, pressures in left and right sides of the heart need to be measured separately. Measures of pulmonary or right heart circulation consist of right atrium, right ventricle, pulmonary artery and pulmonary wedge pressures. The latter is a measure of reflected left atrial pressure transmitted retrogradely to the catheter via pulmonary veins and is accepted as a true value of left atrial pressure,[1] noting that there is a time lag (or phase shift) of some 50–70 msecs between recordings of left atrium and pulmonary artery wedge pressures.

The left heart system or systemic circulation consists of measures of aortic, left ventricular and occasionally left atrial pressure measured by crossing the mitral valve retrogradely from the left ventricle, which is sometimes possible. Left atrial pressure is usually recorded via the pulmonary artery wedge position or by transseptal puncture from the right atrium, or by crossing a patent *foramen ovale*.

In sinus rhythm, right atrium, left atrium and pulmonary arterial wedge pressures are biphasic in contour (i.e. have two distinct waves per heartbeat, Fig. 8.1a) and reflect rise and fall in atrial pressures caused by sequential filling and drainage of blood in the atria. These traces are biphasic because there are no valves separating atria from their filling source, the venae cavae for the right atrium and pulmonary veins for the left atrium. Venous pulse recordings such as superior and inferior venae cavae are also biphasic. Ventricles, which are separated from inflow and outflow ports by valves, reflect only monophasic pressure traces (i.e. one wave per heartbeat, Fig. 8.1b), as do arterial pressures.

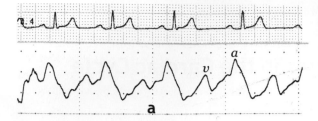

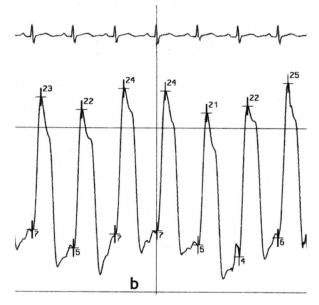

Figure 8.1a. Right atrial pressure waveform showing distinct biphasic trace consisting of repeated 'a' and 'v' waves. The 'a' wave of the atrial pressure trace follows the P wave of the electrocardiogram, the 'v' wave follows the T wave. The downslope of the 'a' wave is the 'x' descent, the downslope of the 'v' wave is the 'y' descent.

Figure 8.1b. Right ventricular presssure showing one deflection per heartbeat. Ventricular diastole aligns with the R wave of the electrocardiogram and corresponds with the 'a' wave of the right atrium.

Left and right heart catheters were once routinely performed for all patients having a cardiac catheter, whether for investigation of ischaemic heart disease or other reasons. In time it was realised that right heart catheterisation was unnecessary for patients presenting only with angina. Right heart catheterisation, either by itself or in conjunction with left heart catheterisation, is now performed selectively for patients presenting with certain conditions such as valvular heart disease, congenital heart disease, sudden cardiovascular death, pericarditis, cardiomyopathy, or heart transplant assessment. Information obtained by these investigations is essential for further clinical management.

The cardiac cycle

The cardiac cycle may be defined as the sequence of events occurring between two consecutive cardiac contractions. Each cycle begins with the right atrium and may be separated into atrial and ventricular components, or according to events in left or right hearts. With each heartbeat, blood returning from the peripheral circulation is channeled by the right ventricle to the lungs for oxygenation and recirculated to the periphery via the left ventricle. A complete description of the cardiac cycle describes changes in electrocardiogram (ECG), blood pressure, volume, blood flow and flow velocity in all cardiac chambers and follows events occurring through both right and left heart systems. The ECG serves as a baseline on which to synchronise different cardiac events.

The cardiac cycle is a continuous cycle that begins with electrical activation of the sinoatrial node. This induces depolarisation and contraction of both atria (P wave of the ECG), followed by stimulation of the atrioventricular node and contraction of both ventricles (QRS complex of the ECG). Before atria or ventricles can contract, however, the chambers must first fill with blood. This description of the cardiac cycle therefore begins with the atrial filling that occurs immediately prior to atrial contraction, and follows the direction of blood flow through the heart.

Right atrium

The key to understanding the haemodynamics of the cardiac cycle lies in understanding the biphasic nature of the atrial pressure waveforms. Blood returns to the right atrium via superior and inferior venae cavae which permit continuous filling of the right atrium during atrial diastole. The right atrioventricular valve (tricuspid) is closed during early atrial diastole, causing atrial pressure and volume to increase as the atrium fills. This pressure increase is evident as an upward deflection of the atrial waveform and is recorded as a 'v' wave (Fig. 8.2a). The tricuspid valve then opens in mid-atrial diastole when the atrium is only partly filled, and blood drains passively from the atrium into the ventricle. Following this decrease in volume load, atrial pressure drops accordingly (seen as the descent of the 'v' wave, Fig. 8.2b). Blood continues to drain freely from venae cavae into the atrium and flows directly across the open tricuspid valve into the right ventricle. With the valve open there is virtually no resistance to flow between atrium and ventricle, therefore pressures in these two chambers will equalise temporarily.

Atrial diastole lasts until the atrium contracts in response to atrial depolarisation at the time of the P wave of the ECG. This causes another small but forceful increase in atrial pressure (seen as the 'a' wave), which empties additional atrial blood into the ventricle (Fig.

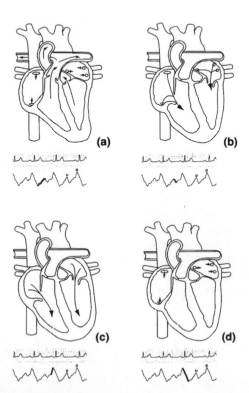

(a)

(b)

(c)

(d)

Figure 8.2. Sequence of events depicting valve opening and closure with corresponding changes in the electrocardiogram and atrial pressure waveform. Passive venous return to the atria causes the upstroke of the 'v' wave during atrial diastole/ventricular systole (a). Opening of the atrioventricular valves allows passive ventricular filling, resulting in a fall in atrial pressure and the downstroke of the atrial 'v' wave (b). Atrial contraction increases atrial pressure, causing the upstroke of the 'a' wave and completing ventricular filling (c). As blood empties from the atria, atrial pressure drops, causing the descent of the 'a' wave as ventricular contraction begins with isovolumetric contraction (d) and closure of all four cardiac valves. The atria refill and the cycle continues anew with (a).

8.2c). Up to 80% of ventricular filling occurs by passive venous drainage across an open tricuspid valve before the atrial contraction or 'atrial kick' occurs. The right ventricle then begins to contract, increasing its pressure relative to the right atrium; the tricuspid valve closes, the atrium relaxes (Fig. 8.2d) and atrial pressure drops (seen as the descent of the 'a' wave). Passive venous return across the tricuspid valve continues with a new 'v' wave (Fig. 8.2a) during ventricular systole and the atrial cycle begins anew with the next 'a' wave.

As each cycle begins with atrial contraction, the 'a' wave is the first upward deflection of the atrial pressure waveform and the 'v' wave follows the 'a' wave in the same beat. As described above, however, each 'a' wave is haemodynamically paired with the preceding 'v' wave, not the one following. This pairing is considered to be part of the same beat of movement of valve leaflets, atrioventricular valve motion and possible regurgitant flow across the valve. Atrial pressure waveforms are reported as an 'a' wave, 'v' wave and mean value (e.g. the right atrial waveform in Fig. 8.1a is reported as 'a' = 5, 'v' = 4 , 'm' = 3), where the value for the 'v' wave is taken from the waveform preceding the 'a' wave. In practice there is usually little difference between any two consecutive 'v' waves.

In sinus rhythm, each atrial depolarisation is paired with a single subsequent ventricular contraction. In atrial fibrillation, however, atrial depolarisation is irregular and exceeds the rate of ventricular contraction; only an occasional atrial depolarisation stimulates a corresponding ventricular beat. On the ECG the rhythm is also irregular, and atrial activity is evident as a series of weak and irregular P waves preceding a single QRS complex. As there is loss of direct atrial contraction, the corresponding atrial pressure waveform shows an absence of 'a' waves, appearing only as a sequence of single 'v' waves.

The c wave

A third wave, the 'c' wave may also be evident as a slight upward deflection during the descent of the 'a' wave. Just after the tricuspid valve closes, ventricular pressure continues to increase from its systolic contraction, causing the valve leaflets to bulge backwards into the atrium. This results in a small pressure increase in the atrial waveform, seen as the 'c' wave. In practice, this third waveform is not clearly apparent and can generally be dismissed. A perfect atrial waveform therefore consists of three upward deflections (the 'a', 'c' and 'v' waves respectively). The downslope of the 'a' wave is called the 'x' descent, while the downslope of the 'v' wave is called the 'y' descent. The same factors identified in atrial pressure waveforms can be identified in the jugular venous pulse, which is transmitted retrogradely from the right atrium.

Left atrium

The preceding description of the right heart cycle applies equally to both right and left heart systems. In the same way that venae cavae fill the right atrium, the left atrium acts as a reservoir for venous blood return during ventricular systole as pulmonary veins fill the left atrium. Passive left atrial filling against a closed mitral valve during ventricular systole forms the left atrial 'v' wave. This is followed by mitral valve opening, then atrial contraction and an 'a' wave. Both left and right atria empty their loads together into each ventricle. Atrial pressure then parallels ventricular pressure until ventricular contraction begins and the mitral valve closes along with the tricuspid valve.

Combined atrial cycle

Right and left atria contract and relax (almost) simultaneously, as do right and left ventricles. The electrical stimulus from the sinoatrial node reaches the right atrium a fraction of a second before the left atrium, creating a slight time lag in left atrial response. Similarly, although the AV node conducts its electrical signal simultaneously along the Bundle of His, for various reasons the left ventricle starts to contract before the right, but right ventricular ejection begins first, lasts longer and ends later than that of the left ventricle. It follows that the mitral valve closes slightly ahead of the tricuspid valve and the aortic valve closes slightly earlier than the pulmonary valve. Such detail can only be appreciated with an echogram (for exact details of timing refer to Fig. 8.7b and subsequent text). Generally, changes in left atrial pressure parallel those of the right atrium, changes in the left ventricle parallel those of the right, and changes in aorta parallel those of the pulmonary artery.

Ventricular cycle

Valves are almost entirely passive structures that open and close according to the pressure difference in chambers on either side of the valve. When the atria begin to fill at the very beginning of atrial diastole, the ventricles are still contracting from the previous systole. The ventricles then relax and ventricular pressure starts to fall. When ventricular pressure falls below that of atrial pressure, the tricuspid and mitral valves are forced open and permit ventricular filling. At first, ventricular pressure increases only slightly with its initial passive atrial inflow. Atrial systole causes a sudden late rise in presssure coincident with a late inflow of blood, seen as a small sharp rise in ventricular pressure at end-diastole. This value is identical to the atrial a wave and is referred to as ventricular end-diastolic pressure or edp (Fig. 8.3). Following atrial systole, ventricular muscles begin to constrict, causing ventricular pressure to rise above atrial pressure and forcing closure of the atrioventricular valves.

End-diastolic pressure (edp)

Left ventricular edp is the pressure in the ventricle immediately preceding ventricular contraction and is called preload. According to the Frank Starling principle, preload is a measure of presystolic muscle fibre stretch, is proportional to ventricular end-diastolic volume, and directly determines the force of cardiac contraction. Aortic end-diastole, the pressure against which the ventricle has to work to open the aortic valve, is called afterload. The higher these respective values, the greater the load imposed on ventricular pumping activity.

Ventricular filling

It should be noted that there are three distinct phases of ventricular filling. The first, early ventricular filling—or rapid filling phase—is an active energy-consuming process resulting

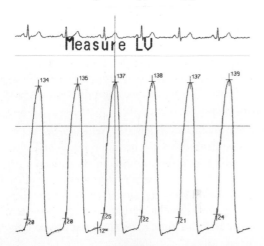

Figure 8.3. Left ventricular pressure waveform showing systole and end-diastole (the 'a' wave). The lower value (12*) indicates the plateau preceding the 'a' wave (see text for explanation). Note that this patient has diastolic values higher than normal, indicating some ventricular impairment.

from relaxation of ventricular forces as the ventricle recovers from systole, and involves uncoiling of the ventricular muscle fibres. Hence, myocardial contraction is not the only energy-consuming period of ventricular activity.[2] The second phase is the period of diastasis consisting of ventricular filling after the preceding uncoiling activity. Diastasis is the passive filling stage that dominates the ventricular filling period. The third phase is the atrial contribution to ventricular filling, or 'a' wave, which boosts passive ventricular filling by forceful atrial contraction and at rest delivers an additional 20–40% volume load to the ventricle.

During diastole, pressure in the ventricle drops to a very low value, not quite reaching zero. The lowest value reached is usually an artifactual downward spike (Fig. 8.1b and Fig. 8.3) and is ignored. True ventricular diastole is therefore taken as the pressure reached immediately prior to systole. The question arises as to what constitutes true ventricular end-diastole. Some operators consider the 'a' wave as their preferred value for end-diastole. The 'a' wave, however, although occurring immediately prior to ventricular contraction and thus a true measure of edp, is a mixture of atrial and ventricular function and cannot be accepted as a true value of ventricular forces. A more accurate measure of passive stiffness of ventricular forces is the plateau before the 'a' wave (see Fig. 8.3). The second phase of ventricular filling, diastasis, is consequently the preferred value for edp. Optimum information can be conveyed by reporting each value individually (e.g. LV = 120/5, 'a' = 9). The post 'a' wave period can also contribute important information about how ventricular muscle accommodates forces generated by filling, but requires more complicated measurement. A mean value for ventricular pressure is physiologically meaningless and is not reported.

The 'a' wave is routinely measured by physiological monitors for both left and right ventricles but because of the dominance of left heart activity, only left ventricular edp is generally evaluated in assessing ventricular performance. The edp may be elevated due to inadequate force of myocardial contraction (systolic dysfunction) or to inadequate relaxation in diastole (diastolic dysfunction).

Left ventricle and aorta

As the left ventricle contracts and left ventricular pressure exceeds that of the aorta, the aortic valve is forced open and blood is forcefully ejected from the ventricle. Aortic pressure begins to rise as soon as the aortic valve opens, when ventricular blood enters the aorta. Because the aortic valve is open there is continuity of flow between left ventricle and aorta, and pressure in the two chambers equalises. Thus aortic pressure follows and parallels left ventricular pressure during the ventricular systolic ejection period (Fig. 8.4). Both pressures peak at mid-systole then decline when the force of ventricular contraction diminishes. As these pressures fall, left ventricular pressure drops below aortic pressure and the aortic valve closes, ending the left ventricular ejection period and marking the beginning of diastole.

Timing of valve movement

The dynamics of the system are such that valve movement on left and right sides is not in perfect synchrony. The aortic valve does not close instantly with the fall in left ventricular pressure. There is a very slight time lag during which its forward momentum continues to propel blood forward for a moment. Blood flow slows and even reverses in a rebound effect from elastic arterial recoil, causing the dichrotic notch or incisura in the arterial waveform (this phenomenon results in aortic valve closure slightly later than would be expected from a fall in pressure alone). Because of residual arterial tone, aortic pressure drops only

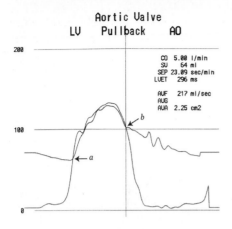

Figure 8.4. *Left ventricular and aortic pressures demonstrating point of opening of aortic valve when left ventricular pressure exceeds aortic pressure (arrow a) and point of closure of aortic valve at dichrotic notch (arrow b) when ventricular pressure again falls below aortic presssure. The ventricular ejection period is the time interval between points a and b. Ventricular diastole begins at b.*

gradually during ventricular diastole, until the next ventricular contraction again opens the aortic valve. A brief period of isovolumetric ventricular contraction ensues, which coincides with closure of both mitral and aortic valves. Aortic valve closure is easily recognisable as the dichrotic notch on aortic waveforms, although fluid-filled catheter systems can be affected by artifactual distortions which can introduce additional unidentifiable notches.

Pressure equalisation

As described, during the period of atrial drainage into the ventricles when atrioventricular valves (mitral and tricuspid) are open there is unrestricted flow between atria and ventricles. Haemodynamically, since blood is a fluid and exerts pressure equally in all directions, pressure equalises between the two cardiac chambers. This means that for a brief period during ventricular diastole pressure in the atrium (and hence in the pulmonary wedge) is identical to pressure in the ventricle (see Fig. 8.5), as the atrioventricular valves (mitral and tricuspid) are both open during ventricular diastole. Pressure equalisation is best observed when pressures in both chambers are recorded simultaneously.

A similar situation exists between any two cardiac chambers separated by an open valve: pressure in each chamber will momentarily equilibrate until the valve closes again. Thus aortic systolic pressure will be identical to the left ventricular systolic trace when the aortic valve is open and there is continuity between ventricle and aorta during the ventricular systolic ejection period (as shown in Fig. 8.4). The same applies to pulmonary artery and right ventricular systolic values, for the semilunar valves (aortic and pulmonary) are open during systole.

Pulmonary cycle

As with the left ventricle and aorta, the pulmonary valve opens when right ventricular pressure exceeds pulmonary artery pressure and closes when ventricular pressure again falls below pulmonary artery pressure. Pulmonary valve opening, which slightly precedes aortic valve opening, marks the beginning of the right ventricular systolic ejection period (which lasts until the pulmonary valve again closes). Apart from the slight asynchrony in timing of valve movement, right heart dynamics parallel those of the left side.

Isovolumetric contraction

Isovolumetric (or isovolumic or isometric) contraction is the period between closure of the atrioventricular valves (mitral and tricuspid) and opening of the semilunar valves (aortic

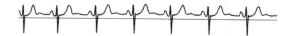

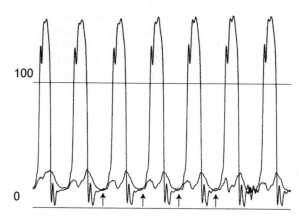

Figure 8.5. *Synchrony between left ventricle and pulmonary wedge pressures measured at the same magnification. Note pressure equalisation when the mitral valve is open (arrows) prior to atrial systole.*

and pulmonary), and represents a period of myocardial contraction marked by a sudden sharp increase in ventricular pressure without change in ventricular volume (Fig. 8.6). This occurs because, as ventricular contraction begins, both inlet and outlet ports to the ventricles are closed, which serves to build up pressure reserve in the ventricles. Myocardial contraction without this initial head of pressure would reduce propulsive velocity of blood flow, velocity of ventricular wall motion during contraction and the force of ventricular contraction. Consequently blood is ejected forcefully from the ventricles when the atrioventricular valves first open. Both the speed of propulsion and ventricular ejection pressure reach a peak during early systole then decline, although at different rates. Rate of change of pressure with respect to time (dP/dt) is another variable that can be recorded automatically by computer and is a measure of efficiency of myocardial contraction, particularly for the left ventricle.

Isovolumetric relaxation

Isovolumetric relaxation is the period between closure of the semilunar valves and opening of the atrioventricular valves and is the diastolic equivalent of isovolumetric contraction. Ventricular pressure continues to drop sharply following aortic and pulmonary valve closure at the end of the systolic ejection period, when mitral and tricuspid valves are also closed (Fig. 8.6). Ventricular volume is unable to change and therefore remains constant while pressure drops to its diastolic value and myocardial muscles relax. When ventricular pressure drops below atrial pressure, mitral and tricuspid valves open and the atrial cycle begins again.

Complete cardiac cycle

The entire cardiac cycle can be summarised by a series of charts, as shown in Fig. 8.7a and b. All events are synchronised with the electrocardiogram, which also serves as a means of timing cardiac events. Like all electrocardiogram recorders, modern computer monitors print paper at a selected rate, which can be used to calculate timing of specific events such as ventricular ejection period or diastolic filling period.

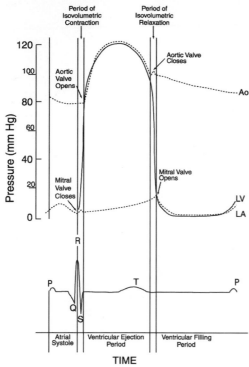

Figure 8.6. Superimposed left ventricular, aortic and left atrial pressures illustrating periods of ventricular and atrial systole and diastole in relation to valve opening and closure with the electrocardiogram. Note the periods of isovolumetric contraction and relaxation, when all four cardiac valves are closed. Ao=aorta; LV=left ventricle; LA=left atrium.

Heart sounds

Valve motion causes a series of characteristic heart sounds that can be detected by auscultation or phonocardiography, as described in Fig. 8.7b. The atrioventricular valves close with a loud slap at the very beginning of ventricular systole: this is called the first heart sound. The aortic and pulmonary valves close audibly when systole ends: this is called the second heart sound. To a certain extent the first and second heart sounds may be split, due to asynchronous closure of the mitral/tricuspid or aortic/pulmonary valves. This splitting is more marked on inspiration and is usually never wide (< 0.03 secs). Wide splitting of the second sound may occur in right bundle block, pulmonary stenosis, atrial septal defect, or anomalous pulmonary venous drainage (the last two causing fixed splitting). Paradoxical splitting of the second sound may occur in tetralogy of Fallot, *truncus arteriosus* and conditions where valve closure is extremely limited, as in severe calcific stenosis.

Increased loudness of the first heart sound may be noted in mobile mitral or tricuspid stenosis, when the valve is pliable, a short PR interval, and during sinus tachycardia. A loud second sound may occur in systemic hypertension (aortic valve closure), or pulmonary hypertension (pulmonary valve closure).

A third or fourth heart sound is referred to as an added or extra sound, and these occur during diastole. The third heart sound is less distinct and represents the end of the rapid filling phase of the ventricular filling period in early diastole (just prior to the begining of diastasis) and results from vibrations of the ventricular wall. The fourth heart sound occurs before the first and is caused by atrial systole into a poorly compliant left ventricle. Extra heart sounds are always abnormal, apart from the third which may be normal in children. The combination of an extra heart sound in a patient with tachycardia is called a gallop rhythm.

Interference with laminar blood flow across a valve, such as occurs with incomplete opening or closure of valve leaflets, can cause turbulence that may be identified as an audible heart murmur or a palpable vibration ('thrill'). Murmurs and thrills can be used by

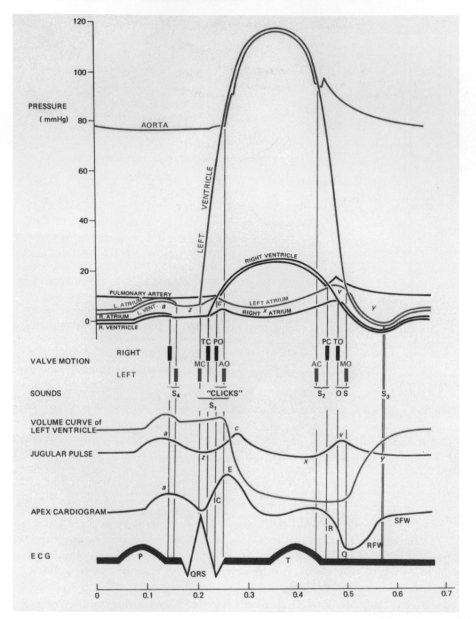

Figure 8.7a. *Diagram of the cardiac cycle, showing the pressure curves of the great vessels and cardiac chambers, valvular events and heart sounds, left ventricular volume curve, jugular pulse wave, apex cardiogram (Sanborn piezo crystal), and the electrocardiogram. For illustrative purposes, the time intervals between valvular events have been modified. Valve motion:* **MC** *= mitral component of the first heart sound;* **MO** *= mitral valve opening;* **TC** *= tricuspid component of the first heart sound;* **TO** *= tricuspid valve opening;* **AC** *= aortic component of the second heart sound;* **AO** *= aortic valve opening;* **PC** *= pulmonic valve component of the second heart sound;* **PO** *= pulmonic valve opening;* **OS** *= opening snap of atrioventricular valves; Apex cardiogram:* **IC** *= isovolumic or isovolumetric (isochoric) contraction wave;* **IR** *= isovolumic or isovolumetric (isochoric) relaxation wave;* **O** *= opening of mitral valve;* **RFW** *= rapid filling wave;* **SFW** *= slow-filling wave. (Reproduced with permission of McGraw Hill from* Hurst's The Heart, Arteries and Veins.[3] *Plate 2.)*

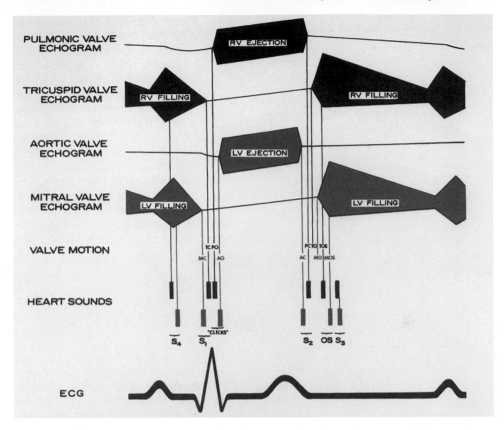

Figure 8.7b. Timing of events in the cardiac cycle: Schematic presentation of the relationships between electrical and mechanical events and heart sounds during the cardiac cycle. The right atrium starts to contract before the left atrium but the left ventricle starts to contract before the right ventricle does; right ventricular ejection begins before left ventricular ejection and ends later than left ventricular ejection does. *MC* = mitral component of the first heart sound (*S1*); *TC* = tricuspid component of the first heart sound (*S1*); *PO* = pulmonic valve opening; *AO* = aortic valve opening; *AC* = aortic component of the second heart sound (*S2*); *TO* = tricuspid valve opening; *TOS* = tricuspid opening snap; *MOS* = mitral valve opening snap. Time intervals are not necessarily in proportion. (Reproduced with permission of McGraw Hill from Hurst's The Heart, Arteries and Veins.[3] Plate 3.)

the cardiologist to detect turbulence arising from valve stenosis or incompetence (leaking) and are invaluable in diagnosing valve disease. Identifying heart sounds is a highly skilled craft of cardiology that requires considerable experience to perfect.

Left heart pressure recordings

Typical pressure recordings for a left heart (diagnostic) catheter are shown in Fig. 8.8. Aortic and/or ventricular pressures are recorded prior to coronary angiography and ventriculography to obtain baseline values. Following ventriculography, pullback measurements from ventricle to aorta are routinely taken to note changes in edp and to quantify possible aortic stenosis. (The illustration used in Fig. 8.4 is a computer-generated overlay of ventricular and aortic pressure traces from two different heartbeats to illustrate absence of an aortic gradient on pullback).

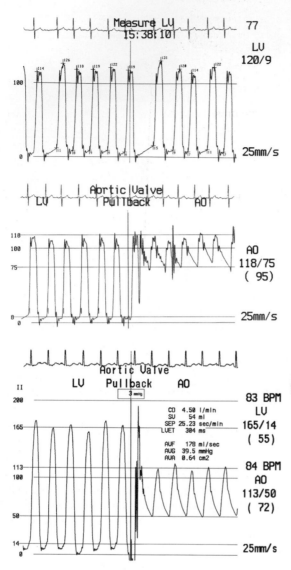

Figure 8.8. Left heart pressures taken during cardiac catheterisation. Note inotropic increase in LV systole following a prolonged diastolic filling period. Pullback measurements from left ventricle to aorta following ventriculography determine presence or absence of aortic stenosis by identifying systolic pressure differences across the aortic valve. Even with atrial fibrilllation, this patient clearly has the same systolic value for ventricle and aorta, indicating absence af aortic stenosis.

Figure 8.9. Pullback pressures from left ventricle and aorta from a patient with aortic stenosis. Note the peak-to-peak gradient across the aortic valve, measured at 52 mmHg (165-113). Size of gradient is directly related to severity of stenosis. The symbols and figures indicate automatically derived computer calculations. The mean aortic valve gradient for this patient is shown below.

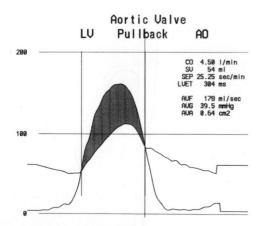

Figure 8.10. Superimposed left ventricular and aortic pressures from separate heartbeats on pullback from the same patient with aortic stenosis as in Fig. 8.9. Mean aortic valve gradient (39.5 mmHg) is calculated as the value of the area bounded by the two curves (shaded region).

The following are key features to note with left heart pressures:

1. Systole, diastole and mean values are required for aorta and other arteries.
2. Systole and end-diastole are required for left ventricle. An edp of 12 or more for the 'a' wave is considered abnormal.
3. Note any difference in systole between ventricle and aorta on pullback. A patient with an intact aortic valve will have the same systolic value for both chambers.
4. It is physiologically impossible for aortic pressure to be greater than ventricular pressure on pullback. If this were noted it would be due to artifact, such as respiratory variations, pressure damping or a sudden change in blood pressure. It is commonly seen if LV pressure has not fully recovered from the negative inotropic effect of contrast, in which case the pullback should be delayed until pressure is stable.
5. An aortic systolic pressure value lower than that of left ventricle indicates aortic stenosis.
6. Leaking valves are routinely evaluated by angiography rather than by pressure. An unusually wide arterial pulse pressure is often associated with a leaking aortic valve.

Aortic stenosis

Systolic differences between left ventricle and aorta caused by aortic stenosis can be readily evaluated on catheter pullback by comparing pressures obtained from the preceding ventricular beats with subsequent aortic beats. Severity of aortic stenosis is determined by magnitude of the pressure difference across the aortic valve on pullback (Fig. 8.9) and is referred to as a peak-to-peak gradient (i.e. the difference between systolic values of ventricle and aorta). Computerised systems will also calculate a mean aortic valve gradient, which is a measure of the area bounded by the two curves when aortic and ventricular pressures are superimposed (Fig. 8.10). Measurements should be taken during the same heartbeat by two catheters recording pressures simultaneously from ventricle and aorta. This is not routinely done because it involves inserting the second catheter via a separate arterial sheath. In practice (as in Fig. 8.10) the mean aortic valve gradient is obtained by superimposing selected aortic and ventricular beats on pullback, although there will always be minor differences in pressure, heart rate, systolic ejection and diastolic filling times with each individual beat. It is also possible to use double lumen catheters to record simultaneous left ventricular and aortic pressure tracings, permitting consecutive beat-by-beat evaluation of aortic stenosis.

Alternatively, aortic valve gradients can be obtained by simultaneously recording left ventricular pressure directly from the catheter in the left ventricle, and femoral artery pressure (in lieu of aortic pressure) from the side port of the groin sheath (Fig. 8.11a) prior to ventriculography. This permits accurate computerised measurement of an aortic valve gradient using pressures taken during the same heartbeat (Fig. 8.11b) and eliminates potential problems from using two central catheters.[4,5] Simultaneous ventricular and aortic (or femoral or brachial) pressures from the same heartbeat can be corrected for time lag by aligning aortic end-diastole with the upstroke of left ventricular pressure, as in Fig. 8.11c. This will give a true measure of the mean gradient across the valve, provided additional correction is also made for slight pressure differences that can exist between femoral artery and aorta. This intrinsic difference (i.e. either the mean difference between femoral and aortic pressure, or simply the average systolic difference between the two pressures) can be detected following pullback, when aortic and femoral pressures are superimposed (Fig. 8.11d). If femoral systolic pressure is higher than aortic, the intrinsic difference should be added to the mean valve gradient (or subtracted if femoral pressure is lower than aortic). This procedure eliminates artifactual variations induced by superimposing measurements

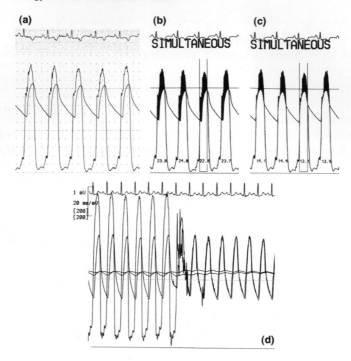

Figure 8.11a-d. Simultaneously recorded pressures from left ventricle and femoral artery from a patient with aortic stenosis. In a and b, the mean gradient across the valve is 23.2 mmHg. Figure 8.11c, which is corrected for the time lag between ventricle and femoral artery, shows that the actual gradient between left ventricle and femoral artery is 13.6 mmHg. In Fig 8.11d, left ventricular, aortic and femoral artery pressures recorded on pullback from left ventricle for another patient with aortic stenosis are shown. In this example aortic systole is 162 mmHg and femoral artery systole is 164 mmHg. As femoral systole is 2 mmHg higher than aortic, this intrinsic difference of 2 mmHg must be added to the mean aortic valve gradient (as measured between femoral artery and left ventricle). In this case the intrinsic difference is inconsequential but greater differences are commonly encountered. Scale is 0-200 mmHg.

taken from separate heartbeats on pullback alone and is particularly helpful when the length of the cardiac cycle is variable, as in atrial fibrillation or with frequent premature beats.

Ultimately it is not the size of the gradient across the valve that determines prognosis and treatment of a stenotic valve but rather size of the opening across the valve, i.e. the valve area. Valve area is derived from the Gorlin formula,[6,7] which depends on a number of variables such as heart rate, cardiac output and mean aortic valve gradient at the time of measurement. It follows that variations in any or all of these values will affect the derived value for aortic valve area. During right heart catheterisation, cardiac output is calculated prior to ventriculography, whereas the valve gradient is calculated by catheter pullback after ventriculography, when blood pressure, heart rate, periphereal vascular resistance and cardiac output can change unpredictably. Combining these variables indiscriminately in the Gorlin formula may yield unreliable results for aortic valve area.

Thus, simply by using an aortic valve gradient derived from the pressure difference between femoral artery and left ventricle, the cardiac output, valve gradient and heart rate can all be measured during the same steady state prior to ventriculography to yield accurate valve areas, within the limits of cardiac catheterisation.[4,5]

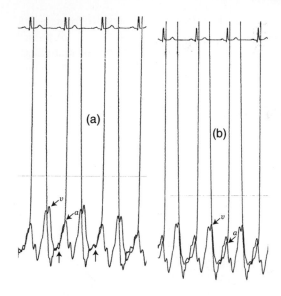

Figure 8.12a and b. *Simultaneous pressure recordings from left ventricle and pulmonary wedge from a patient without mitral stenosis. Figure 8.12a is unedited. Note identical a wave values in both ventricle and pulmonary wedge, indicating absence of a mitral gradient. Note also the overlapping descent of the 'v' wave in Fig. 8.12b (which is corrected for time lag) with the downslope of the left ventricular waveform, and equilibration of both pressure traces during the period of mitral valve opening (vertical arrows). Scale is 0-40 mmHg.*

The Gorlin formula for calculating aortic valve area is

$$A = \frac{CO/(SEP \times HR)}{VC \times \sqrt{AVG}}$$

where CO = flow across the valve (cm³/min), SEP = mean systolic ejection period (sec/beat), HR = heart rate (bpm), VC = valve constant (44.3 for aortic valve) and AVG = mean aortic valve gradient (mmHg). In practice, an abbreviation of this formula (A = CO (L/min)/√AVG) can be used to quickly calculate an approximate valve area, given the other variables cancel to a value of 1.0.[8]

Right heart pressure recordings

For right heart catheterisation or combined left and right heart catheterisation, it is desirable to obtain baseline values by recording right atrium, right ventricle and pulmonary artery pressures prior to ventriculography. The pulmonary artery wedge pressure is taken by advancing the right heart catheter as far as possible until the catheter tip wedges firmly

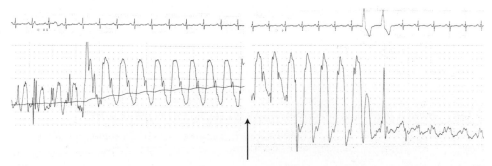

Figure 8.13. *Typical pressure recording of right heart pressures from pulmonary wedge to pulmonary artery, then from pulmonary artery to right ventricle to right atrium. Note that mean wedge pressure cannot be higher than mean pulmonary artery pressure and is roughly the same as diastolic pulmonary artery pressure. Blood samples for Fick calculations can be collected from pulmonary artery and ventricle, then the right side pullback is completed by withdrawing the catheter to right atrium. Scale is 0-40 mmHg.*

at the arterioles, effectively plugging flow and recording the reflected pressure from the left atrium. After the catheter is advanced to the wedge position, it is customary to record wedge pressure simultaneously with left ventricular edp, usually on a magnified scale. Both transducers should be re-zeroed prior to this recording, ensuring both are at mid-chest level and set on the same gain (see Fig. 3.1). This is essential to accurately quantify possible mitral stenosis, as small errors in zeroing transducers or in catheter position may falsely indicate the presence of a significant mitral gradient.

Figure 8.12a and b illustrate a simultaneous tracing of pulmonary arterial wedge and left ventricular pressures for a patient with a normal mitral valve, where wedge pressure directly overlaps ventricular diastolic pressure, indicating absence of mitral stenosis. Pulmonary artery wedge pressure is routinely measured as a substitute for left atrial pressure, introducing a time lag which, as shown in Fig. 8.12b, is easily corrected by computer.

A right heart pullback records the change in pressure from wedge position to pulmonary artery to right ventricle to right atrium (Fig. 8.13). The right heart pullback can be interrupted to collect blood samples from left ventricle and pulmonary artery along with Douglas bag samples for calculations of cardiac output by Fick principle, or by thermodilution. It is good laboratory practice to calculate cardiac output for comparison by both methods. The Fick principle is considered more accurate, particularly for low output states, but only if correct procedures are followed (simultaneous collection of blood and respiratory gas samples). Convenience, ease of use and improved catheter design have resulted in a preference by many cardiologists for the thermodilution technique over the Fick method to determine cardiac output.

The following are key features to note with right heart pressures:

1. Pulmonary arterial wedge pressure cannot be greater than pulmonary artery pressure.
2. Damping artifacts are commonly encountered. As a guide, mean wedge pressure is generally the same as diastolic pulmonary artery pressure.
3. For sinus rhythm, wedge pressure is biphasic, showing both 'a' and 'v' waves; for atrial fibrillation the 'a' wave is absent.
4. Large 'v' waves are expected with severe mitral insufficiency but are also seen with mitral stenosis or shunts.
5. As for aortic stenosis, pulmonary stenosis will show a systolic pressure gradient across the pulmonary valve on pullback.
6. Simultaneous tracings are not generally required for evaluating tricuspid stenosis. Elevated right atrial pressure relative to right ventricular edp on pullback is sufficient.
7. Right heart pressures may be elevated depending on presenting symptoms, such as pulmonary hypertension or pulmonary oedema.
8. A fasting patient can be dehydrated and show falsely low right heart pressures which may mask a pressure gradient characteristic of mitral stenosis.

Table 1. Normal haemodynamic values (mmHg) for a resting adult patient.

	a	v	Mean	Systole	Diastole	Mean
RA	2-10	2-10	0-8			
RV				15-30	0-8	
PA				15-30	3-12	9-16
PAW	3-15	3-12	1-10			
LA	3-15	3-12	1-10			
LV				100-140	3-12	
AO				100-140	60-90	70-105

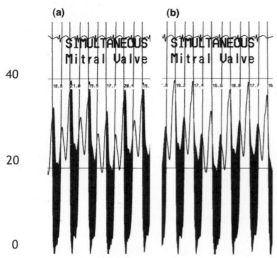

Figure 8.14a and b. *Left ventricle and pulmonary wedge pressures from a patient with mitral stenosis. Left atrial pressure is elevated relative to left ventricular diastolic pressure, causing a pressure gradient across the mitral valve, evident as the shaded area between the two waveforms. Figure 8.14a with a mean gradient of 19.9 mmHg is unedited, Fig. 8.14b with a mean gradient of 18.0 mmHg is corrected for time lag by shifting the wedge trace to the left, such that the downstroke of the 'v' wave overlies the upstroke of the ventricular trace.*

9. Intravascular pressures cannot be negative. If so, transducers should be re-zeroed and reset at mid-chest level. Occasional overshoot may artifactually induce a negative pressure.

10. Movement of the catheter with each cardiac contraction or on pullback (catheter whip) may cause artifactual spikes or exaggerated waveforms to appear. There is provision to compensate for this electronically by introducing low-frequency noise filters.

Pulmonary stenosis

Evaluation of pulmonary stenosis is similar to that for aortic stenosis. Absolute pressure values in the right heart are about one-fourth lower than in the left side but systolic differences across a stenotic pulmonary valve are readily detected on right heart pullback, as for the aortic valve.

Mitral stenosis

The mitral valve is open during ventricular diastole, as discussed, when ventricular pressure is low. Pressure gradients across the mitral valve are also correspondingly low, unlike systolic pressure gradients generated across the aortic valve, which are readily apparent. A simple pullback recording is therefore inconclusive in diagnosing mitral stenosis. To accurately measure mitral stenosis, left atrial and left ventricular pressure are simultaneously recorded to display the area bounded by the two curves. As with the mean aortic valve gradient, the computer calculates this area and applies a variation of the Gorlin formula to derive the size of the gradient across the valve. If a cardiac output is known, mitral valve area is automatically calculated as well.

The Gorlin formula for calculating mitral valve area is:

$$A = \frac{CO/(DFP \times HR)}{VC \times \sqrt{MVG}}$$

where CO − flow across the valve (cm³/min), DFP − mean diastolic filling period (sec/beat), HR = heart rate (bpm), VC = valve constant (37.7 for mitral valve) and MVG = mean mitral valve gradient (mmHG). As for the aortic valve, the abbreviation of this formula ($A = CO$ (L/min)/$\sqrt{MVG}$) can be used to quickly calculate an approximate valve area.

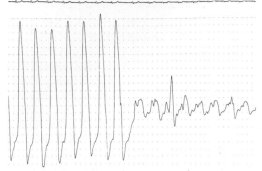

Figure 8.15. Pressure difference between right ventricular end-diastole and right atrium in a patient with tricuspid stenosis. Note elevation of right atrial pressure in this condition, clearly evident during simple catheter pullback. The exact value of the tricuspid gradient can be quantified by overlapping right ventricular and atrial pressures (as shown in Fig. 8.14 for mitral stenosis). Scale is 0-40 mmHg.

Figure 8.14a and b illustrate a simultaneous tracing of pulmonary artery wedge and left ventricular pressures for a patient with severe mitral stenosis, where wedge pressure is markedly elevated relative to left ventricular diastole. The area bounded by the two curves is shown to be 19.9 mmHg in Fig. 8.14a but reduces to 18.0 mmHg in Fig. 8.14b when corrected for time lag. It is essential to measure ventricular and wedge pressures simultaneously as even small variations between different beats can introduce unacceptable errors. This is not a problem if left atrial pressure is measured directly by transseptal puncture. Individual beat variations are not as critical when dealing with the large values that can occur with aortic gradients. A gradient of 7 mmHg across a mitral valve is considered severe, whereas a gradient of 60 mmHg or more is severe across an aortic valve.

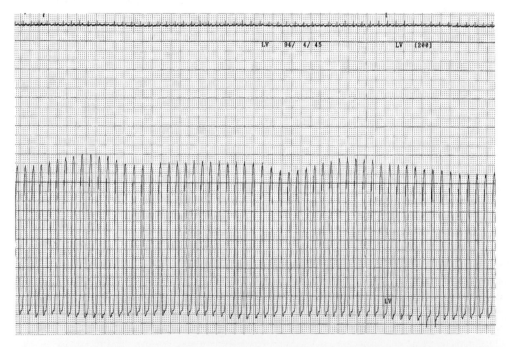

Figure 8.16. Mayer waves. These are cyclic pressure fluctuations in left ventricular trace caused by sympathetic neural changes in arterial tone and are slower than the respiratory rate.

Tricuspid stenosis

This is relatively uncommon but is routinely checked with every right heart pullback. If required, a computer generated overlay ('splice') of right atrial and ventricular pressures can be produced on a magnified scale for evaluation, using traces from separate heart-beats. Generally, however, tricuspid gradients are readily detected and quantifying their exact size is unnecessary (Fig. 8.15).

Rhythmic pressure fluctuations

Inhalation and exhalation have a secondary effect on blood pressure. A negative intratho-racic pressure draws air into the lungs, increases venous blood return to the right heart, causing pooling of blood in the lungs, and lowers arterial blood pressure by decreasing left ventricular filling, thereby decreasing cardiac output. A positive intrathoracic pressure re-sulting from exhalation causes a drop in venous return, with reduced pooling in the lungs. This results in increased left ventricular filling, with an increase in cardiac output and an increase in arterial pressure. These forces can induce cyclic fluctuations in pressure wave-forms in both left and right heart tracings, and can be reduced by asking patients to stop breathing mid-breath.

　　　Other forms of cyclic pressure variations may occur. These are under control of the vasomotor centre of the *medulla oblongata* and are caused primarily by sympathetic neural regulation of vessel tone,[9] resulting in arterial vasoconstriction and vasodilatation. The vasomotor centre may induce slow rhythmic changes in arterial tone, evident as cyclic arterial pressure fluctuations that occur at the same frequency as respiration (Traube-Hering waves), or independently of respiration and at a slower rate (Mayer waves, Fig. 8.16).

Valve insufficiency

Unlike stenotic valves, an incompetent or leaking valve does not induce pressure gradients across adjacent chambers, although artifactual flow-related gradients can occur, and char-acteristic changes in pressure waveforms can be identified. Diagnosis of valve insufficiency therefore relies primarily on auscultation with a stethoscope, angiography and echocardiography, rather than pressure readings alone. Colour doppler echocardiography can quantify valve incompetence by measuring factors such as regurgitant flow and regur-gitant fraction.

Interpretation of data

Correct diagnosis by cardiac catheterisation depends largely on the accuracy of measuring instruments. Care must be taken to ensure accurate and regular calibration and mainte-nance of equipment by a reliable operator, as well as maintaining satisfactory laboratory standards. As with other diseases, cardiac disorders are evaluated from a variety of tests of which catheterisation is only one. Disputes can arise from artifacts which, despite high standards of practice, cause unexpected errors to occur. With invasive cardiology, accurate interpretation of data relies as much on clinical assessment as on data collection from instrumentation.

References

1.   O'quin R, Marini JJ. Clinical commentary. Pulmonary artery occlusion pressure: clinical physiology, measurement, and interpretation. *Am Rev Respir Dis* 1983; **128**:319-26.
2.   Grossman W, Mclaurin LP. Diastolic properties of the left ventricle. *Ann Int Med* 1976; **84**:645-53.
3.   Alexander RW, Shiant RL, Fuster A, et al. (eds). *Hurst's the heart, arteries and veins.* 9th edn. New York: McGraw-Hill, 1998.
4.   Feldman T, Laskey W. Editorial comment. Alchemy in the cath lab: Creating a gold standard. *Cath and Cardiovasc Diag* 1998; **44**:14-15.
5.   Degeratu F, Kreulen T. Calculation of the aortic valve gradient from the left ventricular and aortic-femoral pairs of pressure waveforms. *Cath and Cardiovasc Diag* 1998; **44**:9-13.
6.   Gorlin R, Gorlin G. Hydraulic formula for calculation of area of stenotic mitral valve, other cardiac valves and central circulatory shunts. *Am Heart J* 1951; **41**:1-29.
7.   Baims DS, Grossman W. *Cardiac catheterisation, angiography and intervention,* 5th ed. Baltimore: Williams and Wilkins 1996.
8.   Hakki AH *et al.* A simplified valve formula for the calculation of stenotic cardiac valve areas. *Circulation* 1981; **63**:1050-5.
9.   Berne RM, Matthew NL. *Cardiovascular physiology,* 3rd ed. St. Louis: Mosby 1977.

Further reading

Green JH. *Basic clinical physiology,* 3rd ed. Oxford: Oxford University Press 1978.
Nara RR. *Blood pressure.* Biophysical measurement series. Redmond: Spacelabs Medical Inc 1993.
Kern MJ. *The cardiac catheterisation handbook,* 3rd ed. St. Louis: MosbyYear Book Inc 1995.
Rudd M. *Basic concepts of cardiovascular physiology.* Massachusetts: Hewlett Packard medical electronics division 1973.

Chapter 9

Physiological Interpretation of Pressure Waveforms

Geoffrey S. Oldfield

Interpretation of pressure waveforms involves careful and continued calibration of pressure transducers, physiological reporting devices and cardiac output modules. There may also be times when the accuracy of automatic equipment needs to be checked by manual methods. When interpreting data, consideration must be given to heart rate and cardiac rhythm, pressure scale and recording speed, the waveform of normal physiology related to the cardiac chamber being examined, the disease state under investigation, and the differential diagnosis. This chapter deals with the most common conditions likely to be encountered:

1. Pulsus alternans.
2. Ventricular ectopy.
3. Stenotic lesions: aortic stenosis, mitral stenosis, pulmonary stenosis, tricuspid stenosis, intraventricular pressure gradients.
4. Regurgitant lesions: aortic, mitral, tricuspid, pulmonary.
5. Left ventricular end diastolic pressures (LVEDP).
6. Pulmonary artery wedge (PAW) pressure, pulmonary capillary wedge (PCW) pressure and their relationship to pulmonary vein and left atrial (LA) pressures.
7. Constrictive pericarditis, restrictive cardiomyopathy, cardiac tamponade.
8. Nitrates.

Pulsus alternans

This is alternating strong and weak beats, with every second pulse reduced in amplitude (Fig. 9.1). It is recorded in aortic and left ventricular (LV) pressure tracings and indicates severe myocardial impairment from left ventricular damage. It is often made evident following a ventricular ectopic beat and is seen in cardiomyopathy, ventricular failure from systemic hypertension, ischaemic heart disease and aortic stenosis. When the alteration in pressure is greater than 20 mmHg it can be detected by palpation in the large arteries. Beats with the lower pressure wave have a lower pulse pressure and slower upstroke in the aortic tracing, whilst in the LV tracing there is a delayed early relaxation phase. In patients with pulsus alternans in the LV trace there is usually no change in PAW pressure or in pulmonary artery (PA) pressure, although pulsus alternans can be seen simultaneously or independently in the right ventricular and PA traces.[1] If mitral regurgitation is present, alternating large 'v' waves may be seen in the PAW trace, the large 'v' wave corresponding to the higher aortic pressure.

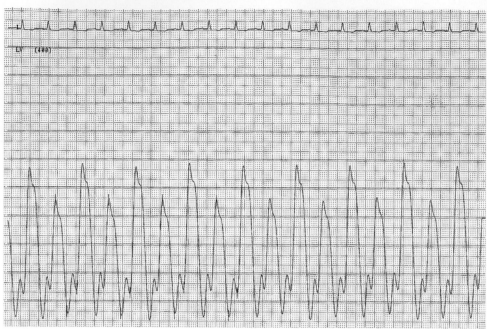

Figure 9.1. *Pulsus alternans shown for a left ventricular pressure trace. Note the regular sequence of alternating strong and weak beats.*

The underlying mechanism for pulsus alternans was originally considered to be related to changes in contractility from inflow pressures, left ventricular end diastolic pressure (LVEDP) and left ventricular volume (Frank Starling curves).[2] It is now believed to result from localised or patchy electromechanical dissociation in the myocytes resulting from variation in calcium movement in the sarcoplasmic reticulum of the myocytes.[3] The changes in traces associated with pulsus alternans may be augmented in aortic regurgitation or following administration of nitroglycerine, which decreases venous return.

Heart rate plays a role in determining the significance of pulsus alternans in heart failure. At heart rates of 50 bmin it is an indicator of significant failure, but if a tachycardia exists (> 100 bpm) its significance decreases as heart rate increases. When not obvious, pulsus alternans becomes prominent following an ectopic beat.[1,4]

Ventricular ectopy

In the normal heart, a ventricular ectopic beat shows a sharp fall in systolic pressure in the left ventricle and aorta, has a shortened diastolic filling period, and results in a prolonged diastolic filling period for the post-ectopic beat. The post-ectopic beat itself has a slower dP/dt, presumably as a result of reduced peripheral resistance and afterload that follow the prolonged diastolic post-ectopic period. In the absence of cardiac or peripheral vascular disease, this may also result in a reduction in LV systolic and aortic pressure during the post-ectopic contraction, in spite of a greater LV volume and force of myocardial contraction. In contrast, in aortic stenosis or in the damaged heart with left ventricular failure, systolic pressure and dP/dt are enhanced or accentuated following an ectopic beat. This is thought to be due to an elevated afterload caused by high peripheral vascular resistance that prevents aortic run off, and increased inotropism from the post-ectopic pause. Similarly, in valvular

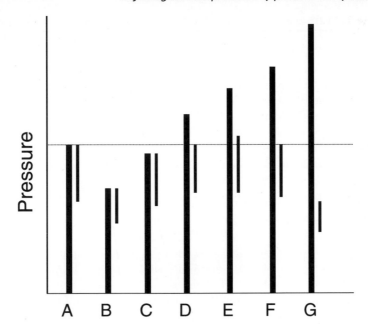

Figure 9.2. Examples of left ventricular and aortic pressure changes with ventricular ectopy. Heavy line represents ventricular pressure, thinner line aortic pressure. (A) Normal sinus beat. (B) Ventricular ectopic beat. (C) Post-ectopic beat. (D) Sinus beat with aortic stenosis. (E) Post-ectopic beat with aortic stenosis. In valvular or membranous sub-valvular aortic stenosis, a post-ectopic beat shows potentiation of left ventricular and aortic pressures, with an increased gradient and increased aortic pulse pressure. (F) Sinus beat with hypertrophic obstructive cardiomyopathy (HOCM). (G) Post-ectopic beat with HOCM, showing ventricular potentiation and elevated pressure gradient (Brockenbrough effect). The horizontal line represents an arbitrary normal systolic value.

aortic stenosis, left ventricular pressure, aortic pressure, the aortic valve gradient and pulse pressure are all elevated following an ectopic beat.

With hypertrophic obstructive cardiomyopathy (HOCM), aortic pressure falls following a premature ventricular beat. This is the Brockenbrough effect (Fig. 9.2). To assist with diagnosis, pressures may need to be recorded with an ectopic during the valsalva manoeuvre, which increases the LVEDP and potentiates the appearance of the Brockenbrough effect.[5] This occurs because the increased inotropic effect of the augmented LV filling is offset by an increase in LV outflow tract gradient. Thus, intraventricular pressures rise markedly but aortic pressure falls.

Stenotic lesions

Aortic stenosis

This is one of the most common valve abnormalities requiring haemodynamic study in the adult in the western world. The most frequent cause is senile calcific aortic stenosis (AS) of a trileaflet valve. Stenosed bicuspid valves are occasionally seen uncalcified in young adults, while calcific bicuspid valves are seen from middle age onwards. There are several ways to evaluate the severity of AS with modern physiological recording equipment. Basically, two techniques are used, depending on whether one or two pressures are recorded:

Technique 1. Pullback from left ventricle to aorta: A pigtail or multi-purpose catheter is introduced into the left ventricle and withdrawn to the aortic root while recording pressures continuously (as explained in Chapter 8). It is usual practice to record 10 consecutive left ventricular and aortic pressure traces. Manual or electronic superimposition of pressure traces can be performed to calculate the gradient across the valve. The 'peak-to-peak' gradient measured by this and other techniques closely approximates the mean stenotic valve gradient, as illustrated in Figs 8.9 and 8.10.

This technique should not be used in atrial fibrillation or if frequent ectopics are present, as waveforms with similar R–R intervals are required for manual calculation.

Technique 2. Simultaneous recording of LV and aortic pressures. This can be performed in a variety of ways, as described in a, b, c and d below:

a) with a single femoral puncture using a double lumen catheter in which the distal lumen (with end and side holes) measures LV pressure and the proximal lumen (side holes) measures aortic pressure (as shown in Fig. 9.3a); or

b) by using a Brockenbrough catheter to cross the inter-atrial septum and advancing into the left ventricle to measure pressure whilst simultaneously recording aortic pressure with a pigtail catheter (also as in Fig. 9.3a); or

c) by using two femoral punctures and two catheters, one in the LV, the other remaining in the aortic root (also as in Fig. 9.3a); or

d) with a single femoral puncture, using a large sheath (e.g. a 6F pigtail catheter with a 7F sheath). The catheter is introduced into the left ventricle and the femoral/iliac arterial tracing recorded via a side port. This technique is not as accurate as with the preceding methods but is used in some laboratories. In pressure waveforms (LV and arterial) visualised with this technique, there is a time delay of some 40 msec in the upstroke of the aortic/iliac pressure trace compared with the LV trace (as shown in Fig. 9.3b). Realignment can be performed electronically by some physiological recording equip-

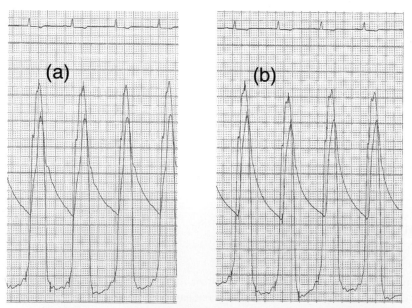

Figure 9.3. Simultaneous pressure traces in left ventricle and central aorta (a), and left ventricle and distal aorta (b) in a patient with aortic stenosis. The time lag of the distal aortic trace relative to the left ventricular trace is clearly evident in (b). This can be corrected by electronically shifting the aortic trace slightly to the left.

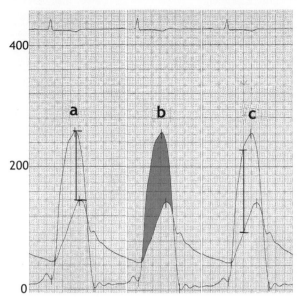

Figure 9.4. *Simultaneous pressure traces of left ventricle and central aorta showing the three common methods for quantifying aortic stenosis. The peak-to-peak gradient (a) is measured by cardiac catheterisation. The mean aortic gradient (b) is calculated as the area between the two curves. The instantaneous gradient (c) is the value measured by echocardiography. The instantaneous gradient is greater than the peak-to-peak gradient, which approximates the mean gradient.*

ment, but it has been shown by Folland *et al.*[6] that only a slight (9 mmHg) overestimation of aortic valve gradient is made if realignment is not performed.

If pressure traces are realigned an underestimation of aortic valve gradient will be made, as the iliac/femoral pulse wave usually has a slightly higher pressure (8–10 mmHg) and dP/dt of the upstroke than the central aortic root, caused by reflection of waveforms from the periphery. Whenever this technique is used a 'pullback' recording as described above should be performed following left ventricular interrogation. If a left ventriculogram is performed the catheter should be flushed carefully and the operator should wait a few minutes after the left ventriculogram for the haemodynamic effect of the contrast agent to wear off. The need for 'pullback' recording is to correlate the two techniques. Normally, femoral artery systolic pressure is greater than that of the aorta. Many elderly patients have co-existent peripheral vascular disease that dampens the iliac/femoral waveform, exaggerating the gradient between left ventricle and the femoral artery. Comparison with the pullback gradient makes this evident. Presence of coexistent aortic regurgitation precludes use of this technique, as it causes amplification of the peripheral pulses with increased systolic pressure and increased pulse pressure, thus falsifying the gradient.

The abovementioned techniques essentially provide either a peak-to-peak gradient (shown in Fig. 9.4a) or a mean aortic valve gradient (shown in Fig. 9.4b). A third value, the instantaneous gradient, is measured by echocardiography (Fig. 9.4c). As indicated, the peak of the aortic pressure trace is delayed with respect to the peak of the left ventricle (the slow rise in dP/dt in the aortic trace is due to outflow obstruction caused by AS). It is this delay between the Ao and LV peaks that generates the difference between the peak-to-peak and the instantaneous gradients.

The upstroke of the aortic pressure waveform varies between patients with normal valves and those with significant aortic stenosis. The anacrotic notch is a notch on the upstroke of the arterial pulse, indicating severe AS. As the severity of aortic stenosis increases, the anacrotic notch appears earlier on the upstroke of the aortic trace and the upstroke (dP/dt) in general slows. The anacrotic notch represents the point of maximal stroke volume and maximal peak flow velocity. At the end of this point 80% of the blood has been ejected from

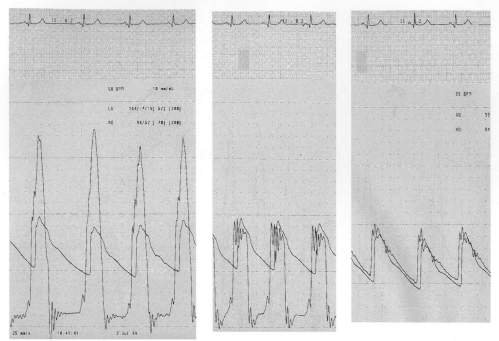

Figure 9.5. *Simultaneous pressure traces of left ventricle and aorta, showing the presence of an intraventricular gradient during a continuous pullback recording from the ventricular apex to the aortic arch*

the left ventricle. If aortic pressure is recorded peripherally the anacrotic notch will be lower on the upstroke of the waveform than if recorded centrally.

Changes evident with aortic stenosis in the LV waveform are increased LVEDP and a prominent 'a' wave. The former is related to the Frank Starling principle initially but may, in severe aortic stenosis, reflect LV failure. The force of atrial contraction is increased due to increase in LV work resulting from an increased LV mass, LV systolic pressure and prolonged systolic ejection period. The increased atrial 'a' wave is often best seen in the LA or PAW traces and protects against pulmonary congestion in the face of increased ventricular compliance and failure. The peak of the left ventricular trace becomes rounded rather than flattened.

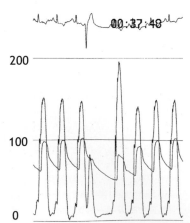

Figure 9.6. *Simultaneous traces of pressure in left ventricle and femoral artery for a patient with hypertrophic obstructive cardiomyopathy (HOCM) showing accentuation of the pressure gradient on a post-ectopic beat (the Brockenbrough effect).*

Variants of aortic stenosis

Aortic stenosis may be evident as valvular, subvalvular or supravalvular stenosis. If subvalvular, it may be classified as membranous AS or as HOCM. Unlike the situation with the first two variants, simultaneous left ventricular and aortic traces will diagnose valvular and supravalvular stenosis, but not subvalvular aortic stenosis. A pullback tracing from the LV apex to the arch of the aorta is required for this, as well as for detecting intraventricular gradients (Fig. 9.5).

An ectopic can usually differentiate intraventricular gradients, including distinguishing HOCM from membranous subvalvular AS (Fig. 9.6). The intraventricular gradient (HOCM) shows the distinctive Brockenbrough effect, while subvalvular membranous AS shows the same haemodynamics as valvular AS.

With intracavitary (or intraventricular) gradients occurring lower in the ventricle, the LV pressure waveform may have a 'bitten off' appearance that is due to catheter entrapment. Operators should be alert to this possibility.

At times other techniques such as a Valsalva manoeuvre or administration of nitroglycerine may be required for differentiation of the types of subvalvular aortic stenosis. In supravalvular aortic stenosis a slow withdrawal to the aortic arch using an end-hole catheter identifies the gradient as being above the valve. Techniques described above for AS can be used to obtain simultaneous recordings as required.

Note the Gorlin formula for aortic stenosis[7] (see also Chapter 8):

$$AVA = \frac{CO/(SEP \times HR)}{44.3 \times \sqrt{AVG}}$$

where AVA = aortic valve area, CO = cardiac output (i.e. flow across the valve), SEP = systolic ejection period, AVG = aortic valve gradient, HR = heart rate. When cardiac output is calculated at the same time that pressure gradients are measured, aortic valve area can be calculated with this formula, an automatic process with modern physiological monitoring systems. If significant regurgitation is present with a leaking valve, valve area calculations are not valid as CO (i.e., forward flow) is not equal to flow across the valve (this includes

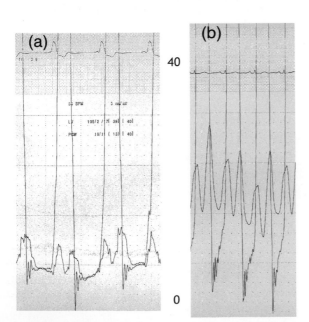

Figure 9.7. Comparison of simultaneous left ventricular and pulmonary artery wedge pressure (PAW) for a patient with a normal normal mitral valve (a), and for one with a stenosed mitral valve (b). Note diastolic equalisation of pressures in (a) and elevation of PAW pressure in (b).

both forward and retrograde flow across the valve, and cannot be measured by catheterisation alone).

Mitral stenosis

This is normally due to rheumatic fever although it may occasionally be due to degenerative disease in some elderly patients. The hallmark pressure waveform finding of mitral stenosis occurs with the simultaneous recording of LVEDP and either LA or PAW pressure at the same gain setting (usually a scale of 0–40 mmHg) (Fig. 9.7). In the normal patient the LV diastolic pressure and PAW/LA diastolic pressures overlap, but with mitral stenosis left atrial pressure is greater than LV diastolic pressure. The left atrial pressure waveform may be obtained directly by transeptal puncture using the Brockenbrough catheter. If recording LA and LVEDP simultaneously (via atrial septal puncture), the pressure traces should overlap exactly. Any variation in 'a' wave pressure, or even during early diastole, indicates some degree of stenosis. Note that when using PAW pressure and LVEDP these traces do not overlap in early diastole, even in the normal patient.

As so many patients with mitral disease are in atrial fibrillation, the 'a' wave is often not present on LVEDP, PAW or LA recordings. When the patient with mitral stenosis remains in sinus rhythm there is a gradient between the 'a' wave of the LV diastolic and PAW or LA pressure. Thus, presence of an 'a' wave gradient (or, if in atrial fibrillation, an end diastolic gradient) is the haemodynamic hallmark of mitral stenosis.

The haemodynamics of mitral stenosis may be mimicked by those of an atrial myxoma, a benign atrial tumour arising from the atrial wall. The tumour may encroach on the mitral valve and cause obstruction to left ventricular inflow. At times, it is difficult to differentiate atrial myxoma from mitral stenosis if not clinically suspected. However, differences occur in the pulmonary artery wedge pressure, where mitral stenosis has a slow 'y' descent and atrial myxoma a normal 'y' descent. Also of note is that in left atrial pressure tracings, both 'a' and 'v' waves in mitral stenosis are increased but the 'x' wave is slow (decreased dP/dt)

Most patients with mitral stenosis present with dyspnoea on effort and these patients have elevated PAW pressures and, more importantly, elevated pulmonary capillary pressure, which causes the symptoms. Pulmonary artery pressures are often only mildly elevated (passive pulmonary hypertension). At times these symptoms are replaced by listlessness and fatigue. Haemodynamically the latter patients have much higher PA pressures, higher pulmonary vein resistance and slightly higher PAW and LA pressures, with a much lower cardiac output. Such patients develop what Grossman refers to as 'second stenosis' from pulmonary vascular disease affecting distal arterioles and the capillary bed (active pulmonary hypertension).[8] The cause of these reactive changes is uncertain. The latter group shows clinically and on the electrocardiogram (ECG) the signs of pulmonary hypertension and right ventricular pressure overload. When the active pulmonary hypertension becomes severe, prognosis is worsened.

Note the Gorlin formula for mitral stenosis:

$$MVA = \frac{CO(DFP \times HR)}{37.7 \times \sqrt{MVG}}$$

where MVA = mitral valve area, CO =cardiac output (ie. flow across the valve), DFP = diastolic filling period, MVG = mitral valve gradient, HR = heart rate. As for aortic valve area, this calculation is automatically derived by modern physiological monitoring systems. Similarly, CO cannot be used to calculate mitral valve area in the presence of a regurgitant valve.

Pulmonary stenosis

Pulmonary stenosis in its various forms is the most common congenital anomaly in cardiology. A gradient between right ventricle (RV) and PA of ≥ 5 mmHg is required to make such a diagnosis and is easily confirmed by catheter pullback. Calculation of valve area is made using the equivalent Gorlin formula for aortic stenosis. In the presence of left to right shunts pulmonary stenosis is frequently present. A modification of the Gorlin formula can be used to quickly calculate the size of the gradient and evaluate the need for intervention. Using the abbreviated formula:

$$PVA = \frac{CO}{\sqrt{PVG}}$$

where PVA = pulmonary valve area, PVG = pulmonary valve gradient, CO = cardiac output (i.e. flow across the valve). For example, for a given pulmonary valve area, if there is a 2:1 shunt, when the shunt is closed the cardiac output is halved, so the $\sqrt{PVG}$ is also halved. If the PVG is 80 mmHg, then $\sqrt{80} = 9$. Halving 9 gives 4.5, therefore the new mean gradient $= 4.5^2 = 20$ mmHg. Thus, after closure of the shunt the new mean PVG = 20 mmHg and intervention on the valve is not required.

Tricuspid stenosis

This complication is nearly always rheumatic, but may rarely be seen in carcinoid tumour (although tricuspid incompetence is more frequent), tricuspid atresia in congenital heart disease, and right atrial (RA) tumours and myxomas. It also results increasingly from stenosis of prosthetic valves implanted for prior tricuspid regurgitation. When due to rheumatic heart disease it is always associated with rheumatic mitral valve disease and often with rheumatic aortic valve disease.

The hallmark finding of tricuspid stenosis is a diastolic gradient across the tricuspid valve associated with a large 'a' wave in the RA pressure trace when in sinus rhythm that is at times almost as high as the right ventricular (RV) systolic pressure, and a slow 'y' descent on the RA pressure trace. However, most of these patients are in atrial fibrillation at the time of catheterisation, so RA and RV traces traces both lack an 'a' wave. As in mitral stenosis, there is an end diastolic gradient, with the RA pressure trace well above that of end diastole on the RV trace (see Fig. 8.15). Systemic venous congestion (liver, gut, peripheral oedema) occurs early in tricuspid stenosis, with gradients as low as 5 mmHg; cardiac output is substantially reduced at rest with little or no rise with exercise.

Exhalation reduces and may even abolish the gradient and so exercise, infusion of normal saline, deep inspiration or even atropine may be required to demonstrate the gradient. Adequate demonstration requires two catheters, one in the RA and the other in the RV, or else a double lumen catheter. To calculate stenotic valve area the Gorlin formula is used as for mitral stenosis.

Regurgitant lesions

Aortic regurgitation

This is leakage of blood from the ascending aorta into the LV during diastole and is usually progressive and chronic, although at times it may be sudden or acute. Forward blood flow is reduced by an amount equivalent to the regurgitant fraction. The degree or amount of regurgitation depends upon:

1. Size of the valve opening.
2. Diastolic duration (filling period).
3. Diastolic aortic pressure.

When it is mild, aortic regurgitation initially occurs in early diastole, but as it becomes more severe the regurgitation progresses throughout diastole. LV filling in this instance is due to a combination of normal blood flow across the mitral valve and blood leaking from the aortic root (regurgitant fraction). Stroke volume, or flow across the aortic valve per heartbeat, is therefore not equivalent to the forward cardiac output (normal cardiac output = heart rate x stroke volume; cardiac output with aortic regurgitation = heart rate x stroke volume minus regurgitant fraction). Cardiac output with aortic regurgitation is thus a measure of effective systemic flow (i.e. forward flow minus regurgitant flow). Without aortic regurgitation, cardiac output is the same as forward flow, whether measured by Fick or thermodilution methods. It is not possible to quantify the regurgitant component by cardiac catheterisation.

Significant aortic regurgitation is said to exist when the leaking valve area is ≥ 0.5 cm^2.[8] It is associated with increased systolic LV pressure from increased stroke volume and low diastolic pressure in the aortic root (from regurgitation) giving a widened pulse pressure. When the heart starts to fail, the ejection fraction begins to fall and the left ventricular end diastolic and end systolic volumes rise. On echocardiography this is indicated by an increased LV internal diameter in systole of ≥ 5.4 cm. In severe chronic aortic regurgitation the excessive regurgitant fraction leads to partial closure of the mitral valve (restriction of inflow orifice) owing to LV pressure exceeding LA pressure in mid diastole.[9] This may be seen on echocardiography and may cause a mitral diastolic murmur (Austin Flint murmur) even in the absence of mitral valve disease.

Acute versus chronic regurgitation

In acute aortic regurgitation, the ventricle is usually of normal or only slightly increased dimensions and systolic pressure and pulse pressure tend to be in the normal range. If severe, the LVEDP rises rapidly, causing a greater increase in left atrial pressure than occurs for a similar degree of chronic regurgitation. In chronic aortic regurgitation, simultaneous pressure recordings of LV and iliac via a femoral sheath show a much higher systolic pressure in the peripheral arterial trace than in the central aortic root pressure; this is further exaggerated in acute aortic regurgitation.

Presence of an atrial 'a' wave in the aortic pressure trace in diastole has high specificity for acute aortic regurgitation.[10]

Mitral regurgitation.

Mitral regurgitation is failure of the mitral valve to prevent retrograde blood flow from the LV to the LA during systole and may be acute or chronic. The mitral valve consists of a large anterior and smaller posterior leaflet and its integrity depends upon the mitral valve annulus, the *chordae tendinae* and the two papillary muscles. The commonest cause of chronic mitral regurgitation is rheumatic heart disease in underdeveloped or third world countries, whereas mitral valve prolapse and myocardial ischaemia are more frequent in the western world. Dilated cardiomyopathy is frequently associated with chronic mitral regurgitation and it is often difficult at presentation to determine whether the problem is mitral regurgitation leading to left ventricular failure, or cardiomyopathy with mitral regurgitation.

Acute mitral regurgitation occurs in infective endocarditis, acute myocardial ischaemia (often causing acute pulmonary oedema), flail mitral leaflets and rupture of *chordae tendinae* or papillary muscle (ischaemic). Some 'acute' causes may be considered to be more 'acute-on-chronic', e.g. a longstanding history of mild mitral valve prolapse with new-onset rupture of *chordae* or flail leaflet, or recurrent endocarditis.

One of the differentiating features of acute versus chronic mitral regurgitation is the chamber size, especially that of the LA. In acute mitral regurgitation, left atrial size is usually normal echocardiographically, as is the LV, although in the ageing western population both left ventricular and left atrial size are influenced by other factors (e.g. hypertension) and may be slightly enlarged.

In chronic mitral regurgitation the left ventricle ejects blood antegradely into the high pressure central system and retrogradely into the low pressure left atrial and pulmonary systems. The major determinant of regurgitation is the effective orifice size.

The hallmark pressure trace of mitral regurgitation is an increased 'v' wave in the PAW pressure or LA trace which reflects LA filling in systole and early LA emptying ('y' descent) in early diastole. Grossman and others[8,11,12] suggest the 'v' wave may be increased in any cause of LV failure, as the 'v' wave reflects the pressure-volume relationship of the left atrium. Thus in chronic mitral regurgitation the atrium expands and the 'v' wave increases only slightly over a long period, whereas in acute mitral regurgitation the 'v' wave is much higher for the same degree of mitral regurgitation and the patient is more symptomatic. Other conditions which can effect this pressure-volume relationship are those which affect LA volume (large left to right shunt) and compliance [ischaemic or rheumatic fibrosis, infiltrative disease (amyloid, sarcoid, haemochromatosis)]. Thus the factors affecting the 'v' wave are:

1. The volume of blood entering the left atrium during ventricular systole from the pulmonary bed and that regurgitating from the left ventricle, and the rate of filling.
2. Left ventricular contraction.
3. Systemic vascular resistance.
4. Extra-cardiac compression.
5. Cardiac rhythm.

A 'v' wave of at least twice the mean LA or PAW pressure indicates severe mitral regurgitation, and if it is more than three times the left atrial mean pressure then severe mitral regurgitation is almost certainly present.[8] As chronic mitral regurgitation progresses and regurgitant volume increases, the LA and left atrial appendage dilate, as does the LV. As the LV simultaneously empties into both aortic root and LA, factors that affect systemic

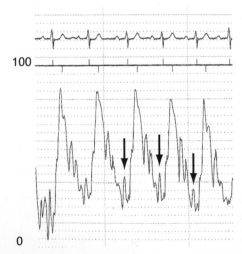

Figure 9.8. *Pulmonary artery (PA) trace from a patient with severe mitral regurgitation, showing retrograde transmission of 'v' waves (arrows) to the PA pressure trace.*

100

0

vascular resistance either worsen or alleviate the regurgitant volume. This is the reason for use of vasodilatory agents (nitrates) and ACE inhibitors in providing symptomatic relief to patients with mild chronic mitral regurgitation.

In severe mitral regurgitation or in acute or acute-on-chronic mitral regurgitation, the 'v' wave may be seen in the PA pressure trace due to transmission through the pulmonary vascular bed but, owing to a delay in transmission, is seen in the descending limb of the PA pressure (Fig. 9.8). Severe mitral regurgitation with failing LV systolic functions may at times have a normal 'v' wave due to the capacitance of the LA and decreased LV systolic pressure (LA pressure-volume loop).

As mentioned above, at presentation of a patient in cardiac failure with significant mitral regurgitation, it is at times difficult to determine whether the patient has severe mitral regurgitation and a failing left ventricle, or a dilated cardiomyopathy with moderate to severe mitral regurgitation due to stretching of the mitral valve annulus and *chordae tendinae*. Generally, if the 'cv' wave is greater than 50 mmHg it relates to valvular pathology[14] and the height of the 'v' wave does not always correspond to the severity of mitral regurgitation. It may relate more to acuteness (see above). Others consider that if a separate 'c' wave is present in the PAW tracing then incompetence is not severe.

Tricuspid regurgitation

Most commonly, tricuspid regurgitation is due to right ventricular and tricuspid annular dilatation, often referred to as functional tricuspid regurgitation. Functional tricuspid regurgitation is due to pulmonary hypertension of any cause, most frequently mitral valve disease or severe left ventricular failure due to hypertensive heart disease, cardiomyopathy or chronic obstructive airways disease. Other causes include pulmonary stenosis and primary pulmonary hypertension.

Tricuspid regurgitation from valvular disease is most commonly seen in infective endocarditis, right ventricular infarction, tricuspid valve prolapse, rheumatic heart disease, trauma, Ebstein's anomaly and rarely in carcinoid syndrome.

The 'cv' wave

No matter what the aetiology, regurgitation is associated with a large systolic wave in the right atrial pressure tracing. The systolic wave is best referred to as a 'cv' wave as its timing precedes the onset of the usual 'v' wave, although it has also been referred to as the 'S' wave. In severe tricuspid regurgitation the 'S' wave mirrors the RV pressure tracing. Grossman[8] considers that if RV systolic pressure is > 60 mmHg then tricuspid regurgitation is functional, whereas if it is ≤ 40 mmHg, it is organic. Organic tricuspid regurgitation requires surgical intervention, whereas functional tricuspid regurgitation may improve with medical treatment.

Pulmonary incompetence

Whereas pulmonary stenosis is always organic and mostly congenital, pulmonary incompetence is mostly functional due to high pulmonary artery pressures. Doppler echocardiography frequently shows physiological pulmonary regurgitation in 'normal' populations. However, once PA pressure rises to ≥ 70 mmHg from any cause, pulmonary regurgitation becomes evident clinically (e.g. chronic obstructive airways disease, mitral valve disease, cardiomyopathy, primary pulmonary hypertension). Organic pulmonary regurgitation is most commonly seen in infective endocarditis, idiopathic pulmonary artery dilatation and, rarely, in carcinoid disease, where plaque formation leads to fibrosis and constriction of the valve and valve annulus.

Left ventricular end diastolic pressure (LVEDP)

The diastolic filling period commences when the mitral valve opens and continues until the end of diastole, when the mitral valve closes (see Fig. 8.7). Note the following:

1. Early ventricular relaxation and dilatation causing low pressures.
2. Rapid inflow through the mitral valve followed by
   a) Slower mitral inflow.
   b) Left atrial contraction.

Various disease processes affect the left ventricular diastolic wave pattern and LVEDP. The end diastolic pressure (EDP) is a relationship between pressure inflow across the mitral (and at times aortic) valve and the distensibility and compliance of the left ventricle itself. Distensibility and compliance are not the same thing. Distensibility (i.e. filling capacity) relates to the upward/downward movement (the systolic component) of the LV pressure volume curve where the slope remains unchanged, as can happen in angina pectoris and in treatment with nitroglycerine. Compliance (i.e. stiffness) involves the shape and slope of the LV pressure volume curve, so in these two conditions the slope remains the same; however, in angina the entire curve is displaced upwards, whereas with nitroglycerine it is displaced downwards.

Factors affecting LV distensibility

(1) Intrinsic myocardial left ventricular problems such as:
  (a) LV hypertrophy — includes myocyte hypertrophy and increased fibrosis.
  (b) Abnormal left ventricular wall structure with infiltration (amyloid, sarcoid, haemochromatosis, fibrosis ischaemia/infarct).
  (c) Drug effects (hypercalcaemia, beta blockers, calcium antagonists).
(2) Extramyocardial problems such as: constrictive pericarditis, cardiac tamponade, external compression (tumour, pneumothorax, chronic lung disease [emphysema]), drug effects (e.g. nitroglycerine), right atrial pacing.
(3) Interaction of ventricles.
  (a) RV pressure overload (primary pulmonary hypertension).
  (b) RV volume overload (large left to right shunt).

Effects of supine exercise

In normal patients there is little or no rise in LVEDP with exercise, and stroke work index rises. In the abnormal ventricle, even if LVEDP is 'normal' at onset of exercise, LVEDP will rise with exercise. The effect on stroke work index is variable and may fall or rise, while PA and PAWP increase with exercise. Pulmonary vascular resistance falls in the absence of cardiovascular disease and rises in the abnormal patient.[15]

Effects of right atrial pacing

This technique has been used in many laboratories as a diagnostic aid in coronary artery disease and valvular disease to assess the need for intervention. There are two techniques:

1. Fixed-rate pacing at rates of 120–160 per min for 10 minutes[16] and
2. Incremental increases in heart rates of 2–3 minutes each until atrio-ventricular block or symptoms occur.[17] The LVEDP falls in normal patients and is related to a fall in end diastolic volume (stroke volume) but rises in abnormal hearts, especially if myocardial ischaemia is induced. The rise in EDP may relate to changes in compliance secondary to contracture of the ischaemic segment of myocardium, or else impairment of segmental

relaxation. Immediately after pacing, abnormal ventricles respond with an abrupt increase in EDP relative to that of the normal population.

Post-ventriculographic changes in LVEDP

The normal LV has an EDP of 3–12 mmHG. Following ventriculography, depending on the contrast used, there can be a small rise in EDP of 5–10 mmHg in normal patients. In patients with an abnormal left ventricle the rise can be as high as 20–23 mmHg. Injection of contrast causes decreased inotropy, reducing LV and aortic systolic pressure, decreasing the peripheral vascular resistance and resulting in peripheral vasodilation.

Nitroglycerine

Vasodilation by nitroglycerine causes peripheral pooling of blood and a decrease in stroke volume and end diastolic pressure. Heart size may also decrease from a decreased stroke volume. A fourth heart sound, if present, may disappear and the 'v' wave of mitral regurgitation decreases.

Constrictive pericarditis

The LVEDP in constrictive pericarditis (see below) has a typical 'dip and plateau' or 'square root sign' pressure pattern. In early diastole there is significant dip or drop in pressure. This is followed by a rapid rise in pressure from mitral inflow, then the pressure plateaus until atrial contraction at end diastole. The RVEDP and LVEDP in constrictive pericarditis are the same (see below).

The relationship of PAWP and PCP to pulmonary vein and LA pressure

When measuring right heart pressures, the PAWP measurement is generally taken as an approximation for LA pressure. This is possible because wedging a catheter in the PA blocks flow to the distal artery, causing the catheter tip to detect the LA pressure conducted retrogradely via the pulmonary veins.

It is necesary to draw a distinction between pulmonary artery wedge pressure (PAWP) and pulmonary capillary pressure (PCP), which are often used interchangeably but incorrectly.[18,19]

PAWP is the pressure measured by occlusion of a pulmonary artery and may vary according to the site of occlusion. The site of venous pressure measured is the segment supplied by the occluded arterial vessel and is considered to be the point where a vein with no flow adjoins veins with flow. The larger the artery occluded, the larger the vein measured, i.e. the farther away from the capillary bed and the closer to the left atrium. It is also important to note that the pressure recorded by a Swan-Ganz catheter is not necessarily the same as that recorded by a 5F or 7F Cournand catheter, where it is considered that the diameter of the vein measured is the same as that of the artery occluded. PCP is the pressure at the capillary level, not the peripheral arterial or proximal venous level of the PAWP; it is also higher, forcing blood flow through to the left atrium.[20]

It is the PAWP that is generally measured during cardiac catheterisation, and which is taken as an approximation for LA pressure. This is because in most situations there is no flow across the mitral valve in end diastole. Thus pressures in the LVEDP, LA and pulmonary vein (PV) equilibrate, particularly as there is little resistance to flow across the normal pulmonary veins into the normal heart in the horizontal plane (so normally PAWP = LA

= LVEDP). It is this phenomenon that permits PAWP, or the PA occlusion pressure, to be used as an approximation for both LV diastole (EDP, or filling pressure) and for pulmonary venous pressure.

In some diseases the pulmonary veins are affected, causing a rise in pulmonary vascular resistance. Here the PCP and pulmonary vein pressure are elevated even though the PAWP may be normal when measured by a Swan-Ganz catheter (a Cournand catheter would show a higher pressure), as in veno-occlusive disease, central pulmonary oedema, hypovolaemic shock or infusion of adrenergic agonists.[21-24] PAWP usually equates to left ventricular diastolic pressure and is a factor in determining the LV end diastolic volume (preload in the Frank-Starling equation). However the LV end diastolic volume is determined by transmural ventricular distending pressure, which is the LVEDP minus the juxta-cardiac pressures and ventricular compliance. One of the commonest causes of variation in juxta-cardiac pressure is positive end expiratory pressure (PEEP) and severe emphysema. Ventricular compliance is influenced most commonly by myocardial ischaemia and hypertension and less frequently by pericardial diseases. It should also be noted that height of the catheter tip relative to the horizontal LA level can affect PCP measurements; the higher the position (particularly if an upper respiratory lobe is selected), the lower arterial and venous pressures become relative to alveolar pressure.[24]

The PAWP does not always equilibrate with left ventricular end diastolic pressure. In some situations:

1. LA pressure inaccurately reflects LVEDP (mitral stenosis, *cor triatriatum*, severe mitral regurgitation, acute myocardial infarction, hypertension, hypertrophic cardiomyopathy and occasionally dilated cardiomyopathy).

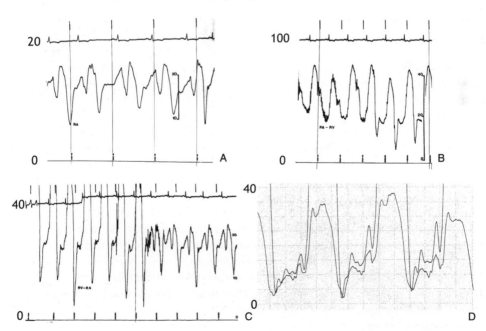

Figure 9.9. Right heart pressure traces from a patient with constrictive pericarditis. Note elevated atrial pressure in (A), with a characteristic 'M' pattern. There is also general equalisation of diastolic pressures, as shown in (B) for the pulmonary artery and right ventricle, and in (C) for the right ventricle and right atrium, and in (D) for right and left ventricles. Note also the 'dip and plateau' or 'square root' configuration in (D).

2.   The pulmonary vein pressure inaccurately reflects LA pressure (veno-occlusive disease, atrial myxoma, central pulmonary oedema, infusion of adrenergic agonists, large left-to-right shunts).

3.   Pulmonary artery wedge pressure inaccurately reflects pulmonary vein pressure (large left-to-right shunts, high output heart failure [thyrotoxicosis], chronic obstructive airways disease, PEEP and artifacts.)

If a large pulmonary artery is used to measure PAWP (via a Swan-Ganz catheter), collapse of the distal artery may mean that neither the PCP nor the PV pressure is measured. This results in pulmonary alveolar pressure being directly transmitted to the catheter tip instead.[24] Loss of "a" or "v" waves or marked respiratory variation in the pressure trace indicates that the catheter is too proximal and needs to be repositioned appropriately.

Constrictive pericarditis

This is the result of a thickened fibrotic pericardium preventing appropriate diastolic filling of the left and right ventricles. As the pericardium consists of visceral and parietal portions, these usually become fused and act as one. In Third World countries tuberculosis is likely to be the commonest cause, but in the Western world the most common cause is idiopathic, followed by viral infection, then other causes such as radiotherapy, chronic renal failure (especially dialysis patients), connective tissue disorders (rheumatoid arthritis, SLE), cancer and surgery.[25–27]

The development of signs of constrictive pericarditis is often slow and easily missed until the late stage, when calcification of the pericardium may have occurred. Treatment involves surgical removal of the pericardium, although this may not be possible in patients where it is a late complication of coronary artery bypass grafting, when symptomatic treatment with diuretics may be tried initially.[28]

The constricting effect of the thickened fibrotic pericardium affects all chambers of the heart equally, impairing diastolic filling and causing a rise in diastolic pressures. When recordings of right and left ventricular pressures are made simultaneously on the same gain settings, the diastolic portion of the traces should overlap exactly or within 5 mmHg.

Due to other factors, however, such as coexistent mitral or tricuspid valve disease, atrial pressures may not always be equal. At times, if the patient has been aggressively treated with diuretics, mean atrial filling pressure may be low and the ventricular characteristics may be missing. Thus when constrictive pericarditis is suspected and RA pressure is ≤ 12 mmHg, a rapid infusion of 1000 ml saline should be given. This elevates pressures, bringing right and left ventricular pressure traces into equilibrium, confirming the diagnosis in such cases.[29]

Atrial pressure traces show high pressures (≥ 15 mmHg) with rapid 'x' and 'y' descents (similar to atrial septal defect [ASD], restrictive cardiomyopathy) giving an 'M' or 'W' pattern (Fig. 9.9). The 'a' wave is elevated and particularly steep.

Atrial contraction occurs into a ventricle that will not expand further against pericardial constraint; this leads to a steep 'x' descent, and a steep and deep 'y' descent occurs as the atrium abruptly empties into the diastolic ventricle.

Normally on inspiration, intra-thoracic and intra-pericardial pressures fall, causing increased venous return to the right atrium, with a slight increase in right ventricular size. There is also a slight decrease in left ventricular size due to (a) decreased pulmonary venous return to LA from pooling of blood in the lungs, and (b) a slight bulge from the interventricular septum into the LV. The consequent left ventricular changes lead to a fall in systolic blood pressure of up to 10 mmHg.

Inspiration with constrictive pericarditis leads to a paradoxical rise in RA mean pressures, exaggerating the 'y' descent. This is clinically seen in the neck veins as a rise in jugular venous pulse (JVP) with a clear 'y' descent, referred to as Kussmaul's sign, which is also seen in restrictive cardiomyopathy, right ventricular infarction and pulmonary embolism.

Kussmaul's sign in constrictive pericarditis is based on the fact that in these patients, negative intra-thoracic inspiratory pressure is not transferred through the thickened fibrotic pericardium to the intra-pericardial space and right ventricle, so blood flow through the right ventricle to the lungs remains constant (not increasing). This causes the increased systemic venous return to accumulate in the right atrium, seen in the neck as a rise in JVP. As inspiration normally causes a decrease in LV stroke volume, the aortic component of the second heart sound (A2) occurs a little earlier, and P2 is delayed due to increased venous return of blood to the lungs. With constrictive pericarditis, because of fixed right-sided flow, on inspiration P2 does not move and A2 occurs much earlier than expected as a result of the augmented decrease in LV stroke volume, thus causing the sudden wide splitting of A2/P2 with the first post-inspiratory beat.[30]

In the ventricular traces an 'early dip and plateau' or 'square root' configuration in diastole is apparent. The early dip is normal, but because of pericardial constraint the ventricles fill rapidly and ventricular filling stops abruptly in early diastole, causing a flat or plateau pattern on the pressure trace (Fig. 9.9). On auscultation a 'pericardial knock' may be heard in early diastole, coinciding with the abrupt cessation of flow into the ventricles.

Restrictive cardiomyopathy

Restrictive cardiomyopathy may be caused by haemochromatosis, amyloid and metabolic storage diseases or it may be idiopathic. At times, presentation may occur years before a diagnosis can be made histologically.

Differentiation from constrictive pericarditis can sometimes be very difficult. Clinical findings can be the same with tachycardia, raised systemic venous pressure with Kussmaul's sign, normal systolic contraction of the ventricles and reduced stroke volume. Whereas in constrictive pericarditis the myocardium is usually normal, in restrictive cardiomyopathy it is the myocardium itself which, due to infiltration of amyloid, iron or fibrosis, causes impaired diastolic filling. The LVEDP is usually higher than the RVEDP, rather than equivalent as in pericardial constriction. These pressures are exaggerated by exercise. Generally, in restrictive cardiomyopathy, pulmonary artery pressures are elevated ($\geq$50 mmHg) and the EDP is usually less than one-third the right ventricular systolic pressure[31] (Table 9.1).

Even careful examination of haemodynamics may not differentiate between constrictive pericarditis and restrictive cardiomyopathy. Echocardiography can help by demonstrating increased LV mass, normal pericardial thickness (also demonstrated by C. T. scanning), thickening of the inter-atrial septum and valve leaflets in infiltrative disease or restrictive cardiomyopathy (as compared to constrictive pericarditis). Cardiac, rectal and

Table 9.1. Summary of basic haemodynamic differences between constrictive and restrictive pericarditis, where clinical signs are the same.

Constriction	Restriction
LVEDP may be >1/3 systolic pressure	LVEDP usually < 1/3 systolic pressure
RV systolic pressure < 50-60 mmHg	RV systolic pressure > 50-60 mmHg
EDP equal in all chambers (may need saline infusion	EDP varies from chamber to chamber (does not equalise with saline infusion)

Table 9.2. The three phases of cardiac tamponade

	Phase 1	Phase 2	Phase 3
Intrapericardial pressure (ITP)	<RA but RA is increased	Equal to RA but less than PAWP	Equal to RA and PAWP (both increased)
Pulsus paradoxus	Rarely seen	Occasionally seen	Always seen
Pressure/flow changes	Pressure changes only	Pressure/some flow changes	Severe pressure and severe flow changes
Effects of pericardiocentesis	1. ↓IPP, ↓RA, ↓PAWP	1. ↓IPP, ↓RA, ↓PAWP	1. ↓IPP, ↓↓RA, ↓PAWP
	2. Minor reduction in the exaggerated inspiratory decrease in arterial systolic pressure	2. Large reduction in the exaggerated inspiratory decrease in arterial systolic pressure	2. Reversal to normal inspiratory decrease in systolic pressure
	3. No change in cardiac output	3. Slight increase in cardiac output	3. Marked increase in cardiac output

skin biopsies are also helpful in diagnosing infiltration. In cases of amyloidosis, lupus erythematosus, radiation induced cardiac disease or heart transplantation with rejection, it may still be impossible to differentiate the two, as these diseases affect the myocardium and pericardium causing fibrosis/infiltration, and may also cause substantial pericardial effusions. Under these circumstances, it may be necessary to perform open thoracotomy with open biopsy of the myocardium and pericardium to help with the diagnosis.

Cardiac tamponade

This may be acute from trauma or cardiac rupture (ischaemic), or chronic from neoplasm, viral pericarditis, chronic renal failure or collagen vascular disorders. Haemodynamically, the pericardial collection of fluid, blood or pus causes a rise in intra-pericardial pressure that in turn restricts diastolic function. In acute form (trauma), only small amounts of fluid are necessary, whereas in chronic form (neoplasia, uraemia) the gradual rise in volume and pressure leads to stretch of the pericardium and a more gradual rise in intrapericardial pressures. Thus, much larger fluid volumes are seen before tamponade develops. The clinical consequences of a pericardial effusion therefore depend on the rate of fluid collection and the compliance of the pericardium. The fluid volume is not so important. In the author's experience, 190 ml caused severe tamponade when the right ventricle was perforated during right ventricular biopsy for dilated cardiomyopathy, and more than 1.2 L were removed from a patient with idiopathic pericardial effusion with tamponade (presumed viral). Reddy *et al.*[32] have described three phases of cardiac tamponade—phase one showing pressure but not flow changes, phase two showing mild to moderate pressure and flow changes, and phase three showing severe pressure and flow changes (Table 9.2).

Patients with trauma that has caused tamponade with only small amounts of pericardial fluid frequently demonstrate Beck's triad[33] of (a) progressive elevation of JVP, (b) progressive systemic arterial hypotension and (c) a small quiet heart. These patients require urgent surgical consultation. With the more chronic development of effusion and tamponade, intra-pericardial volumes are usually larger and percutaneous pericardiocentesis is appropriate if the echo free space is ≥10 mm.[34] Most units now introduce a pigtail catheter into the pericardial space, allowing (a) pressure measurement and (b) prolonged drainage to assess re-accumulation. Echocardiography is used in the diagnosis of pericardial effusion and tamponade. Right atrial and right ventricular diastolic collapse occurs through all phases of tamponade and so does not indicate severity. Ultrasound guidance is also commonly used during pericardiocentesis.

Pulsus paradoxus

Pulsus paradoxus is a non-specific finding. Initially described by Kussmaul in constrictive pericarditis, but the mechanisms vary when it is found in cardiac tamponade, severe emphysema and severe pulmonary embolism.

As already mentioned, during normal inspiration, pooling of blood in the lungs during deep inspiration results in less blood flowing to the left side of the heart, and consequently less blood is pumped into the systemic circulation. If this results in a fall in systolic pressure >10 mmHg, it is called pulsus paradoxus. This is in fact a misnomer, as pulsus paradoxus is simply an exaggeration of a normal physiological finding, not a paradox.

In tamponade, inspiration leads to a marked decrease in intra-pericardial pressure but is equally transmitted to both right and left ventricles. This causes increased venous return with an increase in right ventricular stroke volume, causing the interventricular septum to bulge into the left ventricle. Increased pooling of blood in the lungs results from a decreased gradient from the pulmonary artery to the left ventricle (pulmonary vascular resistance) causing a substantial fall in left ventricular stroke volume and systolic pressure, with an associated decrease in pulse pressure.

In constrictive pericarditis, pulsus paradoxus is frequently seen only in one or two beats on inspiration, where both aortic systolic and diastolic pressures fall. It occurs because the thickened, fibrotic pericardium prevents changes in intra-thoracic pressure being transferred to the intra-pericardial space and the cardiac chambers. Inspiration causes a fall in PAWP and PCP but not in LVEDP, which remains the same. Flow to LV decreases and stroke volume decreases, leading to a decreased systolic pressure. Intramural pressures do not alter throughout.

In severe emphysema and severe pulmonary embolism, pulsus paradoxus results from:
a) transfer of significantly negative intra-thoracic pressures to the lungs, pulmonary artery and right heart, so that the right ventricular stroke volume pools in the lungs, leading to a decrease in left ventricular stroke volume;
b) some transfer of the negative intra-thoracic pressure to the aorta and great vessels, and
c) pulmonary hypertension, which may actually prevent an inspiratory increase in venous return transferring to the pulmonary artery and lungs.

Nitrates

These drugs are commonly used in the catheterisation laboratory and for ischaemic heart disease to prevent angina.

Nitroglycerine is a potent peripheral vasodilator (reducing preload), but is also an arterial and coronary dilator affecting both preload and afterload. Nitrates cause venous pooling, leading to decreased LVEDP, stroke volume and heart size. Arterial dilatation causes decreased arterial pressures and decreased systemic vascular resistance (afterload).

Cardiac output usually falls but may remain unchanged when significant cardiomegaly is present and nitrates are administered. In the normal heart, LVEDP may fall to sub-optimal filling ranges, but in the enlarged heart, when LVEDP is significantly elevated, nitrates reduce the LVEDP to normal levels.

Mitral regurgitation

Administration of nitroglycerine reduces the degree of mitral regurgitation, and in so doing, reduces the 'v' wave of the PAWP. The reduction of mitral regurgitation is related to (a) reducing systemic arterial pressure (afterload), which also reduces the regurgitant fraction; (b) decreasing heart size, and (c) improved myocardial perfusion. If the regurgitation is related to myocardial ischaemia affecting either papillary muscle or global myocardial function, reduction of ischaemia and improvement in function of the mitral apparatus is likely.

Clinically, with nitroglycerine the murmur of rheumatic mitral regurgitation or papillary muscle dysfunction becomes quieter or diminished, whereas that of mitral valve prolapse occurs earlier and may become pan-systolic.

Aortic regurgitation

With aortic regurgitation administration of nitrates reduces the regurgitant fraction with a decrease in systolic pressure (afterload). As a result of this, the regurgitation impinging upon the anterior leaflet of the mitral valve is lessened. Any Austin Flint murmur noted will soften or disappear. Contrary to this, because of decreased systemic vascular resistance in mitral stenosis, the gradient across the mitral valve increases and the diastolic rumble of mitral stenosis increases in intensity and duration. This is potentiated by accompanying tachycardia, increasing cardiac output and raising left atrial pressure.

Hypertrophic obstructive cardiomyopathy/idiopathic hypertrophic sub-aortic stenosis

In hypertrophic obstructive cardiomyopathy (HOCM), reduction in systemic arterial pressure by nitrates causes an increased gradient from left ventricle to aorta. There is also increased inotropism of the left ventricular outflow tract and tachycardia caused by the nitrates, which also cause an increase in intensity and duration of the murmur associated with HOCM. Similarly, in valvular aortic stenosis, the tachycardia associated with the nitrates increases the intensity of the aortic stenotic murmur.

References

1. Hada Y, Wolfe C, Craige E. Pulsus alternans determined by biventricular simultaneous systolic time intervals. *Circulation* 1982; **65:**617–26.
2. Gleason WL, Braunwald E. Studies on Starling's Law of the heart. VI. Relationship between left ventricular end-diastolic volume and stroke volume in man with observations on the mechanism of pulsus alternans. *Circulation* 1962; **25**:841–8.
3. Verheught FWA, Scheck H., Meltzer RS, Roelandt J. Alternating atrial electromechanical dissociation as a contributing factor for pulsus alternans. *Br Heart J* 1982; **48**:459–61.
4. Hess OM, Surber EP, Ritter M, Krayenbuehl HP.Pulsus alternans: its influence on systolic and diastolic function in aortic valve disease. *J Am Coll Cardiol* 1984; **4**:1–7.
5. Brockenbrough EL, Braunwald E, Morrow AG. A Haemodynamic technic for the detection of hypertrophic sub-aortic stenosis. *Circulation* 1961; **23**:189–194.
6. Folland ED, Parisi AF, Carbone C. Is peripheral arterial pressure a satisfactory substitute for ascending aortic pressure when measuring aortic valve gradients? *J Am Coll Cardiol* 1984; **4**(6):1207–12.
7. Gorlin R. & Gorlin G. Hydraulic formula with the calculation of area of stenotic mitral valve, other cardiac valves and central circulatory shunts. *Am Heart J* 1951; **41**:1–29.
8. Grossman W. Profiles in valvular heart disease. In: Baim DS, Grossman W (eds). *Cardiac catheterisation, angiography and intervention.* 5th ed. Baltimore: Williams and Wilkins 1996, pp735–56.

9. Mann T, McLaurin L, Grossman W. Craige E. Assessing the haemodynamic severity of acute aortic regurgitation to infective endocarditis. *New Engl J Med* 1975; **293**:108–13.
10. Godlewski KJ, Talley JD, Morris GT. Acute aortic insufficiency. In: Kern MJ (ed). *Haemodynamic rounds*: interpretation of cardiac pathophysiology from pressure wave form analysis. New York: Wylie-Liss 1993.
11. Pichard AD, Kay R, Smith H *et al.* Large V waves in the pulmonary wedge pressure tracing in the absence of mitral regurgitation. *Am J Cardiol* 1982; **50**:1044–50.
12. Fuchs RM, Heuser RR, Yin FCP, Brinker JA. Limitations of pulmonary wedge V wave in diagnosing mitral regurgitation. *Am J Cardiol* 1982; **49**; 849–54.
13. Haskell RJ, French WJ. Accuracy of left atrial and pulmonary artery wedge pressure in pure mitral regurgitation in predicting left ventricular end diastolic pressure. *Am J Cardiol* 1988; **61**:136–41.
14. Beck W. personal communication. UCT 1981.
15. Khaja F, Parker JO, Ledwich RJ *et al.* Assessment of ventricular function in coronary artery disease by means of atrial pacing and exercise. *Am J Cardiol* 1970; **26**(2):107–16.
16. Parker JO, Khaja F, Case RR. Analysis of left ventricular function by atrial pacing. *Circulation* 1971; **43**:241–52.
17. Sowton GE, Cross VD, Frick MH, Balcon R. Measurement of the angina threshold using atrial pacing. A new technic of the study of angina pectoris. *Cardio Vasc Res* 1967; **1**:301–7.
18. Wiedemann HP. Wedge pressure and pulmonary veno-occlusive disease. *New Engl J Med* 1986; **315**:1233.
19. Holloway H, Perry M, Downey J *et al.* Estimation of effective pulmonary capillary pressure in intact lungs. *J App Physiol: Resp Env Exer Physiol* 1983; **54**; 846–51.
20. Zidulka A, Hakim TS. Wedge pressure in large vs. small pulmonary arteries to detect pulmonary venoconstriction. *J App Physiol* 1985;**59**:1329–32.
21. Shaffer AB, Silber EN. Factors influencing character of pulmonary arterial wedge pressure. *Am Heart J* 1956; **51**:522–32.
22. Walston A, Kendall M E. Comparison of pulmonary wedge pressure and left atrial pressure in man. *Am Heart J* 1973; **86**:159–64.
23. Wiedemann HP, Matthay MA, Matthay RA. Cardiovascular-pulmonary monitoring in the intensive care (part I). *Chest* 1984; **85**:537–49.
24. O'Quin R, Marini J. Pulmonary artery occlusion pressure: clinical physiology, measurement and interpretation. *Am Review Respir Dis* 1983; **128**:319–26.
25. Cameron J, Oesterle SN, Baldwin JL, Hancock EW. The etiologic spectum of constrictive pericarditis. *Am Heart J* 1987; **113**(2)354–60.
26. Marsa R, Mehta S, Willis W, Bailey L. Constrictive pericarditis after myocardial revascularisation: report of three cases. *Am J Cardiol* 1979; **44**:177–83.
27. Cohen MV, Greenberg MA. Constrictive pericarditis: early and late complication of cardiac surgery. *Am J Cardiol* 1979; **43**:657–61.
28. Ayzenberg O, Oldfield GS, Stevens JE, Beck W. Constrictive pericarditis following myocardial revascularisation. *Sth Afr Med J* 1984; **65**:739–41.
29. Bush CA, Stang JM, Wooley CF, Kilman JW. Occult constrictive pericardial disease: diagnosis by rapid volume expansion and correction by pericardiectomy. *Circulation* 1977; **56**(6):924–30.
30. Beck W, Schrire V, Vogelpoel L. Splitting of the second heart sound in constrictive pericarditis, with observations on the mechanism of pulsus paradoxus. *Am Heart J* 1962; **64**(6):765.
31. Shabetai R, Fowler NO, Fenton JC. Restrictive cardiac disease. Pericarditis and the myocardiopathies. *Am Heart J* 1965; **69**:271–80.
32. Reddy TS, Curtiss El, Uretski BF. Spectrum of hemodynamic changes in cardiac tamponade. *Am J Cardiol* 1990; **66**:1487–91.
33. Beck CS. Two cardiac compression triads. *JAMA* 1935; **104**:714.
34. Krikorian JG, Hancock EW. Pericardiocentesis. *Am J Med* 1978; **65**:808–14.

Chapter 10

Coagulation and the Coagulation Cascade

John Boland

Haemostasis

Haemostasis is the body's mechanism for preventing blood loss following vascular injury. Primary haemostasis includes mechanisms such as vasoconstriction, adhesion of opposing vessel surfaces and formation of a primary platelet plug at sites of injury. These mechanisms alone may be sufficient to staunch blood loss from very small vessels such as capillaries. More severe damage results in secondary haemostasis, with aggregation of platelets and activation of the coagulation system, leading to blood clot formation.

Coagulation is an extension of haemostasis and results from interaction between blood vessels and platelets with various circulating plasma proteins, or coagulation factors. There have been many excellent reviews and detailed monographs[1-6] on the pharmacology, biochemistry and physiological activity of platelets and coagulation factors and This information will not be repeated here. This presentation briefly reviews the coagulation process and describes current concepts in the coagulation cascade.

Platelets

Vascular injury results in exposure of collagen to the circulation. Immediately following injury, and directly as a result of contact with exposed sub-endothelial collagen, platelets enlarge, change shape, grow pseudopods, adhere to vessel walls at the site of injury, release their granular contents and aggregate to form a haemostatic plug (a sequence of events referred to as platelet activation, adhesion, release, aggregation and agglutination stages).[6] A flow chart indicating platelet activity and its role in haemostasis and subsequent coagulation is illustrated in Fig. 10.1. The platelet membrane selectively binds coagulation factors XI, IX, VIII, V and X to its phospholipid surface and provides a localised surface for many reactions in the coagulation cascade.[3,7] This helps to restrict coagulation activity to a specific location and to enormously accelerate and amplify the entire process. Other platelet activators include thrombin and adrenalin.

Platelets contain granules with various biologically active agents.[8] There are two main types of granule, called alpha granules and delta or 'dense' granules. The more numerous alpha granules contain proteins (including platelet factor 4), coagulation factors (fibrinogen, factors V and VIII) and glycoproteins.[10] Dense granules contain nucleotides (but not DNA), calcium and serotonin. Upon activation, platelets release their granular contents, including adenosine diphosphate (ADP) and thromboxane A2 (TXA2),[11] both of which promote platelet aggregation

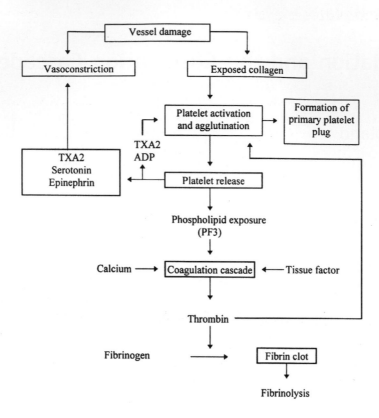

Figure 10.1. *Flow diagram illustrating platelet activity and its role in haemostasis and coagulation.*

in a positive feedback mechanism (Fig. 10.1). The anti-platelet drugs clopidogrel and ticlopidine exert their anticoagulant effects by inhibiting the binding of adenosine diphosphate (ADP) to its platelet receptor, thereby specifically inhibiting ADP-induced platelet aggregation.

Cyclooxygenase is an enzyme that triggers two pathways of arachidonic acid metabolism, one in platelets, the other in endothelial cells. In platelets, enzymatic activity of cyclooxygenase metabolises arachidonic acid (a polyunsaturated fatty acid and component of the platelet phospholipid membrane) into the prostaglandins PGG and PGH2, which are in turn converted by thromboxane synthetase into TXA2. Like serotonin and epinephrine, which are also released from platelets during haemostasis, TXA2 is a potent vasoconstrictor as well as a potent platelet agonist.

Counter to the effects of TXA2, the second pathway of arachidonic acid metabolism in endothelial cells produces prostacyclin, a potent vasodilator and inhibitor of platelet aggregation. Prostaglandins can inhibit platelet function by blocking platelet surface receptors. Like TXA2, prostacyclin is produced by the action of cyclooxygenase on arachidonic acid but is synthesised by vascular endothelium and smooth muscle cells, not platelets; it acts by increasing intracellular cyclic adenosine monophosphate (AMP) levels. Cyclooxygenase is therefore instrumental in generating both prostacyclin from endothelium (platelet inhibition) and TXA2 from platelets (platelet stimulation). These conflicting physiological effects of TXA2 and prostacyclin (along with other physiological and biochemical interactions) serve to regulate and restrict the procoagulant effect of platelets, thus limiting coagulation activity to a specific location.

Aspirin and platelet activity

Aspirin, a powerful platelet antagonist, exerts its anticoagulant effect by blocking activity of cyclooxygenase (by irreversible acetylation), thus inhibiting production of TXA2 and suppressing a promoter of platelet aggregation. In blocking cyclooxygenase, however, aspirin (and related compounds) also suppress production of prostacyclin, a platelet inhibitor. This dual effect of aspirin, influencing production of both prostacyclin and TXA2, has no effect on other activators of platelet aggregation such as thrombin, collagen or ADP (see chapter 14). Its potential effect as a platelet antagonist is therefore limited. The introduction of low-dose aspirin therapy is an effort to balance the opposing effects of aspirin on platelets and endothelium without compromising its benefits in suppressing platelet activity.

Aspirin and pain relief

Prostaglandins also trigger pain and inflammation as part of the inflammatory response. Aspirin, like other non-steroidal anti-inflammatory drugs, reduces pain and inflammation by lowering prostaglandin levels, which it does by blocking cyclooxygenase (used to produce prostaglandins). There are two known types of cyclooxygenase, called COX-1 and COX-2. COX-1 stimulates platelets and protects the stomach lining by producing a protective layer of mucous; COX-2 triggers pain and inflammation. Aspirin blocks both COX-1 and COX-2. In doing so, prolonged use of aspirin can cause ulcers and internal bleeding. The search for new types of analgesic has resulted in a new family of non-steroidal anti-inflammatory drugs called COX-2 inhibitors, which selectively block COX-2 but not COX-1. COX-2 inhibitors can therefore reduce pain and inflammation without affecting platelet activity.

GPIIb/IIIa antibodies and coagulation

Platelets also have glycoproteins on their surface which act as receptors for several adhesive proteins that enable platelets to bind selectively to vessel walls and each other. There are nine major platelet glycoproteins, numbered I to IX.[9-11] Glycoprotein Ia (GPIa) binds platelets directly to collagen, while glycoproteins Ib, IIb and IIIa (GP Ib, GPIIb, GPIIIa) bind to Von Willebrand factor (VWF, a component of factor VIII plasma protein), which itself has receptors that bind to myofibrils in smooth muscle cells. Glycoproteins fibronectin and vitronectin are also involved in platelet binding. In addition, GPIIb and IIIa form a unique complex that binds fibrinogen, an important component in platelet aggregation. A conformational change of GPIIb/IIIa that follows platelet activation is considered a critical component in facilitating platelet aggregation and subsequent coagulation.[12] The monoclonal antibody Abciximab (Reopro®, Eli-Lily & Co.) and synthetic second and third generation GPIIb/IIIa antagonists such as tirofiban and eptifibatide exert their anticoagulant effect by selectively and irreversibly blocking the GP IIb/IIIa receptor site, thus preventing fibrinogen binding to platelets and inhibiting fibrin formation. Failure of activated platelets to aggregate and bind with fibrinogen via GPIIb/IIIa prevents continuation of the coagulation sequence and is therefore considered the final common pathway for platelet aggregation and eventual fibrin formation. This mechanism is also exploited by a new range of oral GpIIb/IIIa antagonists currently under investigation for their effectiveness in preventing primary and secondary thrombosis following coronary interventions.

The coagulation cascade

Once platelets are activated to aggregation and release stages, coagulation proceeds to completion. The coagulation cascade theory, originally proposed by McFarlane in 1964, is now universally accepted as representing the mechanism of coagulation. It may be defined as a complex series of biochemical reactions, each step of which results in the activation of the next step in the sequence, in a 'cascade' or waterfall effect. The process begins in response to vessel injury and ends with the formation and subsequent dissolution of a stable fibrin clot.

The coagulation factors

Thirteen factors were originally identified and numbered accordingly, with the exception of factor VI (accelerin, or activated factor V) which is not recognised. Table 10.1 lists these and other coagulation components, along with molecular weights and concentrations in blood. By convention, certain factors are usually referred to by name rather than number (tissue factor, prothrombin, fibrinogen, calcium). With the exception of factor III (tissue factor or thromboplastin), coagulation factors normally circulate in plasma in a dormant or inactive state until activated. Activation of circulating factors in the cascade results from specific proteolytic cleavage of polypeptide molecules from the parent plasma protein.

Biochemistry of coagulation factors

Thew biochemistry of coagulation factors has been studied extensively.[13-15] All the factors have been identified as enzyme precursors or cofactors, except for calcium (factor IV), platelet phospholipid (platelet factor III) and fibrinogen, which is basically a substrate with no enzymatic activity. All enzymes in the cascade are serine proteases (proteins with the amino acid serine at the active site), except for factor XIII which is a transglutaminase. Tissue factor, high molecular weight kininogen (HMWK) and factors VIII and V have been designated as cofactors, meaning they participate in reactions, not as enzyme precursors but as catalysts, identifying and localising relevant substrate sites and increasing the catalytic efficiency of their respective activated enzymes.[8]

The biochemical properties of coagulation factors permit their classification into 3 major groups: the fibrinogen, prothrombin and contact groups.[4,5] The **fibrinogen group** consists of factors I, V, VIII and XIII. They all interact with thrombin, are present in plasma but not serum (meaning they are used up during coagulation), they increase during inflammation and pregnancy and do not depend on vitamin K for their synthesis; factors V and VIII lose activity in stored plasma.

The **prothrombin group** includes factors II, VII, IX and X and depends on vitamin K for synthesis. Vitamin K activity permits binding of calcium and phospholipid to form reactive complexes with these factors, an essential process in coagulation. Absence of vitamin K seriously curtails production of thrombin, the crucial element in converting fibrinogen to fibrin. Warfarin exerts its anticoagulant effect by inhibiting manufacture of vitamin K, thus interfering with production of the prothrombin group of factors and indirectly inhibiting production of thrombin. Without thrombin, coagulation cannot proceed to completion. Warfarin does not influence the activity of already-activated factors. It therefore requires a few days to demonstrate its effects and is initially administered in conjunction with heparin. This group also requires calcium for activation, is present in both plasma and serum (except for prothrombin) and remains stable in stored plasma.

The **contact group** consists of factors XI, XII, prekallikrein and HMWK; they are not dependent on vitamin K or calcium and remain stable in stored plasma.

Coagulation pathways

The coagulation system has traditionally been separated into two different pathways: intrinsic and extrinsic.[16] Both pathways follow their own independent sequence of events, then meet at a common point and form a common pathway. The intrinsic pathway is so called

Table 10.1. Basic properties of the major coagulation factors. For historical interest the original outdated names of factors I to XIII have been included.

Component	Factor No.	Active form	Molecular weight	Plasma concentration	
				µg/mL	µM
Fibrinogen	I	Fibrin subunit	330 000	3000	9.09
Prothrombin	II	Serine protease	72 000	100	1.388
Prethrombin					
Tissue factor	III	Cofactor			
Thromboplastin					
Calcium	IV	—	20		
Proaccelerin	V	Cofactor	330 000	10	0.03
Labile factor					
Thrombogen					
A globulin accelerator (ACG)					
Proconvertin	VII	Serine protease	50 000	0.5	0.01
Stable factor					
SPCA					
Autoprothrombin I					
VWF	VIII	Cofactor	330 000	0.1	0.0003
Antihaemophilic A factor (AHF)					
Antihaemophilic globulin (AHG)					
Antihaemophilic factor A					
Platelet cofactor I					
Thromboplastinogen					
Christmas factor	IX	Serine protease	56 000	5	0.08928
Plasma thromboplastin component (PTC)					
Antihaemopholic factor B (AHB)					
Autoprothrombin II					
Platelet cofactor II					
Stuart factor	X	Serine protease	58 800	8	0.13605
Stuart-Power factor					
Autothrombin III					
Thrombokinase					
Plasma thromboplastin antecedent (PTA)	XI	Serine protease	160 000	5	0.031
Antihaemophilic factor C					
Hageman factor	XII	Serine protease	80 000	30	0.375
Contact factor					
Fibrin stabilising Factor	XIII	Transglutaminase	320 000	10	0.03125
Fibrinase					
Fibrinoligase					
Laki-Lorand factor					
Prekallikrein		Serine protease	86 000	50	0.5814
Fletcher factor					
HMWK	Cofactor		110 000	70	0.6363
Fitzgerald factor					
Protein C		Inhibitor	62 000	4	0.0645
Protein S		Inhibitor	69 000	10 (free)	0.1449
Protein Z		Inhibitor	62 000	2.2	0.0355
Fibronectin		Receptor	450 000	300	0.6667
Antithrombin III		Inhibitor	58 000	290	5
Plasminogen			90 000	216	2.4
Urokinase			53 000	0.1	0.001887
Heparin cofactor II	Cofactor	66 000		90	1.3636
Alpha2-Antiplasmin	Inhibitor	63 000		60	0.9524
Protein C inhibitor	Inhibitor	57 000		4	0.0702
Alpha-2 Macroglobulin		725 000		2100	2.8966

because all required factors are contained within the blood. The intrinsic pathway is slower than the extrinsic, taking two to three minutes to induce thrombin formation. Factors unique to this pathway are factors XII, XI, IX and VIII. The extrinsic pathway requires a substance outside the blood, tissue factor, for activation and is faster than the intrinsic. Coagulation time for the extrinsic pathway is 10–20 seconds. Factor VII is unique to this pathway.

The common pathway includes final stages of the coagulation cascade and is shared by both extrinsic and intrinsic pathways. Factors that form the shared common pathway are factors X, prothrombin and fibrinogen (and consequently include thrombin, fibrin and factors VIII, V and XIII). The cascade sequence is shown diagrammatically in simplified form in Fig. 10.2.

Intrinsic pathway

In vitro experiments have demonstrated that the intrinsic pathway can be activated by contact with glass, kaolin, celite, or in general by a negatively charged surface. The process begins by interaction between small amounts of activated factor XII with high molecular weight kininogen (HMWK), which converts the coagulation factor prekallikrein into kallikrein in a positive feedback mechanism. Kallikrein then interacts with HMWK to further activate increasing amounts of factor XII. This reaction is not known to occur *in vivo*, where the inital activation stimulus for factors XII and XI remains unclear,[5,15] although thrombin can activate factor XII. The physiologic significance of the intrinsic pathway *in vivo* is therefore in doubt, but is still relevant in explaining certain phenomena, such as stent thrombosis.

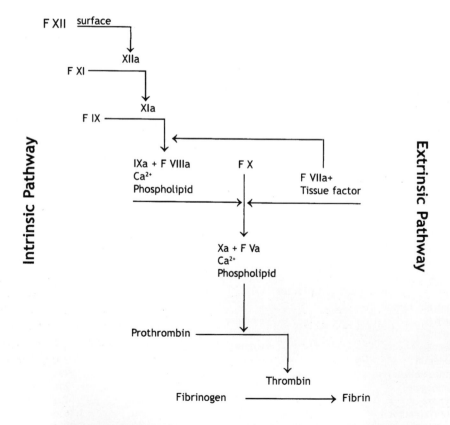

Figure 10.2. *Simplified representation of the coagulation cascade.*

The first step in the classic coagulation pathway is initiated by a contact factor, specifically contact of platelets with exposed collagen in damaged vessels. Activation of platelets then stimulates activity of coagulation factors. A change in molecular configuration stimulates conversion of factor XII into its activated form, designated as XIIa. This activates factor XI into XIa, which then interacts with factor IX to form IXa, which in turn forms a complex (tenase complex) with cofactor VIII, calcium and phospholipid to activate factor X and start the common pathway. Thrombin accelerates this process by stimulating increased production of factors V and VIII in a positive feedback effect.

Extrinsic pathway

Tissue factor (thromboplastin) is expressed on the surface of adventitial cells, which are not normally exposed to the circulation. When a vessel is damaged, tissue factor is exposed and comes into contact with blood. Independently of the intrinsic system, activation of the extrinsic pathway starts by interaction of factor VII with tissue factor which, together with calcium, form a complex to activate factor X. This also begins the common pathway.

Common pathway

Once begun, the common pathway proceeds by interaction between factor Xa and cofactor V which, together with calcium, platelet phospholipid and prothrombin form a complex (prothrombinase complex) to stimulate conversion of prothrombin into thrombin, which then converts fibrinogen into fibrin. Thus, conversion of prothrombin to thrombin by factor Xa can be mediated by either the intrinsic or extrinsic pathways.

Alternative pathway

Because the coagulation cascade was derived largely from *in vitro* experiments, it was originally considered that the intrinsic and extrinsic pathways operated as separate, unrelated events. Evidence now suggests that both pathways operate simultaneously *in vivo*.[5] Furthermore, it has also been demonstrated that the extrinsic pathway can stimulate the intrinsic by directly activating factor IX, which then proceeds to interact with factor VIIIa and activate factor X as described above. This activation of the intrinsic by the extrinsic pathway is known as the alternative pathway. It has also been suggested that activation of factor IX by factor VII dominates the coagulation process *in vivo*.[5]

The preceding description of the coagulation cascade is a simplified version, partly because it excludes positive feedback mechanisms, inhibitors and fibrinolysis. When these and other components are included, a diagrammatic representation of the cascade becomes more complex, as shown in Fig. 10.3.

Fibrin formation

Following conversion of prothrombin into thrombin by factor Xa, fibrin formation occurs by hydrolysis of negatively charged fibrinopeptides A and B from the soluble fibrinogen molecule in plasma. The remaining like-charged monomers of fibrin form weak hydrogen bonds to build a polymer of fibrin sub-units. Thrombin activates factor XIII which, together with calcium, stabilises the growing complex by covalent bonding to form a stable clot, strengthened by trapped inclusions such as platelets and other cells. Clot retraction follows, which further compacts the clot.

Fibrinolysis

Following coagulation, fibrinolysis[15,17] begins by conversion of circulating plasminogen into plasmin, notably by release of tissue plasminogen activator (tPA) from endothelium.

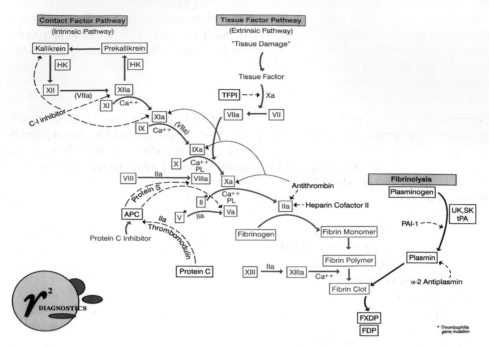

Figure 10.3. *Current status of the coagulation cascade. Note the role of thrombin, the sequential activation of coagulation factors via the two major pathways, and the action of inhibitors (dotted lines). (Reproduced courtesy of R² Diagnostics, Inc. 412 S. LaFayette Blvd, South Bend, IN 46601; Ph: (219) 288-4377; fax: (219) 288-2272; email: r2@enzymeresearch.com).*

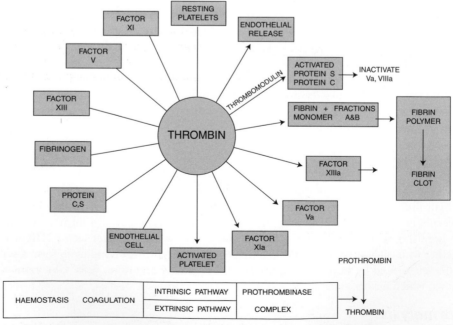

Figure 10.4. *Central role of thrombin in coagulation as an activator of platelets, coagulation proteins and endothelial cells, and in fibrin formation.*

Plasmin induces fibrinolysis by proteolysis of fibrinogen and other proteins into fibrin degradation products. Fibrinolysis is regulated by inhibitors such as a2-antiplasmin and a2-macroglobulin which inactivate plasmin, plasminogen activator inhibitor-1 (PAI-1) which inactivates tPA, and activated protein C which promotes fibrinolysis by targeting inhibitors of tPA.

Thrombin

Thrombin[18] plays a central role in coagulation (Fig. 10.4) as well as participating in other physiological activities such as leucocyte activation. It is a potent platelet agonist, directly promotes fibrin formation and stabilises the fibrin clot by activating factor XIII. It also regulates its own production by a positive feedback effect in generating factors V and VIII in the coagulation cascade. Thrombin also activates protein C which, together with thrombomodulin (a product of endothelium) and protein S, indirectly inhibits thrombin formation by inactivating factors Va and VIIIa. It activates factor XII and is known to activate factor XI *in vivo*. Thrombin also both promotes and inhibits fibrinolysis by promoting release of tPA from endothelial cells, as well as stimulating activity of the tPA inhibitor PAI-1. The antithrombotic/anticoagulant drug enoxaparin (Clexane®, Rhone-Poulenc Rorer) has a double effect on coagulation, inactivating thrombin and inhibiting the activity of prothrombinase (a complex of factor Xa, cofactor V, calcium, phospholipid and prothrombin).

Heparin

Heparin[19] is a naturally occurring anticoagulant and is considered the most effective anticoagulant known. Heparin exerts its anticoagulant effect primarily by potentiating the effect of antithrombin (which inhibits thrombin, factors XIIa, XIa, Xa, IXa and Va) and heparin cofactor-II, which inhibits thrombin. Although an effective anticoagulant in depressing thrombin activity, efficacy of heparin is limited, partly by its inability to inhibit thrombin already bound to fibrin, and because of circulating inhibitors such as heparinase and PF4.

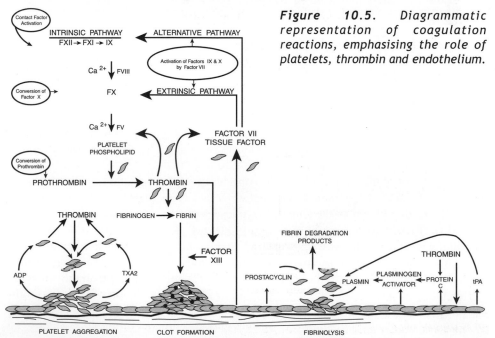

Figure 10.5. *Diagrammatic representation of coagulation reactions, emphasising the role of platelets, thrombin and endothelium.*

Inhibitors and coagulation

Inhibitors play a crucial role in the regulation of haemostasis.[20] They may either inhibit coagulation by selectively blocking pro-coagulant activity, or promote coagulation by restricting activity of anti-coagulants. In the latter sense they can even inhibit other inhibitors (Fig. 10.3). Inhibitors of coagulation include antithrombin, heparin, heparin cofactor-2, proteins C and S, $\alpha 2$ macroglobulin, $\alpha 1$-antitrypsin, C-I inhibitor and tissue factor pathway inhibitor (TFPI-1). Some (e.g. thrombin, protein C) have multiple roles in regulation and can enhance activators or inhibitors.

Physiological regulation

Uncontrolled coagulation, such as occurs in disseminated intravascular coagulation (DIC), is as physiologically untenable as uncontrolled bleeding. The coagulation process is therefore finely regulated by a balance of activators and inhibitors which, together with vascular responses such as vasodilation or vasoconstriction, act in concert to either disperse or restrict the activity of coagulation factors to specific sites.[20] Additional mechanical factors such as differences in shear stress from variations in blood flow between arteries and veins can also influence platelet binding activity. (This mechanism is explained in Chapter 12.) Blood flow itself, regulated partly by vessel diameter, is also effective in restricting or removing activated factors from a local area of injury. There are also important physiological differences between arterial and venous thrombosis. Arterial thrombosis is primarily platelet driven and subject to increased shear stress, whereas venous tghrombosis occurs in an environment of low shear stress and is primarily driven by thrombin activity.

    Another example of balanced coagulation activity, the antagonistic effect of TXA2 and prostacyclin, has already been described, as have examples of positive feedback effects (ADP, TXA2, HMWK and factor XII, thrombin). Indeed, positive feedback mechanisms have widespread application in regulating many biological systems and are well represented in the coagulation cascade.

    Failure of this system of physiological control can lead to an imbalance in the regulation of coagulation, possibly leading to a variety of potential disease states.

Coagulation as a single process

Instead of considering coagulation as a rigid system of discrete pathways with the traditional step-wise conversion of zymogens (inactive precursor plasma proteins) to their derivative enzymes, it has been suggested[7] that the coagulation cascade can be reinterpreted as consisting of only three separable groups of reactions: (i) contact factor activation of factor XIa; (ii) conversion of factor X to Xa via factors IX and VIII, and (iii) conversion of prothrombin to thrombin with resultant fibrin formation (a fourth reaction, activation of factors IX and X by factor VII may also be included).[21]

    The merit of this proposal lies in its consideration of coagulation as an interrelated sequence of simultaneous events that operate *in vivo* to regulate activity of circulating plasma proteins, rather than the somewhat artificial separation into a step-wise sequence of individual reactions. The concept of a cascade, however, is still a useful and simple way of presenting what may otherwise be considered an incomprehensible biochemical process.

    Another way of demonstrating coagulation is to illustrate reactions in diagrammatic form, as in Fig. 10.5. This has the additional benefit of consolidating apparently unrelated events into a unified structure, graphically displaying the interaction of various components. In this illustration the cascade itself is presented as being secondary to the main protagonists of coagulation, which are platelets, endothelium and thrombin.

References

1.   Beutler E, Lichtman MA, Coller BS, Kipps T J (eds). *Williams Hematology,* 5th ed. Part X: Hemostasis and Thrombosis. New York Mcgraw-Hill 1995, 1149-91.
2.   Lee GR, Foerster J, Lukens J, Paraskevas F, Greer JM, Rodger GM (eds). *Wintrobe's Clinical Haematology,* 10th ed. Vol I, Part III, Section 5: Platelets, haemostasis and coagulation. Baltimore: Williams & Wilkins 1999, 615-773.
3.   Hughes-Jones NC, Wickramasinghe SN. Haemostasis, abnormal bleeding and anticoagulant therapy. In: *Lecture Notes on Haematology,* 6th ed. Oxford: Blackwell Scientific Publications 1996, 202-36.
4.   Brown BA. Coagulation. In: *Haematology: Principles and procedures.* Philadelphia: Lea & Febiger 1988, 195-267.
5.   Hoffbrand AV, Pettit JE. Platelets, blood coagulation and haemostasis. In: *Essential haematology,* 2nd ed. Oxford Blackwell Scientific Publications 1996, Chapter 16.
6.   Hutton RA. Normal haemostasis. In: Hoffbrand AV and Lewis SM (eds). *Postgraduate haematology,* 3rd ed. Oxford: Heinemann Professional Publishing 1990, 560-97.
7.   Nemerson Y. Sequence of coagulation reactions. In: Williams WJ *et al.* (eds). *Hematology,* 4th ed. New York: Mcgraw-Hill 1990, 1295-1304.
8.   Ware JA, Coller BS. Platelet morphology, biochemistry and function. In: Beutler E *et al.* (eds). *Williams hematology,* 5th ed. New York: Mcgraw-Hill 1995, 1161-1201.
9.   Stenberg PE, Hill RJ. Platelets and megakaryocytes. In: Lee GR *et al.* (eds). *Wintrobe's clinical hematology,* 10th ed. Baltimore: Williams & Wilkins 1999, 615-60.
10.   Parise LV, Boudignon-Proudhon C, Keely PJ and Naik UP. Platelets in hemostasis and thrombosis. In: Lee GR *et al.* (eds). *Wintrobe's clinical hematology,* 10th ed. Baltimore: Williams & Wilkins 1999, 661-83.
11.   Bithell TC. Platelets and megakaryocytes. In: Lee R *et al.* (eds). *Wintrobe's clinical hematology,* 9th ed. Philadelphia: Lee & Febiger 1993, 511-39.
12.   Eli Lilly Aust. Reopro: Clinical Monograph 1994.
13.   Mann KG *et al.* Molecular biology, biochemistry and lifespan of plasma coagulation factors. In: Beutler E *et al.* (eds). *Williams hematology* 5th ed. New York: Mcgraw-Hill 1995, 1206-26.
14.   Bithell TC. Blood coagulation. In: Lee R *et al.* (eds). *Wintrobe's clinical hematology* 9th ed. Philadelphia: Lee & Febiger 1993, 566-615.
15.   Greenberg CS, Ortner CL. Blood coagulation and fibrinolysis. In: Lee GR *et al.* (eds*). Wintrobe's clinical hematology* 10th ed. Balltimore: Williams & Wilkins 1999, 684-764.
16.   Jesty J, Nemerson Y. The pathways of blood coagulation. In: Beutler E *et al.* (eds). *Williams hematology* 5th ed. New York: Mcgraw-Hill 1995, 1227-38.
17.   Francis C, Marder V. Mechanisms of fibrinolysis. In: Beutler E *et al.* (eds). *Williams hematology* 5thed. New York: Mcgraw-Hill 1995, 1252-60.
18.   Topol EJ, Serruys PW. *Current review of interventional cardiology,* 2nd ed. Philadelphia: Current Medicine 1995.
19.   Fiore L, Daykin D. Anticoagulant therapy. In: Beutler E *et al.* (eds). *Williams hematology* 5th ed. New York: Mcgraw-Hill 1995, 1562-84.
20.   Bauer K, Rosenberg R. Control of coagulation reactions. In: Beutler E *et al.* (eds). *Williams hematology* 5th ed. New York: Mcgraw-Hill 1995, 1239-52.
21.   Comp PC. Control of coagulation reactions. In: Williams WJ *et al.* (eds). *Hematology* 4th ed. New York: Mcgraw-Hill 1990, 1304-12.

Chapter 11

Formation and Progression of Atherosclerosis

Brian J. Nankivell

Structure of atherosclerotic plaque

Symptoms and events in coronary atherosclerosis begin with plaque.[1-5] Atherosclerotic plaque represents a focal pathological lesion within the intima and media of medium to large arteries (Table 11.1). Lesions are usually composed of a lipid core surrounded by extracellular matrix and collagen associated with intimal cells that have proliferated within the arterial wall, and immune cells such as macrophages and T-lymphocytes (Fig. 11.1a). Plaque can be classified into different types according to its structure.[2] American Heart Association (AHA) types IV and Va have a lipid core covered by a fibrous cap composed of a densely woven pattern of type I collagen, surrounding smooth muscle cells that produce matrix proteins. These plaques are capable of bearing considerable tensile stresses without rupture. Some 'mature' plaques without a lipid core (AHA type Vc) are stronger still. Plaque is capable of gradually reducing vascular blood flow and causing symptoms (e.g. exertional angina) or it may suddenly rupture resulting in vessel thrombosis and distal organ infarction (e.g. acute myocardial infarction, Table 11.2).

Table 11.1. Differences and similarities between the two major types of human vascular disease, atherosclerosis (atheroma or plaque) and arteriosclerosis

Feature	Atherosclerosis	Arteriosclerosis
Significance	pathological	'ageing process' of artery
Arterial wall pathology		
Intima	+++	+
Media	+ - ++ (late)	+++
Structure	complex	diffuse hypertrophy
Lipid deposits	frequent	no
Lesion distribution	focal & patchy branching vessels (turbulence)	diffuse, most vessels
Arteries affected	carotid, coronary, renal femoral & infra-renal aorta	thoracic aorta & central arteries
Vessel characteristics		
Compliance	normal	reduced (stiff vessels)
Conduit function	impaired	normal until late
Events & rupture	common	rare
Important risk factors	cholesterol, smoking, age	age, diabetes, hypertension

1a: STABLE

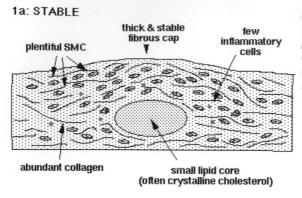

Figure 11.1a, b. Characteristics of typical stable (1a) and unstable (1b) plaque, characterised by differing amounts of lipid core, extracellular matrix and fibrin cap, collagen, macrophages and T-lymphocytes.

1b: UNSTABLE

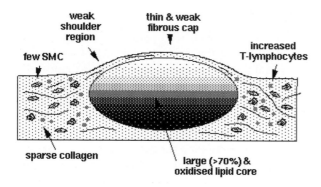

Table 11.2. Clinical effects of plaque in different arterial systems, according slow hindrance to vessel blood flow (haemodynamic impairment) or events such as plaque rupture with arterial thrombosis and distal infarction.

Arterial system	Haemodynamic impairment	Plaque rupture (+/- vessel thrombosis)
Cerebral	vertebrobasilar ischaemia*	transient ischaemic attack ('ministroke'), cerebrovascular accident ('stroke')
Coronary	exertional angina (exertional chest pain)	unstable or crescendo angina acute myocardial infarction
Renal	renovascular hypertension	ischaemic atrophy renal infarction
Mesenteric	'mesenteric angina' (abdominal pain after food)	acute bowel infarction
Lower limb	intermittent claudication (exertional calf pain)	acute vascular insufficiency of the leg, gangrene
Onset of symptoms	slow and gradual	sudden
Vascular impairment	transient	permanent
Organ damage	nil	infarction

Key: * Four cerebral arteries supply the brain (2 carotid and 2 vertebral arteries), and have excellent cross circulation via the circle of Willis, resulting in fewer cases of ongoing symptomatic cerebral ischaemia.

Arteriosclerosis

In contrast with atherosclerosis, arteriosclerosis (Table 11.1) is a diffusely distributed abnormality of the media, is found in central and medium-sized arteries, and is often a consequence of vascular ageing, diabetes, hypertension or renal failure. In patients with renal failure and accelerated vascular disease, arteries are characterised by fibrosis and calcification of the media and intima, with very little lipid. Because arteriosclerosis causes a stiff and non-compliant vessel it is frequently associated with hypertension, but does not usually interfere with the conduit function of the blood vessel (Table 11.2). Atherosclerosis and arteriosclerosis often co-exist in the same patient. As plaque is responsible for the majority of vascular syndromes, this chapter concentrates on atherosclerosis.

Epidemiology of atherosclerosis

Atherosclerosis is one of the most prevalent fatal diseases in Western societies, causing one half of all deaths. By early adult life, most individuals will have begun to form coronary plaque, which in some cases may be quite severe and advanced.[1,6] When the coronary arteries of young (and otherwise fit) men killed in action in war were examined, the beginnings of cardiac atheroma were found. Atheroma formation is a slow process, usually evolving without symptoms over decades and presenting later in life with the syndromes of acute cardiac and cerebral vascular insufficiency.

Traditional risk factors

Epidemiological studies have identified risk factors for coronary heart disease and, by implication, for its associated condition, atheromatous plaque.[2,7] Longitudinal studies (such as Framingham), carried out over several decades, produce the most reliable data. [7] Cross-sectional studies of a group at a single time-point produce a 'snapshot' of risk factors, but are less informative. Risk is expressed as an 'odds ratio' or a 'relative risk', and studies show that a combination of genetic and environmental risk factors shape an individual's response to the development of atherosclerosis. These risk factors are broadly divided into those that are modifiable (e.g. smoking habits, dietary fat intake), or unmodifiable (e.g. family history or patient's sex), and should be evaluated in all patients with vascular disease and corrected where possible.

Risk factors for atherogenesis

Family history of early (below 65 years) coronary disease
Male sex
Smoking (cigarettes > pipe & cigars > passive)
Dyslipidaemia
    Total cholesterol level
    Low-density lipoprotein (LDL) cholesterol level
    Total cholesterol/high-density lipoprotein (HDL) cholesterol ratio
    Lipoprotein (a)
    Fasting triglycerides*
Hypertension (both systolic and diastolic)
Diabetes mellitus and impaired glucose tolerance
Obesity (body weight, body mass index, waist/hip ratio etc.)/sedentary occupation
Gout or hyperuricaemia
Left ventricular hypertrophy*

Inflammatory markers (fibrinogen VII, C-reactive protein, PAI-1, hypoalbuminaemia, white blood cell count etc.)*
Hyperinsulinaemia†
Homocysteinaemia*
Chronic infections (e.g. *C. pneumoniae*)†

Protective factors

Female sex (until menopause)
High HDL cholesterol level
Vegetarian diet
Other diets (fish intake, omega-3 fatty acids, Mediterranean diet)*
Alcohol (red wine and other types of alcohol in moderation)*
Dietary polyunsaturated fatty acid intake†
Dietary antioxidant intake (Vitamin E, Vitamin C, garlic etc.)†

Key: * probable; † speculative factors (awaiting further evidence)

Diabetes mellitus and hypertension

Diabetic patients frequently have widespread vascular disease related to their increased number of risk factors (such as obesity and hyperlipidaemia), but also to an additional effect of hyperglycaemia, which can induce widespread vascular abnormalities including protein glycation.[8,9] Diabetic vascular disease is characterised by diffuse and smooth arteriosclerosis interspersed with patchy atheromatous plaque, and microvascular disease reflected by retinopathy, nephropathy, dermopathy, peripheral and autonomic neuropathy. When diabetic patients develop microalbuminuria, a marker of microvascular disease, their cardiac death-rates increase dramatically, possibly due to disease within the microcirculation of the heart or the coronary vasa vasorum (small vessels that supply the coronary arteries themselves with blood).

Hypertension also increases cardiovascular risk, especially when associated with older age or other risk factors such as diabetes mellitus.[7,9] Antihypertensive treatment reduces the event rates by 16%–45%, but does not normalise the risk entirely. Indeed, most vascular events occur in normotensive individuals.

Dyslipidaemia and cholesterol

Serum cholesterol may help initiate fatty streaks and plaque, influence the composition of the lipid core and affect plaque stability. [2,10] When small, dense particles of LDL cholesterol are combined with low levels of protective HDL cholesterol, vascular event rates are increased.[2,7,9-11] LDL is oxidised in vascular endothelial cells to a highly injurious product that results in dysfunction of large arteries and resistance vessels, including loss of vascular dilation and constriction as well as thrombosis and inflammation, particularly during plaque rupture.[10] Lipid-lowering agents do not correct angiographic stenosis but exert their benefit by stabilisation of a complex atheromatous lesion, depletion of the core of lipid content and reduction of inflammatory stimuli.[6] HMG Co-A inhibitors (e.g. pravastatin, simvastatin, fluvastatin, atorvastatin and cerivastatin) substantially reduce hepatic cholesterol synthesis and cardiovascular event rates in high risk individuals[10,11] without any cardiac history ('primary prevention' studies) or after a cardiac event[11] has occurred ('secondary prevention' trials). Marked reductions in rates of acute myocardial infarction, cardiac death and cerebrovascular accidents by lipid lowering agents indicate that we should actively treat at-risk patients.

Novel risk factors

Epidemiological studies fail to identify up to 50% of the causes of coronary vascular disease, suggesting that other possible causative factors may be responsible.[7]

Homocysteine

Homocysteine is an intermediate metabolite of the sulphur-containing essential aminoacid, methionine, that is produced after excessive dietary intake.[12] It is cleared by a urinary pathway and a remethylation process, which require vitamin cofactors to operate (pyridoxine-vitamin B_6, cyanocobalamin-vitamin B_{12}, and folic acid). Patients with inherited homocysteinuria, a rare disorder of metabolism associated with massive increases of blood homocysteine, experience early and accelerated atherogenesis and thromboembolic episodes. A Western diet high in protein (containing methionine) and low in fresh vegetables and fruit (to supply the essential vitamins to help clear accumulated homocysteine) may increase levels in the general population and contribute to atherogenesis. Some studies have shown that fasting serum homocysteine powerfully and independently predicts increased atherosclerosis and death from ischaemic heart disease, at risk levels comparable to that of smoking and hypercholersterolaemia.[12] It is increasingly being used to screen patients with premature or unexplained atheroma (as well as for venous thrombosis) and can be treated by supplementary folic acid and/or vitamins B_6 and/or B_{12}.

Fibrinogen and inflammatory markers

Human atherosclerotic plaques have all the hallmarks of inflammation, which in turn can destabilise plaque.[1,6] Plaques that rupture often have greater leucocytic infiltrates, which may impair the strength and stability of the fibrous cap and its resistance to rupture. Activated T-lymphocytes within atheroma produce interferon-gamma, which inhibits collagen production by vascular smooth muscle cells. Other inflammatory cytokines such as interleukin-1, tumour necrosis factor a and its cell surface homologue (CD-40 ligand) can increase proteolytic enzyme generation from macrophages and smooth muscle cells, which can further weaken the overlying extracellular matrix.[1,6,13] Serum markers of inflammation that have been associated with increased cardiovascular events include fibrinogen, C-reactive protein, PAI-1, hypoalbuminaemia and white blood cell count.

Infections and atheroma

Infective agents have also been recently implicated in atherogenesis,[1,14] including *Chlamydia pneumoniae*, and also cytomegalovirus, Helicobacter and the oral pathogens *Porphyromonas gingivalis* and *Streptococcus sanguis*. *C. pneumoniae* is an intracellular obligate pathogen that can persist inside macrophages and endothelial cells. Evidence for a role of *C. pneumoniae* includes serological studies linking increased relative risk in patients with IHD, autopsy identification of the agent in atherosclerotic plaques and fatty streaks, culture from diseased coronary arteries, and preliminary success with antimicrobial therapy by roxithromycin and azithromycin in unstable angina and IHD patients.[14] *C. pneumoniae* infection may occur via the lung (where it can also cause an atypical pneumonia), with infected lung macrophages travelling to activated endothelial cells to initiate plaque, or alternatively 'infect' established plaque. Long-term trials are underway to determine if these agents cause or exacerbate plaque, or are only 'innocent bystanders'.

Natural history of atherosclerosis

Formation of atherosclerosis results from an intricate interaction between diverse patho-logical factors such as lipid metabolism, blood coagulation elements, cytokines and haemodynamic stresses. Endothelial cells, smooth muscle cells and macrophages also have important roles in the genesis of atherosclerosis, by increased expression of adhesion mol-ecules, secretion of cytokines that increase inflammation, activation of matrix metalloproteinase enzymes and by expression of tissue factor within plaque.[1,6,13]

Initiation and progression of atheroma

Areas of turbulence or arterial shear stress damage and activate endothelial cells, increas-ing expression of homing receptors (such as e-selectin) or adhesion molecules (such as ICAM-1). Slowing and trapping of circulating monocytes and inflammatory cells is fol-lowed by diapedesis through to the subendothelial layer.[1,6] The earliest vascular lesions are fatty streaks (Fig. 11.2), which consist of intimal extracellular lipid deposits, T-lympho-cytes and macrophages. Activated T-cells appear early in plaque formation and can se-crete both soluble and contact-dependent mediators, which coordinate further atherogen-esis. Monocytes differentiate into macrophages (literally 'big eaters') which ingest lipid to become 'foam cells'. Macrophages can oxidise LDL cholesterol and secrete growth and proliferative factors. Migration and proliferation of smooth muscle cells from the media then follow.[6,10]

Plaque gradually increases in size and becomes more complex with time, occurring in increased numbers of coronary and other arteries, and especially in areas of high turbu-lence such as arterial branch points. One method of plaque growth and angiographic progression is by subclinical plaque disruption, followed by a healing response with prolif-eration of smooth muscle cells and collagen deposition.[2] Activation of inflammatory cells and death of masses of lipid-laden foam cells within the plaque result in large deposits of extracellular lipid forming the core of plaque. Advanced plaque is a heterogeneous mixture

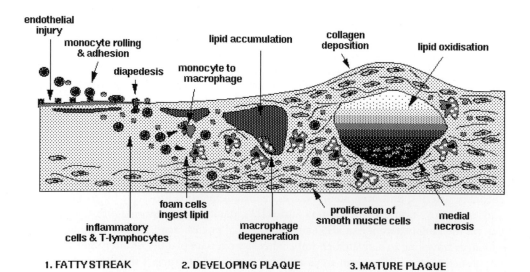

Figure 11.2. Formation and progression of atheromatous plaque, from its beginning as a fatty streak and evolving into mature and complex plaque.

of varying amounts of lipid, collagen, protein and calcium resembling gruel (atheroma is Greek for 'porridge').

Arterial response to plaque

Although a growing plaque occupies space, pathology studies have shown that the lumen is not always compromised.[1,15] The arterial wall is not a static structure, it can remodel itself to accommodate expanding plaque without compromising its lumen. It does this by increasing its external diameter. Part of this process involves medial atrophy, allowing the plaque to bulge outwards through a ruptured internal elastic lamina, and extruding from the arterial wall. Arterial enlargement is a focal and local response to the development of atherosclerotic plaque, and functionally important stenosis of coronary vessels is usually delayed until the lesion exceeds 40% of the internal elastic lamina diameter.[15] This process was first observed in monkeys fed an atherogenic diet, and later confirmed in human studies of femoral intravascular ultrasound and post-mortem coronary plaque studies.[15] Intra-mural plaque may evolve for decades before causing any clinical symptoms, and the rate of change depends on local conditions within the vessel wall. Patients with vessels that actively form plaque or generate new lesions on repeat coronary angiography have greater event rates and a worse prognosis.

Atherosclerosis and clinical disease

Acute coronary syndromes

Our view of atheroma and its role in acute events has changed. Coronary thrombosis and myocardial infarction were originally thought to occur at sites of high-grade stenosis. Recent studies have indicated that the more numerous non-stenotic lesions were the most vulnerable, and responsible for most acute events.[1,3,4] A change in vessel character from stable to unstable plaque may present as an acute coronary syndrome such as unstable angina or acute myocardial infarction, on a background of a previously stable angina or an asymptomatic patient (Table 11.2).

Unstable angina is heralded by change in the pattern or frequency of angina, prolonged angina, frequent anginal episodes within a 24-hour period, resting or nocturnal angina. It is caused by either erosion of the endothelial surface[4] or rupture of an unstable coronary plaque inducing local coagulation, with intermittent partial occlusion of the vessel and distal ischaemia.[3,10] Clot dissolution by the fibrinolytic system or by therapeutic heparin follows, with cardiac reperfusion. When a thrombosis around an unstable plaque fails to disassociate and extends, complete coronary occlusion usually proceeds to a completed myocardial infarction, depending on collateral perfusion.

Unstable plaque and plaque rupture

Plaque stability is a critical factor determining catastrophic vascular events such as myocardial infarction, unstable angina or cerebrovascular accidents.[1] This stability factor underscores the great clinical diversity of presentations of an individual with atherosclerosis. A young man may suddenly die during exercise from an 'insignificant' lesion that ruptures and causes death, in a coronary circulation that otherwise is not greatly diseased. In contrast, an elderly patient with widespread vascular disease of coronary, cerebral, carotid, aorta and lower limb arteries, with extensive but stable atherosclerosis, may die of other causes. So while the presence of atheroma is a necessary prerequisite, it is plaque stability that is critical to final outcome as it determines future events and ultimate mortality.[3-5]

Thrombosis of a disrupted plaque causes most acute coronary events, and the structure of plaque governs its physical integrity.[1,3-5] The extracellular matrix of the fibrous capsule overlying the thrombogenic core of the atheroma is of particular importance. Stable atheroma generally have thick fibrous caps overlying the soft thrombogenic lipid core, which is smaller and less oxidised than lesions that have ruptured (Fig. 11.1a). The fibrous cap becomes weakened either by decreased synthesis of extracellular matrix, increased degradation of the matrix, or both. The cytokine interferon-gamma produced by T-lymphocytes can inhibit smooth muscle cell synthesis of collagen, which is an important component of the fibrous cap.[1,6] Matrix metalloproteinases are a family of enzymes that can further degrade collagen, elastin and proteoglycans of the extracellular matrix and can further weaken the plaque.[13]

Unstable and dangerous plaques are characterised by thin fibrous caps, large lipid cores, macrophages in the critical shoulder region and depletion of structurally important smooth muscle cells (Fig. 11.1b). Such lesions are prone to rupture, allowing blood to contact the highly thrombogenic material within the lipid core of the plaque, precipitating thrombosis.[1,5] Plaques vulnerable to disruption often do not produce flow-limiting stenoses or symptoms that may announce their presence (e.g. with exertional angina). These lesions are often asymptomatic, are not detected on exercise or pharmacological stress testing, and are not regarded as 'significant' by coronary angiography. Angiography only defines the vessel lumen, and may significantly underestimate the extent of vascular disease when compared with coronary intravascular ultrasound, which visualises plaque within the arterial wall.[16] Currently we do not have good tests to identify potentially unstable atheroma before it becomes clinically evident.

Restenosis and the pathogenesis of vascular injury

One of the major limitations of interventions such as angioplasty is the risk of restenosis, despite the use of primary stenting and anti-platelet agents such as ticlopidine. When the vessel wall is injured by angioplasty, it can initiate a healing inflammatory response resulting in further stenosis or restenosis.

Originally, arterial smooth muscle cell proliferation was thought responsible for restenosis, from the response of acute carotid arterial injury in the rat that gave rise to the multi-wave model of restenosis. However, this simple model of arterial injury in a rat differs from coronary angioplasty of diseased human vessels, which already contain abundant smooth muscle cells and leucocytes. Strategies that have targeted smooth muscle replication have failed in clinical trials. Recent evidence suggests that human restenosis depends less on neointimal hyperplasia (smooth muscle proliferation appears more indolent), but rather is due to constrictive remodelling and adventitial scarring. Accumulation of extracellular matrix and failure of the damaged vessel to 'remodel' outwards to maintain its increased calibre following interventional arterial dilatation results in a smaller vessel lumen and restenosis.[1]

Primary angioplasty is sometimes performed in patients with an acute myocardial infarction whose 'culprit' lesions underlying the thrombus are often not critical. The healing response of the angioplastied vessel in this case may be beneficial. In some instances the benefit of angioplasty may be from stimulation of smooth muscle replication and collagen synthesis, reinforcement of the plaque's fibrous cap, and conversion of an 'unstable' plaque to a more stable one.

References

1. Davis MJ. Stability and instability: Two faces of coronary atherosclerosis. *Circulation* 1996; **94**:2013–21.
2. Stary HC, Chandler AB, Dinsmore RE *et al*. A definition of advanced types of atherosclerotic lesions and a histological classification of atherosclerosis: A report from the Committee of Vascular Lesions of the Council of Atherosclerosis. American Heart Association. *Circulation* 1995; **92**:1355–74.
3. Farb A, Burke AP, Tang AL *et al*. Coronary plaque erosion without rupture into a lipid core: a frequent cause of coronary thrombosis in sudden death. *Circulation* 1996; **93**:1354–63.
4. Falk E. Unstable angina with a fatal outcome: dynamic coronary thrombosis leading to infarction and/or sudden death. *Circulation* 1985; **71**:699–708.
5. Richardson P, Davis M, Born G. Influence of plaque configuration and stress distribution on fissuring of coronary atherosclerotic plaques. *Lancet* 1989; **2**:941–44.
6. Libby P, Schoenbeck U, Mach F *et al*. Current concepts in cardiovascular pathology: the role of LDL cholesterol in plaque rupture and stabilisation. *Am J Med* 1998; **104**:14S–18S.
7. Flack JM, Neaton J, Grimm R *et al*. Blood pressure among men with prior acute myocardial infarction. Multiple Risk Factor Intervention Trial Research Group. *Circulation* 1995; **92**:2437–45.
8. Turner RC, Millins H, Neil HA *et al*. Risk factors for coronary artery disease in non-insulin dependent diabetes mellitus: United Kingdom Prospective Diabetes Study (UKPDS: 23). *BMJ* 1998; **316** (7134):823–8.
9. Homma S, Ishii T, Tsugane S, Hirose N. Different effects of hypertension and hypercholesterolemia on the natural history of aortic atherosclerosis by the stage of intimal lesions. *Atherosclerosis* 1997; **128**:85–95.
10. Selwyn AP, Kinlay S, Libby P, Ganz P. Atherogenic lipids, vascular dysfunction, and clinical signs of ischaemic heart disease. *Circulation* 1997; **95**:5–7.
11. 4S group. Randomised trial of cholesterol lowering in 4444 patients with coronary heart disease: the Scandinavian Simvastatin Survival Study (4S). *Lancet* 1994; **344**:1383–89.
12. Wald NJ, Watt HC, Law MR *et al*. Homocysteine and ischaemic heart disease: results of a prospective study with implications regarding prevention. *Arch Intern Med* 1998; **158**:862–7.
13. Galis Z, Sukhova G, Lark M, Libby P. Increased expression of matrixmetalloproteinases and matrix degrading activity in vulnerable regions of human atherosclerotic plaque. *J Clin Invest* 1994; **94**:2493–2503.
14. Davidson M, Kuo CC, Middaugh JP *et al*. Confirmed previous infection with Chlamydia pneumoniae (TWAR) and its presence in early coronary atherosclerosis. *Circulation* 1998; **98**:628–33.
15. Glagov S, Weisenberd E, Zarins C *et al*. Compensatory hypertrophy of human atherosclerotic coronary arteries. *N Eng J med* 1987; **316**:1371–75.
16. Mintz GS, Painter JA, Pitchard AD *et al*. Atherosclerosis in angiographically normal coronary artery reference segments: an intravascular ultrasound study with clinical correlations. *J Am Coll Cardiol* 1995; **25**:1479–85.

Chapter 12

Thrombosis, Heparin and Laboratory Monitoring of Heparin Therapy

Steven Faddy

Thrombosis

Thrombosis has been described as the pathologic process resulting from the inappropriate initiation and propagation of the coagulation system.[1] Thrombosis occurs as the result of endothelial damage or alteration of blood flow characteristics. Once a thrombus forms in a blood vessel, a series of positive feedback mechanisms may assist in continued growth of the clot until it completely occludes the vessel. In the case of the coronary arteries, this can have dire consequences. Acute coronary conditions such as myocardial infarction and unstable angina are usually the result of thrombosis secondary to rupture of atherosclerotic plaque.[2]

Normal endothelium has a number of properties that inhibit thrombus formation (antithrombotic properties), or that promote thrombus formation in response to injury (prothrombotic properties). Normal haemostasis is a delicate balance between these properties, maintaining uninterrupted blood flow under normal circumstances and promoting clot formation in response to injury. Pathologic thrombus formation can result either from the inhibition of antithrombotic properties or induction of prothrombotic properties.

The pathology giving rise to thrombosis can be broadly grouped into three categories: (i) abnormalities in endothelial function, (ii) changes in blood flow characteristics and (iii) abnormalities in blood components (including platelet function and anomalies in the coagulation and fibrinolytic systems). Abnormalities in one or more of these groups can initiate and propagate thrombus formation.

Endothelial function

The common antithrombotic and prothrombotic properties of normal vascular endothelium are listed in Table 12.1. Normal endothelium inhibits thrombus formation by a number of mechanisms. Prostacyclin (Prostaglandin I_2) is produced by endothelial cells and released into the blood stream, causing inhibition of platelet activation and inducing vasodilation via an increase of cyclic AMP. Endothelium-derived relaxing factor (EDRF, nitric oxide), which inhibits platelet activation and induces vasodilation by increasing cyclic GMP, is another molecule produced and secreted by endothelium. Other antithrombotic agents such as Ecto-ADPase and thrombomodulin are not released into the blood but are expressed on the surface membrane of the endothelial cell. Thrombomodulin is a protein which, in response to binding with thrombin, activates the naturally occurring anticoagulant Protein C. Heparin sulfate glycosaminoglycans are expressed on the cell surface and catalyse binding of antithrombin III and heparin cofactor II to thrombin and other

Table 12.1. Common antithrombotic and prothrombotic properties of normal vascular endothelium

Factor	Activity
Antithrombotic properties	
Prostacyclin (Prostaglandin I$_2$)	Inhibits platelet activation, promotes vasodilation
Endothelium-derived relaxing factor (EDRF, NO)	Inhibits platelet activation, promotes vasodilation
Thrombomodulin	Binds thrombin, activates Protein C
Glycosaminoglycans	Bind ATIII and heparin co-factor II to thrombin
Tissue plasminogen activator (tPA)	Promotes fibrinolysis
Tissue factor pathway inhibitor (TFPI)	Inactivates factors VIIa and Xa
Receptors for t-PA and uPA	
Ecto-ADPase	
Prothrombotic properties	
von Willebrand factor	Activates platelets, assists coagulation cascade
Factor V	Promotes thrombin generation
Tissue factor	Activates extrinsic pathway
Plasminogen activator inhibitor-1 (PAI-1)	Inhibits fibrinolysis

coagulation proteins, inactivating them and arresting propagation of the coagulation response. Plasminogen activators such as tissue plasminogen activator (tPA) and urokinase (uPA) are produced and released by endothelium in response to a range of stimuli. These molecules bind to fibrin, which allows them to form complexes with circulating or membrane-bound plasminogen. Formation of plasmin results, facilitating fibrinolysis. Tissue factor pathway inhibitor (TFPI) is a membrane-bound protein that inactivates factors VIIa and Xa.

Thrombosis can be promoted in response to disease or injury by the loss (or masking) of the antithrombotic properties of endothelium, or by expression of the prothrombotic properties. A number of pathological states can lead to alterations in the antithrombotic capabilities of endothelium. Atherosclerosis leads to a localised decrease in production of prostacyclin and tPA, while EDRF production is inhibited in patients with hypercholesterolaemia or hypertension. Reduced expression of thrombomodulin and decreased EDRF production have been noted in patients with hyperhomocyst(e)inaemia,[1] which has been identified as a risk factor for atherosclerotic disease in young individuals with a strong family history of coronary artery disease.[2]

In addition to loss of antithrombotic properties, diseased or damaged endothelium can also express a number of prothrombotic properties to promote thrombosis. Tissue factor (factor III) is produced and expressed on the surface of endothelial cells in response to a number of plasma proteins including interleukin-1, tumour necrosis factor and some endotoxins. Expression of tissue factor induces activation of the extrinsic coagulation pathway. Dysfunctional endothelial cells can express factor V on their cell surface and, in response to hypoxia, can express a molecule capable of activating factor X. On exposure to thrombin, endothelial cells produce and secrete von Willebrand factor and plasminogen activator inhibitor-1 into the blood. The action of these molecules is discussed in Chapter 10.

Blood flow

Blood flow patterns within arteries also play a part in maintaining fluidity of blood. Blood flows through arteries in concentric layers called laminae. Layers at the centre of the arterial lumen circulate at a higher velocity and carry heavier particles such as red and white blood cells. Platelets are displaced to the outer layers, which flow with less velocity and approach stasis near the vessel wall. Platelets become trapped in the outer layers and are inhibited from moving into the more central laminae by the relative differences in flow rates. This phenomenon benefits the clotting process by providing a concentration of platelets close to the site of any vessel injury. Low-velocity blood flow near the vessel wall prevents the weak platelet plug from being dislodged before reinforcement by the secondary coagulation pathways.

The difference in flow velocity from its maximum at the centre of the artery to the almost static flow rate near the wall of the artery is known as the velocity gradient. The steepness of the velocity gradient is directly related to the shear rate.[1] The shear rate has been described as the rate at which one layer of fluid moves with respect to the adjacent layers.[3] An increase in shear tends to increase the number of platelets deposited in response to vessel injury.[1] Such increases are typically seen in response to injury in the microvasculature. Decreased shear rates tend to increase the amount of fibrin deposited and are more common in larger veins and vascular pockets. In the heart, such pockets include aneurysms in vessels or the ventricle, and the left atrial appendage of patients with atrial fibrillation.

Arterial thrombosis is brought about by increased flow and high shear and is characterised by a predominance of platelets in the thrombus. Vessel bifurcations are at particular risk of thrombosis because they divide flow patterns. Endothelium at the inner junction is exposed to high flow velocities and the potential for turbulent flow, which dramatically increase local shear forces. Normal endothelium is adapted to withstand these highly prothrombotic effects. Continued exposure and other factors such as hypertension, however, reduce the resistance of endothelium and increase the risk of thrombosis.

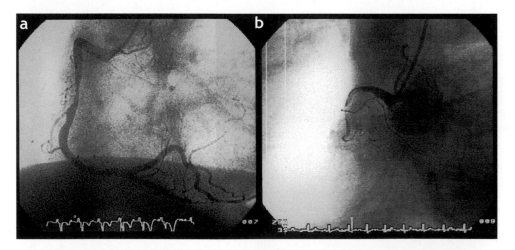

Figure 12.1. Case study of a 60-year-old male who underwent cardiac catheterisation for investigation of recent-onset exertional chest pain. His history included coronary angioplasty to the left circumflex and second obtuse marginal arteries two years previously, and both were found to be free of obstructive disease. The angiogram showed a 70% narrowing in the mid right coronary artery (a). The patient was discharged to be treated medically and placed on the non-urgent waiting list for angioplasty of this lesion. Six weeks later, he began experiencing episodes of unstable angina and was readmitted for angioplasty of the RCA lesion. Initial angiography showed the vessel was occluded proximally by thrombosis (b), with retrograde flow from the left system only reaching the crux. The patient was treated with thrombolytic therapy before angioplasty was attempted.

Once a clot forms it is prevented from growing larger by the antithrombotic properties of the surrounding endothelium. Yet, formation of even the smallest clot will disturb blood flow properties within the artery, leading to turbulent flow patterns and increased shear forces. Endothelial damage is initiated or worsened, and platelet activation and adhesion increase by virtue of increased collision frequency between platelets. The thrombus grows in size and intrudes further into the vascular lumen, worsening the turbulent flow patterns and leading to further growth of the thrombus. This 'snowballing' effect has the potential to continue to enlarge the size of the thrombus until the entire lumen of the artery is occluded.

Clots formed in response to vessel injury are not alone in altering blood flow properties in this manner. Any obstruction, including atherosclerosis, will alter blood flow properties within the artery and promote formation and propagation of a thrombus (Fig. 12.1).

Venous thrombosis is the result of decreased flow and, in some cases, complete stasis of blood. Low rate of blood flow increases venous pressure and causes dilatation of the vessel, the distension inducing endothelial dysfunction. Prothrombotic substances are released and the decreased flow inhibits dilution of these substances, facilitating the initiation and growth of the thrombus. Due to low flow rates, the thrombus is typically rich in red blood cells and fibrin.

This type of peripheral thrombus formation is brought about by several conditions such as immobilised postoperative states and low-output congestive heart failure. In the

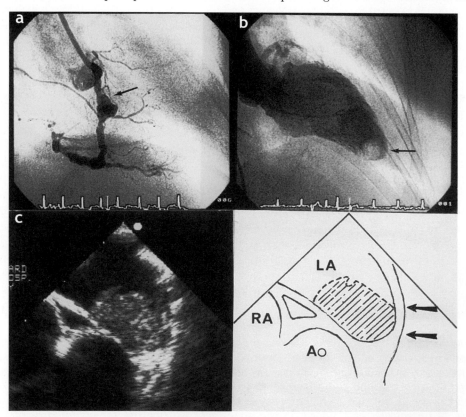

Figure 12.2. *Venous thrombosis in the heart: (a) a partly thrombosed (arrow) aneurysm of the right coronary artery; (b) thrombus (arrow) in an akinetic left ventricular apex; (c) a trans-oesophageal echocardiogram of a thrombus (arrow) in the left atrial appendage of a patient with atrial fibrillation and severe spontaneous echo contrast. LA:left atrium, RA:right atrium, Ao: aortic root.*

heart, this process can manifest as thrombus in an arterial aneurysm (Fig. 12.2a), thrombus in an aneurysm of the ventricle (Fig. 12.2b) or thrombus in the left atrial appendage in patients with atrial fibrillation (Fig. 12.2c).

The same mechanism is responsible for clot formation in catheters and sheaths during cardiac catheterisation. Anticoagulants such as heparin are given during the procedure, primarily to reduce the risk of thrombosis in environments of low shear stress.

Blood constituents

As previously discussed, the coagulation process is a complex and delicately balanced interaction among platelets, vascular endothelium coagulation factors, fibrinolytic proteins and naturally occurring anticoagulants. The pathological process of thrombosis can result from abnormalities in one or more of these groups. Such abnormalities are referred to as prothrombotic or hypercoagulable states. It should be noted that prothrombotic states not only result from excesses or deficiencies of these factors (primary prothrombotic states) but also as the result of abnormalities brought about by a number of disease states (secondary prothrombotic states).[4]

Spontaneous lysis of a thrombus occurs via a variety of mechanisms as outlined above. Whether spontaneous or resulting from thrombolytic therapy, presence of residual thrombus predisposes the patient to recurrent thrombotic occlusion.[2] The presence of fragmented thrombus appears to be one of the most powerful thrombogenic risk factors. Platelet deposition has been shown to be two to four times higher on residual thrombus compared with a severely injured arterial wall.[5]

Thrombosis and atherosclerosis

Atherosclerosis alone is rarely fatal.[6] Acute coronary and cerebrovascular conditions are usually the result of thrombosis formed secondary to rupture or fissure of the surface of an atherosclerotic plaque.[2] Clear evidence is beginning to emerge that thrombosis at the site of rupture is an important mechanism in the progression of atherosclerosis, [2] but also that not all plaque ruptures lead to thrombotic occlusion or plaque progression.

Patients with ischaemic heart disease usually have numerous plaques in their coronary arteries. Although only a small number may be identified angiographically, many more can be seen by intra-vascular ultrasound (IVUS). The reason for this is that most plaques do not encroach into the vascular lumen, they undergo compensatory abluminal vascular enlargement or 'remodelling'.[6] Hence, the lumen may remain unobstructed despite the presence of large amounts of atherosclerotic plaque.

Composition of plaque is a greater determinant of the risk of rupture and thrombosis than severity of stenosis. Atherosclerotic plaque contains two distinct components. The atheromatous component forms the core of the plaque and is soft and rich in lipids. The outer sclerotic plaque is collagen-rich and hard. Rupture occurs more frequently in plaques with a large, soft atheromatous component. When spontaneous or mechanically induced rupture of atherosclerotic plaque occurs, the atheromatous core of the plaque is exposed. The atheromatous core is the most thrombogenic component of human atheromatous plaque. [2] Thus, plaques with a large core content are at high risk of leading to acute coronary conditions if rupture occurs.

Any method that could quantify core size and composition would allow identification of plaque lesions, which have a high thrombogenic risk and hence are likely to lead to acute coronary conditions. It may then be possible to treat minor but highly thrombogenic stenoses while leaving more severely stenosed but less thrombogenic lesions. Similarly, lesions at high risk of thrombotic reocclusion could be treated with specific antiplatelet drugs to prevent acute thrombosis following angioplasty.

In most plaques, the sclerotic component accounts for the majority of plaque volume. The collagen contained therein is produced by adjacent smooth muscle cells and is responsible for the mechanical strength of the plaque.[6] Smooth muscle cell proliferation may protect plaques against rupture and these cells are often missing from sites of plaque rupture. Inflammation and macrophage infiltration may weaken the fibrous sclerotic cap, reducing tensile strength of the plaque, predisposing to rupture and leading to thrombosis. In eccentric plaque lesions, the shoulders are at particular risk for active inflammation, concentration of biomechanical and haemodynamic forces, and rupture.[6]

Coronary thrombosis

There appear to be three main factors that determine whether a thrombus will form at the site of plaque rupture and how severely the process will affect the coronary circulation. First, severity of stenosis plays a part by altering blood flow characteristics and increasing local shear forces. The second and perhaps the major determinant is the composition of exposed plaque, with the soft atheromatous core more likely to evoke a prothrombotic response. Third, the delicate balance between the antithrombotic and prothrombotic properties of endothelium and blood may promote or impede a thrombotic response to plaque rupture.

Other factors play a role in coronary thrombosis. The apparently non-random onset of acute coronary syndromes (unstable angina, myocardial infarction) have led some to suggest that catecholamines may play a part in platelet activation and thrombin generation. Increased frequency of these conditions is associated with early mornings[2,6,7] (particularly the first half hour after waking), Mondays,[6] winter months and cold days,[6,8] emotional stress,[2,6,8] vigorous exercise[6,8] and eating.[8] There is increasing evidence of enhanced platelet reactivity in smokers.[2] It has been suggested that this, too, is due to catecholamine stimulus, since cessation of smoking results in a sharp decrease in acute vascular events. The pathophysiology behind this relationship is unclear, but may be due to plaque disruption (surges in sympathetic tone produce sudden increases in blood pressure, heart rate, contraction and coronary flow), thrombosis (platelet aggregation and thrombin generation promoted by circulating catecholamines) and vasoconstriction (occurring locally around plaque lesion).[6]

Other studies are showing increasing evidence of relationships such as hypercoagulability in patients with progressive coronary disease, enhanced platelet reactivity at the site of vascular damage in experimental hypercholesterolaemia, and enhanced platelet reactivity in young patients with a strong family history of coronary artery disease.[2]

Heparin

Heparin molecules are heterogenous mixtures of sulphated simple chain polysaccharides of variable length that bond covalently to a polypeptide matrix to form the macromolecule heparin proteoglycan. The functional domain of the heparin molecule consists of regular segments of trisulphated disaccharide units interspersed between variable lengths of saccharide chains. Variations in the saccharide sequence of the functional domain determine the biological activity of the molecule. The various biological functions of heparin include suppression of aldosterone secretion, activation of lipoprotein lipase and inhibition of smooth muscle hyperplasia.[9]

Heparin is not absorbed well by the gastrointestinal tract, so it must be given by either intravenous or intramuscular injection. It is inactivated by the liver and excreted by the kidneys in urine. The half-life has been reported to be approximately one hour[10] but others have shown that the half-life increases with increasing dose.[11-13]

Heparin does not possess any anticoagulant properties, it acts as a co-factor. The anticoagulant and antithrombotic properties of heparin result from binding with a naturally occurring plasma protein, antithrombin III (ATIII). This is achieved when the functional domain of the heparin molecule is made up of a unique pentasaccharide (known as the ATIII binding site). When heparin binds to ATIII it induces a conformational change in the ATIII molecule, exposing an arginine molecule that is essential in the binding of thrombin. ATIII in its native form is capable of binding thrombin but when bound to heparin becomes about 1000 times more efficient at binding thrombin.[9,14]

The heparin molecule 'snares' thrombin by electrostatic binding at some point along the saccharide chain. The captured heparin molecule then migrates along the heparin chain until it is bound by antithrombin III. The ATIII-thrombin complex dissociates from the heparin chain and is cleared by the reticuloendothelial system. The heparin chain is left to bind another ATIII molecule and be re-used.

The heparin-ATIII complex has both antithrombotic and anticoagulant activity. The anticoagulant effect results from its direct scavenging effect on thrombin described above, and is more readily seen when full therapeutic doses of heparin are given to treat ongoing thrombosis.[9] At low prophylactic doses given to prevent thrombosis, the antithrombotic effect of heparin appears to be more important. Heparin prevents generation of thrombin, and hence coagulation, by inhibiting activated factors XI, IX and more importantly, factor X, thereby slowing a large part of the coagulation cascade responsible for thrombin production.

Activated factor II (thrombin) is an appropriate molecule to target in attempting to prevent or reverse thrombus formation. It is responsible for activating the final step in the coagulation cascade, conversion of fibrinogen to fibrin. If thrombin is removed, activation of any part of the coagulation cascade will not result in clot formation. As discussed earlier, thrombin has a number of positive feedback mechanisms for its own production. It is able to activate factors V and VIII and can activate platelets that facilitate activation of the coagulation system and, ultimately, generation of thrombin. Inhibition of this enzyme impedes these positive feedback mechanisms and prevents further clot formation.

Following spontaneous or chemically induced lysis of a thrombus, thrombin may become exposed to circulating blood, leading to activation of platelets and coagulation factors and culminating in further thrombosis. The antithrombin activity of heparin is limited for three major reasons.[2] First, residual thrombus contains thrombin bound to fibrin, which is poorly accessible to the heparin-ATIII complex and requires about 20 times more heparin for inactivation compared to unbound thrombin.[15] Second, platelet-rich arterial thrombus releases large amounts of platelet factor 4 which inhibits heparin. Third, the fibrin II monomer, formed by the action of thrombin on fibrinogen, is also an inhibitor of heparin. Hirudin, a naturally occurring compound derived from leech saliva, has antithrombin properties and is at least 10 times smaller than the heparin-ATIII complex. It has no natural inhibitors. As such, it is more accessible to thrombin bound to fibrin, and may prove to have a clinically useful role in this situation.

Heparin is manufactured in two basic forms: unfractionated and low molecular weight heparin (LMWH). Unfractionated heparin chains vary greatly in length, averaging around 50 monosaccharide units per chain (average molecular weight 15 000). Heparin chains containing the ATIII binding site account for less than one third of all chains in commercially produced preparations made from porcine or bovine intestinal mucosa or bovine lung.[9] Low molecular weight heparins are produced from unfractionated heparin by controlled enzymatic depolymerisation of the unfractionated heparin chain and have a molecular weight of less than 6000.

Low molecular weight heparin has a half-life two to four times longer than unfractionated heparin, allowing subcutaneous administration once per day; it also has a higher bioavailability than unfractionated heparin, allowing more accurate dosing based on body weight. LMW heparin possesses a lower antithrombin activity than unfractionated heparin as evidenced by its lack of effect on the activated partial thromboplastin time (APTT), but has greater effect on inhibition of factor Xa.

The antithrombin activity of the heparin-ATIII complex is proportional to the mean chain length of the heparin molecule. Anti-Xa activity is not dependent on chain length. Unfractionated heparin and LMW heparin exhibit comparable efficacy *in vivo*, suggesting that anti-Xa activity may play an important role in the action of LMW heparins.[9] It has also been suggested that LMW heparins contain an abundance of chains without the ATIII binding site, which exert their effect not by binding heparin but by neutralising inhibitors such as platelet factor 4, which otherwise block the ATIII binding sites on heparin chains. LMWH may also stimulate the release of tissue factor pathway inhibitor.[9]

Excretion of heparin varies according to the type of heparin used. The higher molecular weight heparins, which possess the majority of antithrombin activity, bind to endothelial cells and monocytes. Endothelial cells internalise and depolymerise these chains, eventually releasing lower molecular weight heparin chains. This may explain the apparent preservation of anti-Xa activity for some time after antithrombin activity begins to diminish.[9] LMW heparins are cleared mostly by the kidneys and the half-life may be prolonged in patients with underlying renal pathology such as chronic renal failure. Patients with acute pulmonary embolism have been shown to have an enhanced rate of heparin excretion.

An increased prothrombotic potential has been noted in some patients following cessation of intravenous heparin therapy. Becker *et al.*[16] found thrombin generation to be greatest among patients in whom heparin was ceased abruptly, compared with those who were weaned off the infusion over 12hours. Watkins *et al.*[17] measured fibrinopeptide A (FPA), a marker of thrombin activity, in the coronary circulation of patients having undergone percutaneous interventions. They demonstrated a significant increase in FPA levels several hours after cessation of therapy. Although the underlying mechanism of rebound prothrombotic activity is unknown, tissue factor and the extrinsic coagulation pathway have been implicated as likely culprits.[9]

Laboratory monitoring of heparin therapy

Heparin has the effect of slowing down the intrinsic pathway of the coagulation cascade. When utilising heparin therapy it is necessary to closely monitor the level of anticoagulation. Although some authors suggest there is no correlation between over-heparinisation and risk of bleeding, [9,18–20] any detected increase in laboratory clotting times resulting from heparin therapy generally receives prompt medical evaluation. Under-anticoagulation may block the desired therapeutic effect of clot prevention or lysis.

Several laboratory tests exist for monitoring therapeutic heparin administration. Each has relative advantages and disadvantages. Unlike tests for other therapeutic drugs such as digoxin, quinidine or antimicrobials, assays for anticoagulant therapy do not test the direct concentration of drug in the blood, but rather the overall effect of the drug on the coagulation system. In doing so, these assays take into account the action of the drug on coagulation factors, the body's response to the drug (such as rate of excretion) and the ability of other factors to antagonise the drug (such as replenishment of coagulation factors by the liver or the amount of ATIII available to bind thrombin). Tests of heparin anticoagulation are only screening tests of the intrinsic pathway. They start with activation of factor XII and end with clot formation. An extended test result indicates inhibition of one or more coagulation factors, but does not identify which one(s).

Activated partial thromboplastin time (APTT)

The most commonly used test is the activated partial thromboplastin time (APTT). The closely controlled conditions under which the test is performed, standardisation of reagents and methods, and the frequency with which the assay is requested make this test the gold standard in monitoring of heparin therapy.

The target APTT for a patient on therapeutic heparin should be 1.5 to 2.5 times the mean of the normal range for the institution.

As the preferred method, the APTT is highly standardised. Each laboratory standardises its normal range with respect to heparin sensitivity and constantly monitors this sensitivity with multiple-level quality control samples. The results are highly reproducible. Regardless of the method, very precise volumes are used. Current instrumentation possesses extremely sensitive clot detection systems, and most institutions run samples in duplicate to avoid reporting erroneous results.

The APTT is not necessarily appropriate to every clinical setting. It is less sensitive at the higher concentrations of heparin used in coronary angioplasty and cardiopulmonary bypass, where the dose-response has been demonstrated to be non-linear.[15] Most laboratories assign an upper limit above which results are reported as 'greater than' the threshold value.

The APTT has very specific collection requirements. Blood cannot be drawn through heparinised catheters or cannulae. A clean, non-traumatic venipuncture is required to avoid activation of the coagulation cascade by prothrombotic mechanisms. Such activation may initiate the coagulation cascade before the anticoagulant can take effect, resulting in a shorter APTT time because the assay has commenced part way through the cascade or a longer APTT time, because some of the available coagulation factors have been used up prior to the assay. The citrate tube must be filled correctly, as over- or under-filling will alter the dilution factor of 9 volumes blood to 1 volume citrate and render the result invalid.

Obtaining an APTT result is often a time-consuming process. Specimens must be transported to the pathology laboratory and processed by the central specimen reception department. Once in the haematology department, the specimen requires a 10 to 15 minute centrifugation [21] to obtain platelet-poor plasma for analysis. The assay involves an incubation, usually three to five minutes, and the endpoint may not be reached for up to 3 minutes. Quality control results must be verified prior to reporting of test results.

Activated clotting time (ACT)

In settings such as the cardiac operating room or catheter lab, where the delays outline above may be to the detriment of the patient, results are required more promptly. The activated clotting time (ACT) is one test that provides comparable information to the APTT in a much shorter time. The ACT has no specimen preparation, improving the turnaround time for obtaining results. Whole blood is used and is injected directly into a tube containing an activator. A simple clot detection system times clot formation and the microprocessor-controlled solid state electronics ensure accuracy of results. The test is designed to be used as a bedside monitoring test.

The various ACT tests available are sensitive to different levels of heparin anticoagulation. High levels of heparin are used in coronary artery bypass graft (CABG) surgery and coronary angioplasty, moderate levels in extracorporeal membrane oxygenation (ECMO) and haemodialysis, and low levels are used prophylactically after myocardial infarction and some surgical procedures. The type of activator used may affect the degree of prolongation of the ACT. There are a number of activators to choose from, depending on the particular clinical situation and the individual patient.

Diatomaceous earth is used for high levels of heparin. Protease inhibitors such as aprotinin are often administered to patients to reduce post-operative bleeding, particularly during coronary bypass surgery. These agents can prolong an ACT activated by diatomaceous earth.

Kaolin is also used to test high heparin levels. This activator is unaffected by protease inhibitors and is an alternative for patients receiving agents such as aprotinin.

Glass particles are used for moderate levels of heparin. The clotting process is initiated whenever blood is exposed to a foreign surface. Glass beads markedly enhance the surface area available to activate the clotting process.

General surgical specimens and those from patients on low-dose heparin therapy are often tested without an activator. Low levels of heparin permit clotting in a short period without the enhancement of coagulation activators.

A novel use of the ACT was described by Pitney and associates.[22] They used a heparinase additive to counteract the heparin in the sample and provide a current heparin-free baseline ACT. When performed simultaneously with a standard ACT in a dual-chamber analyser, the difference between the two results—the ACT Differential—was shown to correlate more closely to the APTT than to the standard ACT, and was therefore a better indicator of anticoagulation status than the standard ACT.

Several factors may limit the accuracy and usefulness of the ACT. In a properly maintained and operated instrument, accuracy and precision are largely dependent on quality of the specimen. Collection technique is an important factor. As with the APTT, blood must not be collected through heparinised cannulae. The cannula, catheter or arterial sheath must be aspirated before specimen collection to ensure that only whole blood is collected and tested. Inadequate mixing of specimen and activator will also lead to erroneous results. Vigorous agitation is often required to completely dissolve the activator. Other common pitfalls include improper storage of test kits (particularly prolonged exposure to heat), haemodilution, contamination by cardioplegic solutions, hypothermia and platelet dysfunction from a variety of causes.

Comparison of ACT and APTT

Both the APTT and ACT have a clinically useful role in monitoring heparin therapy. The APTT is routinely used for monitoring therapeutic and prophylactic heparinisation, while the ACT is used in special procedures such as angioplasty and coronary artery bypass surgery, which require large doses of heparin. In these procedures the importance of maintaining therapeutic anticoagulation is paramount, and the time delay inherent in processing APTT samples through a central hospital laboratory may not be in the best interest of the patient. The ACT is a bedside test which requires no specimen preparation and provides a faster turnaround of results, allowing a more rapid response to any change in anticoagulation status.

Point-of-care systems are now available for bedside monitoring of APTT. These devices can utilise plasma or whole blood, but are still limited by the finite linear response of the APTT assay.

The ACT is theoretically a more accurate measurement of anticoagulation status, as the patient's own platelets, calcium and phospholipid are used for the clotting process.

The APTT uses standardised concentrations of calcium and phospholipid which may not be representative of the true physiological state of the patient. The APTT is a highly standardised test and subject to strict quality control. Conversely, performance of an ACT is less rigidly structured and, although manufacturers recommend quality control be performed once per shift with dual level controls, quality control is performed on a less regular basis, if at all.

Numerous studies have compared the APTT and ACT for monitoring heparin therapy in interventional cardiology procedures. Some report good correlation[23-24] while others report a poor correlation.[25] Some studies found the ACT a more useful test[23-24,26-29] while others found the APTT to be more useful.[25,27] Several studies have reported finding sub-therapeutic ACT values in patients with APTT values within therapeutic limits. This has led to suggestions that further study is required to investigate risks associated with prolonged use of heparin at therapeutic ACT levels,[30] and even that the ACT should be used as the reference standard.[26]

Bedside APTT assays correlate well with laboratory assays.[27] As with the laboratory assay, some studies have shown that the bedside assay does not correlate well with the ACT[27,31] while others have shown good correlation.[32]

Given that the ACT gives a more linear response to increasing heparin dose, utilises the patient's own calcium, platelets and phospholipid in the assay, and provides a more rapid turnaround of results compared with the APTT, the ACT appears to be the better test for assessment of heparin therapy for interventional cardiology procedures.

References

1. Loscalzo J. Pathogenesis of Thrombosis. In: Beutler E *et al* (eds). *Williams hematology*, 5th ed. New York: McGraw-Hill 1995.
2. Badimon L, Badimon JJ, Fuster J. Pathogenesis of Thrombosis. In: Verstraete M, Fuster V, Topol E (eds). *Cardiovascular thrombosis*, 2nd ed. Philadelphia: Lippincott-Raven 1998.
3. Berne RM, Levy MN. *Principles of physiology*, 2nd ed. St. Louis: Mosby 1996.
4. Bauer KA. The hypercoagulable state. In: Beutler E *et al.* (eds). *Williams hematology*, 5th ed. New York: McGraw-Hill 1995.
5. Badimon L, Badimon JJ. Mechanisms of arterial thrombosis in non-parallel streamlines: Platelet thrombi grow at the apex of stenotic severely injured vessel wall. Experimental study in the pig model. *J Clin Invest* 1989; **84**:134–44.
6. Falk E, Fuster V, Shah PK. Interrelationship between atherosclerosis and thrombosis. In: Verstraete M, Fuster V, Topol E (eds). *Cardiovascular thrombosis*, 2nd ed. Philadelphia: Lippincott-Raven 1998.
7. Roberts R, Morris D, Pratt CM, Alexander RW. Pathophysiology, recognition and treatment of acute myocardial infarction and its complications. In: Schlant RC, Alexander RW *et al* (eds). *Hurst's The heart, arteries and veins.* New York: McGraw-Hill 1994.
8. O'Rourke RA. Chest Pain. In: Schlant RC, Alexander RW *et al* (eds). *Hurst's The heart, arteries and veins.* New York: McGraw-Hill 1994.
9. Fiore L, Deykin D. Anticoagulant Therapy. In: Beutler E *et al* (eds). *Williams hematology*, 5th ed. New York: McGraw-Hill 1995.
10. Hoffbrand AV, Petit JE. *Essential haematology*, 3rd ed. London: Blackwell Scientific Publications 1993.
11. Stein B, Fuster V. Pharmacology of anticoagulants and platelet inhibitor drugs. In: Schlant RC, Alexander RW *et al.* (eds). *Hurst's The heart, arteries and veins.* New York: McGraw-Hill 1994.
12. Olsson P, Lagergren H, Ek S. The elimination from plasma of intravenous heparin: an experimental study on dogs and humans. *Acta Med Scand* 1963; **173**:619–30.
13. Bjornsson TO, Wolfram BS, Kitchell BB. Heparin kinetics determined by three assay methods. *Clin Pharmacol Ther* 1982; **31**:104–13.

14.   Harker LA, Mann KG. Thrombosis and fibrinolysis. In: Verstraete M, Fuster V, Topol E (eds). *Cardiovascular Thrombosis*, 2nd ed. Philadelphia: Lippincott-Raven 1998.

15.   Hirsh J. Heparin. *New Engl J Med* 1991; **324**:1565–74.

16.   Becker RC, Spencer FA, Li Y *et al*. Thrombin generation after the abrupt cessation of intravenous unfractionated heparin among patients with acute coronary syndromes: potential mechanisms for heightened prothrombotic potential. *JACC* 1999; **34**(4):1020–7.

17.   Watkins MW, Luetmer PA, Schneider DJ *et al*. Determinants of rebound thrombin activity after cessation of heparin in patients undergoing coronary interventions. *Cathet Cardiovasc Diagn* 1998; **44**(3):257–64.

18.   Hull RD, Rascob GE, Rosenbloom D *et al*. Heparin for 5 days versus 10 days in the initial treatment of proximal vein thrombosis. *New Engl J Med* 1990; **322**(18):1260.

19.   Hull RD, Rascob GE, Rosenbloom D *et al*. Optimal therapeutic level of heparin therapy in patients with venous thrombosis. *Arch Intern Med* 1992; **152**(8):1589.

20.   Nieuwenhuis K, Albada J, Banga JD, Sixma JJ. Identification of risk factors for bleeding during treatment of acute venous thromboembolism with heparin or low molecular weight heparin. *Blood* 1991; **78**(9):2337.

21.   Dacie JV, Lewis SM. *Practical haematology*. Edinburgh: Churchill Livingstone 1986.

22.   Pitney MR, Kelly SA, Allan RM *et al*. Activated clotting time differential is a superior method of monitoring anticoagulation following coronary angioplasty. *Cath & Cardiovasc Diag* 1996; **37**:145–50.

23.   Simko RJ, Tsung FF, Stanek EJ. Activated clotting time versus activated partial thromboplastin time for therapeutic monitoring of heparin. *Ann Phamacotherapy* 1995; **29**(10):1015–21.

24.   Dougherty KG, Gaos CM *et al*. Activated clotting times and activated partial thromboplastin times in patients undergoing coronary angioplasty who receive bolus doses of heparin. *Catheterization and Cardiovascular Diagnosis* 1992; **26**(4):260–3.

25.   Brack MJ, More RS, Forbat LN *et al*. Monitoring anticoagulation following intracoronary procedures: which method? *International J Cardiol* 1994; **45**(2):103–8.

26.   Nath FC, Muller DWM, Rosenschein *et al*. Heparin monitoring during coronary intervention: Activated clotting time versus activated partial thromboplastin time. *Can J Cardiol* 1993; **9**(9):797–801.

27.   Reiner JS, Coyne KS, Lundergan CF, Ross AM. Bedside monitoring of heparin therapy: Comparison of activated clotting time to activated partial thromboplastin time. *Catheterization and Cardiovascular Diagnosis* 1994; **32**:49–52.

28.   Kunert M, Sorgenicht R, Scheuble L *et al*. Value of activated blood coagulation time in monitoring anticoagulation during coronary angioplasty [German]. *Zeitschrift fur Kardiologie* 1996; **85**(2):118–24.

29.   Varah N, Smith J, Baugh RF. Heparin monitoring in the coronary care unit after percutaneous transluminal coronary angioplasty. *Heart and Lung* 1990; **19**(3):265–70.

30.   Grill HP, Spero JE, Granato JE. Comparison of activated partial thromboplastin time to activated clotting time for adequacy of heparin anticoagulation just before percutaneous transluminal coronary angioplasty. *Am J Cardiol* 1993; **71**(13):1219–20.

31.   O'Neill AI, McAllister C, Corke CF, Parkin JD. A comparison of five devices for bedside monitoring of heparin therapy. *Anaesthesia and Intensive care* 1991; **19**(4):592–6.

32.   Blumenthal RS, Carter AJ, Resar JR *et al*. Comparison of bedside and hospital laboratory coagulation studies during and after coronary intervention. *Cath & Cardiovasc Diag* 1995; **35**(1):9–17.

Chapter 13

Basic Pharmacology of Cardiac Drugs

Aran Maree and Terence J. Campbell

This chapter discusses the major groups of cardiac drugs in use today. It includes drugs that increase the force and/or rate of cardiac contraction (sympatho-mimetic agents) as well as agents that do the reverse. Agents that control blood pressure can act both centrally (centrally acting antihypertensive agents) or peripherally (sympatholytic agents, calcium antagonists, nitrovasodilators). Over time, a wide variety of antiarrhythmic agents has been added to the medical armamentarium. In more recent times, as the mechanisms that cause coronary thrombosis have been clarified, specific antiplatelet, antithrombotic and thrombolytic medications have been introduced. This chapter touches briefly on the fundamental aspects of each of these groups, with the exception of lipid-lowering therapy, which requires more extensive consideration.

Sympathomimetic agents

Adrenergic receptors and the cardiovascular system

Catecholamines and other sympathomimetic agents exert most of their inotropic (force-increasing) and chronotropic (rate-increasing) effects on the myocardium via beta-adrenergic receptors. Alpha adrenoceptor stimulation is capable of producing a positive inotropic effect (about 10% of that seen in response to beta adrenoceptor stimulation).

The β_1-adrenoreceptor subtype is responsible for the cardiac inotropic and chronotropic effects of catecholamines. There is now good evidence for the involvement of β_2-adrenoreceptors in mediating the positive inotropic effects of adrenaline in human atrium, and to a less extent in human ventricle. The involvement of the β_2-receptor appears to be most important in the sinoatrial node, less so in atrial myocardium and even less so in ventricle.

The extracardiac effects of alpha- and beta-receptor stimulation of relevance to cardiovascular pharmacology include the well known vasodilating effect of β_2-adrenergic stimulation. This is most marked in the arterial bed within skeletal muscle. Both $alpha_1$- and $alpha_2$-receptor subtypes appear to mediate vasoconstriction in most arterial systems, with the coronary and cerebral circulations being relatively spared. The actions of alpha-receptor stimulation to promote platelet aggregation may also be of cardiovascular relevance.

At least one other receptor group needs to be considered in the present context. These are the dopamine receptors, which are traditionally subdivided into D_1 and D_2. The D_1-receptor, the receptor of relevance to the present discussion, mediates vasodilatation,

Table 13.1. Complexity of catecholamine activity in the cardiovascular system

Receptors	α	β1	β2	Dopaminergic
ACTIONS	Vasoconstrictor inotropic	Inotropic chronotropic	Inotropic chronotropic vasodilator and inotropic in high doses)	Splanchnic and renal vasodilator (+vasoconstrictor
Noradrenaline	++++	++	0	0
Adrenaline	+++	+++	++	0
Isoprenaline	0	++++	++++	0
Dopamine	0 to +++	++	0	++++
Dobutamine	+ to ++	+++	+++	0

particularly in the renal and splanchnic beds, via the enhanced formation of cyclic adenosine monophosphate (AMP). The D_2-receptor is found in the pituitary gland.

Specific agents

The relative activities of the main sympathomimetic agents in clinical use for the treatment of cardiovascular disorders at present are listed in Table 13.1. This table is meant as an approximate guide to relative activities only and is not quantitative.

Adrenaline

Also known as epinephrine, and produced endogenously mainly in the adrenal medulla, this compound is a potent stimulator of both alpha- and beta-adrenergic receptors and its effects on target organs are complex. Bolus intravenous injections of large amounts (0.5–1.5 mg) tend to produce rapid increases in systolic blood pressure with lesser increases in diastolic pressure. This effect is due to a combination of vasoconstriction (alpha effect), increased contractility and heart rate ($β_1$ and $β_2$ effects), and vasodilatation in skeletal muscle vasculature ($β_2$ effect). With a large bolus, the first two actions tend to predominate, and hypertension is produced. Frequently the direct tachycardia is replaced by an indirect reflex-mediated bradycardia in response to the increase in intra-arterial pressure.

Intravenous infusion of adrenaline at 5–30 mg per minute tends to produce an increase in systolic blood pressure with a decrease in diastolic pressure and generally some increase in heart rate. As the rate of infusion is increased, there is a growing tendency for the vasoconstrictor (alpha) effect to predominate over vasodilatator ($β_2$) and for the diastolic pressure to rise also. Myocardial oxygen consumption and blood lactate concentrations tend to rise considerably. Blood flow to skeletal muscles and the splanchnic bed tends to increase. There is no significant constriction of cerebral arterioles seen, and because of the increased pressure, cerebral blood flow tends to increase. Conversely, renal blood flow tends to fall considerably although there is a corresponding increase in filtration fraction, and glomerular filtration rate (GFR) is only slightly altered. In the presence of background nonselective beta-blockade, only vasoconstriction and increases in systolic and diastolic pressure will be seen with adrenaline.

Noradrenaline

Also known as norepinephrine, this compound is approximately as potent as adrenaline at stimulating $β_1$-receptors. It is a little less potent than adrenaline on the alpha-receptors, and has very little action on $β_2$-receptors. Consequently intravenous infusion (approximately 10 mg/min) tends to produce increases in both systolic and diastolic pressures.

There commonly a reflex slowing of the heart rate in response to the hypertension. Blood flow tends to be reduced to the kidney, liver and skeletal muscle. GFR is initially maintained quite well but falls at higher doses. Coronary blood flow tends to increase. Both adrenaline and noradrenaline are rapidly destroyed in the body.

Metaraminol (aramine)

Metaraminol (or aramine) is a powerful and fairly selective alpha-adrenergic agonist. It leads to widespread vasoconstriction via its alpha-receptor effect. There is relative sparing of the coronary arteries and cerebral arteries because these have few alpha-receptors. It is therefore useful for elevating blood pressure without placing undue strain on myocardial or cerebral blood supply. Metaraminol must be given by intravenous injection or infusion.

Isoprenaline

Also known as isoproterenol, this substance is a potent non-selective beta-adrenergic agonist with negligible alpha-adrenergic effects. Intravenous infusion into humans normally lowers the peripheral resistance via the β_2-adrenergic vasodilating effects of this agent. Mean and diastolic blood pressures fall, although systolic blood pressure may remain unchanged or even rise due to the concomitant inotropic and chronotropic actions of the drug on the heart. Renal blood flow falls in normotensive humans but generally increases in initially hypotensive patients, as a result of the increase in cardiac output and reversal of reflex renal vasoconstriction. Its duration of action is very brief and it is normally administered by intravenous infusion.

Dopamine

This is the metabolic precursor of noradrenaline and adrenaline. Table 13.1 indicates the complex actions of dopamine in the cardiovascular system. Low-dose infusion predominantly leads to D_1 (dopaminergic) stimulation resulting in vasodilatation in the renal, mesenteric and coronary beds. This commonly results in an increase in renal blood flow, GFR and urine flow. These effects are typically seen at infusion rates of 1.5–5 µg/kg/min.

As the infusion rate of dopamine is increased, positive inotropic and chronotropic effects mediated by beta-receptors are increasingly apparent. Dopamine also has the ability to release noradrenaline from nerve endings and this contributes to its actions. Systolic and mean blood pressure tend to rise. Diastolic blood pressure may increase slightly.

At very high infusion rates $alpha_1$-adrenergic vasoconstrictor effects appear and eventually overcome the dopaminergic vasodilating action, resulting in further increases in blood pressure and eventually a reduction in blood flow to vital organs, including the kidneys. Combination therapy with dobutamine, which has vasodilating properties, can help to overcome this tendency to cause vasoconstriction and lead to additive inotropic effects (see below).

Dobutamine

This agent bears some resemblance to dopamine structurally and exerts its effects via both alpha- and beta-adrenergic receptors. It does not release noradrenaline from sympathetic nerve endings nor stimulate dopaminergic receptors. At therapeutic rates of infusion (2.5 to 15 µg/kg/min), dobutamine tends to produce an increase in contractility with relatively less increase in heart rate than seen with other beta-stimulants such as isoprenaline. At the same time the total peripheral resistance and the pulmonary vascular resistance tend not to change much and in fact may fall, leading to a reduction in systemic and pulmonary venous pressures. This is due to a balance between the $alpha_1$-receptor mediated vasoconstrictor actions and the β_2-receptor mediated vasodilating effect. Consequently the cardiac output rises, with little change in peripheral resistance. Dobutamine also increases coronary blood flow secondary to a decrease in coronary vascular resistance mediated by β_2-receptors. In the presence of beta-blockade, the cardiac effects are largely obliterated, and the net result is a largely alpha$_1$-receptor-mediated increase in peripheral resistance. Dobutamine is rapidly broken down enzymatically, with a half-life of about 2 minutes.

Sympatholytic agents

Alpha-adrenergic blocking agents

Alpha-blocking agents are currently used only to a limited extent in cardiology. Prazosin is the most important, and the only example discussed in detail herein. Alpha-blocking agents can be alpha$_1$-selective (e.g. prazosin), alpha$_2$-selective (e.g. yohimbine), or nonselective (e.g. phentolamine and phenoxybenzamine). Non-selective alpha-blockers are basically unsuccessful as antihypertensive agents because of the reflex tachycardia with which they are associated. Phenoxybenzamine is still used in the management of phaeochromocytoma, but the only common cardiovascular application of alpha-blocking agents is the use of prazosin, either for hypertension or as an afterload-reducing agent in cardiac failure.

For most alpha-adrenergic antagonists, the fall in blood pressure produced by vasodilatation is opposed by baroreceptor reflexes, causing increases in heart rate and cardiac output. This effect is more marked if the antagonist also blocks alpha$_2$-receptors on peripheral sympathetic nerve endings. These presynaptic alpha$_2$-receptors normally inhibit excessive release of noradrenaline. Their blockade leads to enhanced release of noradrenaline, resulting in increased stimulation of post-synaptic β_1-receptors, further amplifying the tachycardia.

Prazosin

Prazosin produces most of its effects by blocking alpha$_1$-adrenergic receptors in arterioles and veins. This leads to a reduction in peripheral vascular resistance and also to venodilatation, which can reduce preload and venous return to the heart. There is generally little or no reflex tachycardia.

The popularity of prazosin as an antihypertensive agent has increased somewhat of late because it has been shown to decrease cholesterol and sometimes triglyceride levels, and to increase the HDL/LDL ratio without changing the HDL level.

Beta-adrenergic blocking agents

There are large numbers of these agents currently available and their pharmacology is well covered in standard textbooks. The following is a brief outline of a very large topic, in an attempt to highlight points of major importance to the practice of cardiology.

Beta-blockers were first introduced in 1962 for treatment of arrhythmias and angina, but were soon found to have antihypertensive properties as well. The mechanism of the antihypertensive effect is still essentially unexplained. All beta-blockers are competitive inhibitors of beta-receptors, and structurally similar to catecholamines.

'Cardio-selective' (i.e. β_1-selective) blockers such as metoprolol and atenolol have theoretical advantages over non-selective blockers such as propranolol in patients with peripheral vascular disease, diabetes or asthma. In practice, no beta-blocker is safe in asthmatics.

The more lipophilic beta-blockers, such as propranolol, are probably more prone to cause central nervous system disturbances (such as bad dreams) than the more hydrophilic drugs such as atenolol.

Beta-blockers are generally well absorbed from the gut (90%+), but some (e.g. metoprolol and propranolol) undergo extensive first-pass metabolism. The half-lives of propranolol and metoprolol are two to three hours in acute usage but this may rise to about six hours with chronic use. The half-life of atenolol is about eight hours. Water-soluble compounds such as atenolol tend to be eliminated in urine with minimal metabolism and hence have longer half-lives in renal disease. Lipid-soluble compounds are generally metabolised by the liver and because beta-blockers reduce hepatic blood flow, they tend to increase their own half-lives in chronic use.

Serious side effects include bronchospasm and acute left ventricular failure, both of which may be life threatening. Postural hypotension is not a problem, since the innervation of the alpha-receptor is intact. The 'oculomucocutaneous' syndrome, which caused the withdrawal of practolol, occurs rarely with the remaining beta-blockers. Peripheral vascular disease may be aggravated due to the reduction in blood flow and possibly also due to increased exercise tolerance associated with reduced angina pectoris. 'Minor' side effects may occur. Abdominal discomfort sometimes occurs with large doses of propranolol. A degree of weakness and lethargy can be present and this may intefere with exercise tolerance, particularly for vigorous sports. Central nervous system disturbances are common, mostly reduced sleep requirement and disturbed sleep with or without dreams, which may be bizarre or frightening. Depression may also be a problem. Impotence occurs in about 1–3% of males on long-term beta-blockers. Despite concerns, there is little evidence that beta-blockade causes significant problems in most patients with diabetes mellitus, although beta-blockers may mask the adrenergic symptoms of hypoglycaemia. Beta-blockers tend to have complex effects on plasma lipids. This is particularly true of beta-blockers without intrinsic sympathomimetic activity, which may reduce HDL cholesterol while modestly elevating VLDL cholesterol and triglycerides. Total cholesterol may not change. These altered lipid concentrations may detract from some beneficial effects of the drug in the long term.

It seems likely that the major antiarrhythmic and anti-anginal effects of beta-blockers relate directly to their antagonism to the actions of catecholamines but, as noted above, their mechanism of action in hypertension is unclear. The acute intravenous administration of propranolol, for example, usually causes a decrease in heart rate and cardiac output, but a reflex increase in peripheral resistance with little change in blood pressure. If blood pressure does fall, it is usually not for several hours after the administration of the agent and seems to result from a late reduction in peripheral resistance. It has been postulated that the mechanism is mediated via the central nervous system, but this seems unlikely in view of the fact that, as antihypertensive agents, the less lipid-soluble beta-blockers appear to be as effective as the more lipid-soluble compounds. Beta-blockade significantly inhibits release of renin and this mechanism may well be of particular relevance in patients with high renin hypertension. It has also been postulated that at least part of the antihypertensive action of beta-blocking drugs might be due to presynaptic beta-blockade resulting in inhibition of catecholamine release. Another popular theory is that beta-blockers somehow reset baro-receptors.

Combined alpha- and beta-blockade (labetalol)

This agent which is of some value in the treatment of hypertension is both an $alpha_1$-receptor blocker and a non-selective beta-blocker. Its beta-blocking potency is three to seven times greater than its alpha-blocking action.

Vasodilating beta-blockers: β_1*-blockade plus* β_2*-agonism*

There is considerable interest in this new group of pharmacological agents, which simultaneously exhibit both β_1-antagonism and β_2-agonism. In theory at least, they offer many of the advantages of the traditional beta-blocker with additional peripheral vasodilating effects from the β_2 action on blood vessels in skeletal muscle, without the threat of bronchospasm related to β_2-antagonism. Two such agents are celiprolol and carvedilol. These agents are particularly attractive for the therapy of hypertension and also in the possible use of beta-blockers in treating cardiac failure.

Carvedilol

Carvedilol is now available in Australia for oral use for the management of heart failure. There is no good evidence that it is superior to standard beta-blockers for this indication in terms of efficacy or safety, but it is more convenient to use. At present it is the only beta-blocker officially approved for treatment of heart failure, and for this purpose it is available in very low-dose tablets. It is also possible that its initial vasodilating effect helps overcome the early negative inotropic effects of therapy with beta-blockers in patients with heart failure.

Centrally acting antihypertensive agents

This is an old term that is generally applied to two agents, alpha-methyldopa and clonidine. They act predominantly as agonists on central alpha$_2$-receptors, producing a reduced sympathetic outflow from the brainstem and consequent reduction in blood pressure.

Alpha-methyldopa

It is now known that alpha-methyl-noradrenaline (a metabolite) actually has significant agonist activity and the major mechanism of action of alpha-methyldopa is thought to be due to this metabolite, which subsequently stimulates central alpha$_2$-receptors.

A fall in arterial pressure lasting some 6 to 8 hours after the administration of oral or intravenous alpha-methyldopa is associated with a reduction in vascular resistance, with either no change or some decrease in heart rate and stroke volume. Plasma concentrations of noradrenaline and renin secretion both fall. These reflect the reduced sympathetic tone induced by this agent.

Clonidine

This compound has a very similar mechanism of action to methyldopa. As with methyldopa, clonidine decreases the plasma concentration of noradrenaline and renin. Also, as with methyldopa, an unfavourable side-effect profile has seen clinical use of clonidine fall markedly in the last decade.

Calcium antagonists (calcium channel blockers)

A common fallacy concerning these important drugs is to think of them as a homogeneous group with only minor differences in dosage, kinetics, and side effects. There are in fact quite major differences between the calcium antagonist drugs. By far the most important distinction from a clinical point of view is between the dihydropyridines (nifedipine and related compounds) and the other two pharmacological groups, represented by verapamil and diltiazem (see below). It is therefore potentially quite misleading to refer to calcium antagonists as being useful or not being useful for a given clinical condition, without specifying the particular family of calcium antagonists one means.

Calcium channels are found in a wide variety of tissues throughout the body, and it is therefore not surprising that calcium antagonists exhibit a large number of beneficial or potentially harmful effects. Of major relevance to cardiovascular pharmacology are the effects of these agents on myocardium and vascular smooth muscle. The other actions of calcium antagonists are well covered in standard text books and are not further discussed here.

Calcium channel sub-types

The calcium-selective ion channels on cell membranes relevant to the present discussion can be sub-divided into L-type, T-type and N-type. 'L' stands for 'long-lasting', and these channels are found on nerve and all types of muscle, including myocardium. They are the only group of channels to show significant sensitivity to organic calcium channel antagonists and are the basis of the remaining discussion.

Tissue selectivity

While there are calcium channels in all types of muscle, those in skeletal muscle do not play a major role in triggering contractions. Organic calcium channel antagonists therefore tend to exhibit clinical effects only on cardiac and smooth muscle. Furthermore, there are major differences between calcium antagonists in terms of their relative selectivity for myocardium and for vascular smooth muscle. For example, on a scale that rates verapamil as having roughly equal effects on both muscle types, diltiazem exhibits approximately nine times more effect on vascular smooth muscle than on myocardium, nifedipine approximately 20 times more vascular selectivity, and felodipine (another dihydropyridine) is more than 100 times more vascular-selective.

The vascular-relaxing effects of calcium antagonists tend to be predominantly seen in arteries and arterioles and not on the venous side of the circulation. This is because the former contain a higher proportion of smooth muscle, the tone of which is modulated by calcium, whereas veins depend more on neurogenic and humoral influences. It follows from this that the vasodilating actions of calcium antagonists tend to be seen predominantly as a reduction in cardiac afterload, with little effect on preload.

Verapamil

Verapamil is a synthetic papaverine-like molecule. It is the only member of the phenylalkylamine family in widespread clinical use.

Approximately balanced effects are exerted by verapamil on myocardium and vascular smooth muscle, so that in therapeutic doses its negative inotropic effects tend to be balanced by a decrease in afterload, and the negative chronotropic effects balanced by reflex increases in sympathetic tone. In patients with abnormal hearts, however, verapamil is quite capable of provoking cardiac failure or significant bradycardia.

Verapamil has a number of clinical applications including therapy for hypertension, angina pectoris and a small but important sub-group of tachyarrhythmias in which part of the re-entrant circuit is calcium channel dependent (classically intra-nodal supraventricular tachycardia). More controversial applications of this agent include its use as a possible cardioprotective agent after myocardial infarction, and as therapy for pulmonary hypertension.

Side effects of verapamil include depression of contractility and heart rate already mentioned, constipation due to gastrointestinal smooth muscle relaxation, which can be particularly troubling to the elderly, non-specific tiredness, headache related to vasodilatation and occasionally an irritating pruritis of uncertain etiology. Verapamil also interacts with digoxin, and may produce a marked increase in serum levels of this drug.

Diltiazem

This is the only example of the benzothiazepine family in clinical use. The clinical applications of diltiazem are rather similar to those of verapamil, except that its role in treating angina pectoris is relatively greater, its use in hypertension (at least to date) relatively less, and its application as an intravenous antiarrhythmic agent has not been widespread.

The side effects are mostly predictable, being due either to vasodilatation (resulting in headache or flushing and occasionally hypotension) or from depression of the SA or AV nodes (resulting in bradyarrhythmias or heart block). Diltiazem has less propensity for negative inotropic effects than verapamil, but has certainly demonstrated an ability to provoke or worsen cardiac failure in patients with abnormal myocardium. Diltiazem, like verapamil, may elevate plasma digoxin concentrations 20–60% when these agents are co-administered orally.

Nifedipine

This is the prototype of a number of agents from the dihydropyridine family in clinical use today. Others include nimodipine, amlodipine and felodipine. It is used for the management of angina pectoris, coronary artery spasm and hypertension. More recently it has been investigated as a cardioprotective agent in myocardial infarction and for its possible ability to reverse atherosclerosis.

As mentioned above, the dihydropyridines are basically pure vasodilators in therapeutic doses. Nifedipine is less vascular-selective than some other members of this family, but considerably more so than either verapamil or diltiazem. It does not commonly produce clinically significant negative inotropic or chronotropic effects, but there are reports of this occurring in patients with initially abnormal ventricles.

Because dihydropyridines act via their effects on arterioles and arteries but not veins, nifedipine markedly reduces peripheral resistance and cardiac afterload but has no significant effect on preload.

The major side effects of nifedipine relate to its vasodilating properties and include headache, flushing and ankle oedema. In addition to this, the reduction in peripheral resistance produced by nifedipine frequently leads to symptomatic increases in sympathetic tone which may be associated with palpitations or sweating. This increase in sympathetic tone as a reflex response to the direct action of nifedipine can act as a counteracting influence to the beneficial effects of this agent in myocardial ischaemia. This can lead to worsening rather than improvement in symptoms when the indication is angina pectoris, and has led to the widespread recommendation that nifedipine be combined with a beta-blocker for this application.

The main clinical uses for nifedipine are for myocardial ischaemia, particularly angina pectoris (and particularly if coronary artery spasm is thought to be playing a role), and for hypertension.

Other dihydropyridines

As mentioned earlier, those in clinical use include nimodipine, amlodipine and felodipine. Apart from the relatively experimental use of nimodipine for treatment of cerebral artery spasm in patients with subarachnoid haemorrhage, by far the major use of these agents is as anti-hypertensive drugs.

Amlodipine has a long half-life, allowing once or twice daily dosage and making it attractive for treating hypertension. Calcium channel blockers are generally regarded as contraindicated in patients with heart failure. This may change in the future as new data become available.

Angiotensin converting enzyme (ACE) inhibitors

This group of compounds has revolutionised our thinking about the pharmacotherapy of cardiac failure and hypertension since captopril was introduced in the mid 1970s. In parallel with this, understanding of the renin-angiotensin system has widened markedly in recent years. The classical concept of the renin-angiotensin (R-A) system has been expanded to fit in with growing evidence of a number of local R-A systems within individual organs or tissues, including the heart. In the simplest formulation, renin is released from the juxtaglomerular apparatus of the kidney in response to a perceived reduction in renal perfusion pressure, hyponatraemia, or an increase in sympathetic tone. Renin splits the inactive peptide angiotensin I from its precursor protein angiotensinogen. Classically this occurs in the circulation, and the intravascular angiotensin I is then converted by angiotensin-converting enzyme into the active peptide angiotensin II. This converting enzyme is traditionally thought to reside in the endothelium, particularly in the pulmonary circulation. Angiotensin II acts via a specific receptor to produce a large number of effects on various end organs. These include constriction of smooth muscle, particularly vascular smooth muscle, an increase in sympathetic tone (probably mediated by a presynaptic mechanism), the release of the salt- and water-retaining hormone aldosterone from the adrenal cortex, direct stimulation of the thirst centre in the hypothalamus, release of vasopressin from the posterior pituitary (which in turn produces water retention and further vasoconstriction), increased myocardial contractility and possibly hypertrophy of myocardium and vascular smooth muscle. Angiotensin II has other actions that are not well understood, including a role in blood pressure control within the brain itself. Angiotensin-converting enzyme is also a 'kininase', and as such is responsible for the degradation of a number of circulating vasodilating substances, particularly bradykinin. The clinical importance of this latter function is still under debate.

Side effects

The reported incidence of adverse effects with low dose captopril or enalapril is less than 10% in the series with large numbers of patients.

There are three particular adverse reactions that do appear to be 'class-specific' for all the ACE inhibitors. The first is hypotension, particularly after the first dose of drug. This is seen particularly in patients who are volume- and salt-depleted. In addition, it seems to be less of a feature with the longer-acting ACE inhibitors than with the short-acting captopril.

The second adverse reaction is the development of a cough, which may not begin until some time after the commencement of treatment and is dry, irritating and persistent. The true incidence is uncertain, with reports ranging from 0.2–10% (in the last study the incidence was 14.6% of 109 women and 6% of 100 men). The cough almost invariably resolves within two weeks of discontinuation of ACE inhibitor therapy. Related to this side effect, though much less common, is angioneurotic oedema. As with cough, no predisposing factors have been identified. Angio-oedema usually, but not invariably, occurs within several days of initiation of therapy. When there is symptomatic involvement of the tongue, glottis or larynx, as evidenced by respiratory distress, prompt subcutaneous administration of adrenaline has been recommended, as laryngeal obstruction can occur. It is thought that both cough and angio-oedema may be related to high levels of bradykinin in patients on ACE inhibitors.

The third adverse reaction attributable to ACE inhibitors is an acute deterioration in renal function. This overlaps to some extent with the hypotensive reaction discussed above, although that is not the only mechanism. Angiotensin has a number of effects on the glomerulus, one of which is to maintain vasoconstriction of the efferent arteriole. In many patients with cardiac failure in particular, this vasoconstrictor effect is essential to maintaining adequate glomerular filtration pressure. Patients with bilateral renal artery stenosis are particularly sensitive to this side effect.

As with most new antihypertensive compounds, there is very limited experience in the use of ACE inhibitors to treat hypertension or heart failure in pregnancy. It is well established, however, that captopril is quite toxic to the foetus in sheep, and for this reason ACE inhibitors in general should be avoided if there is any question of pregnancy.

In summary, ACE inhibitors are an extremely useful group of new agents for treating hypertension and cardiac failure. Considerable care needs to be exercised in those with renal dysfunction, the elderly and those with a history of reactions to other ACE inhibitors. The drug should not generally be given in pregnancy. With these provisos, ACE inhibitors provide a useful once-daily treatment for a large number of patients with mild to moderate hypertension. The addition of a single dose of thiazide diuretic has been shown to have a considerable synergistic effect, and provides effective antihypertensive therapy in the majority of patients with mild to moderate hypertension.

Many new agents were released on the Australian market in 1992 and 1993. In general these all have long half-lives, allowing once- or twice-daily dosage. Various other claims have been made for individual agents including improved 'tissue selectivity', referring to the fact that some of these agents have been shown to bind tightly to angiotension converting enzyme localised in tissues, particularly vascular tissues. It has been suggested that this may allow improved local action, which may turn out to be important in preventing the long-term hypertrophy of myocardium and vascular smooth muscles seen in patients with hypertension. This claim remains untested, and apart from the possible advantages of once-daily dosage afforded by some of the newer agents, there appears to be no strong reason for abandoning captopril and enalapril at this stage.

Angiotensin-II antagonists

These agents have somewhat similar actions to the ACE inhibitors but are in fact different in their mechanism of action. They directly antagonise the angiotensin II receptor. In fact, the available agents (which include losartan, irbesartan and several others) all antagonise exclusively the AT_1 angiotensin receptor and have no effect on the AT_2 receptor. ACE inhibitors, on the other hand, decrease stimulation of both receptor types and also lead to increased circulating levels of vasodilating, nitric oxide-releasing substances such as bradykinin. This means that because they do not raise bradykinin levels, angiotensin-II antagonists cause much less cough than do ACE inhibitors. Whether this translates into a clinically relevant difference in terms of efficacy remains to be seen. Several large-scale trials are currently underway.

Nitrovasodilators

The organic nitrates nitroprusside and related compounds have recently been designated as nitrovasodilators. These drugs have been used for clinical management of angina pectoris since soon after nitroglycerine was first synthesized in 1846, but their basic mechanism of action has only been elucidated in the last few years. Their detailed chemistry and pharmacology is well covered in standard textbooks and will not be discussed here. The most commonly used examples are nitroglycerine (or glyceryl trinitrate), isosorbide dinitrate and sodium nitroprusside.

It should be noted that the nitrovasodilators act on all smooth muscle. Bronchial smooth muscle and the muscles of the biliary tract, gastrointestinal tract (including the oesophagus), ureter and uterus may also be affected. Thus, 'angina' due to biliary or oesophageal spasm may also be relieved by nitrates.

Even when chest pain is truly due to myocardial ischaemia, the mechanisms by which nitrates relieve this pain are at least threefold; the commonest effect seen with low-dose nitrovasodilators (especially sublingual and transcutaneous use) is preload reduction due to venodilatation. This can relieve ischaemia by reducing myocardial oxygen demand. Direct dilatation of the coronary arteries is a second important action of these agents. They are not, however, specific coronary artery dilators, and at doses in which this effect is seen they also act to dilate other large arteries. It has recently been recognised that by reducing arterial wave reflection, this mechanism may lead to a significant reduction in afterload, the magnitude of which may be underestimated by monitoring effects on systolic blood pressure recorded in the brachial or radial arteries. Finally, in high doses (generally only seen with intravenous administration), nitrates produce arteriolar dilatation. This leads to a reduction in peripheral resistance which, by reducing afterload, may also contribute to the relief of ischaemia. This last effect can also lead to unwanted falls in blood pressure, and possibly in coronary perfusion.

Unlike the organic nitrates (e.g. glyceryl trinitrate and isosorbide), itroprusside breaks down spontaneously in blood to produce nitric oxide. It non-selectively dilates arteries, arterioles, veins and venules—unlike nitroglycerine, which appears to dilate only vessels greater than about 200 µm in diameter. Smaller vessels apparently lack the metabolic machinery required to break the nitrates down to release nitric oxide. This difference probably explains the observation that nitroprusside can result in redistribution of blood flow away from ischaemic myocardium in patients with coronary artery disease, whereas nitroglycerine appears to do the opposite, mainly by dilating collateral vessels.

Nitrate tolerance

Continuous administration of organic nitrates leads to rapid development of drug tolerance in most patients. In the case of intravenous administration of nitrates, this can generally be overcome simply by increasing the infusion rate. There is good evidence that development of tolerance to transcutaneous nitrate can be largely prevented by the practice of a nitrate-free interval of 10 to 12 hours per day, most commonly during the night). Similarly, it has been shown that tolerance to the clinical effects of isosorbide dinitrate develops with a sustained dosage of 30mg four times daily, but not when the drug is given two or three times daily.

Toxicity and side effects

The vast majority of side effects from use of nitrovasodilators are predictable on the basis of their effects on smooth muscle. Headache is by far the commonest and may be quite severe, although it varies from patient to patient. Postural hypotension and even syncope are relatively frequent. These relate mainly to reductions in preload with a consequent fall in cardiac output rather than to a reduction in afterload. Patients with myocardial ischaemia or cardiac failure frequently have a high initial preload, and hence are less subject to this problem than normal volunteers taking nitrates.

Diuretics

Diuretics are agents that increase production of urine by the kidneys. They comprise a large and heterogeneous group of compounds, but only the more clinically important groups are discussed here. Comprehensive reviews are available in the standard textbooks.

Benzothiadiazides

These are commonly referred to as the 'thiazide' diuretics. At a normal glomerular filtration rate (approximately 125 ml/min) the total extracellular fluid volume is filtered every 100 minutes. Normally well over 99% of this is reabsorbed by the renal tubules. This reabsorption is largely achieved by active transport of electrolyte and other solutes, first into the tubular cell and then from the tubular cell into the extracellular fluid.

By far the most important electrolyte in the present discussion is the sodium ion. Essentially there is only one way of extruding sodium ions from the tubular cell into the extracellular fluid. This is via the Na-K-ATPase pump. There are at least five different mechanisms for reabsorbing sodium from the tubular filtrate into the tubular cell. These include (i) passive diffusion down an electrochemical gradient, (ii) sodium entry coupled to an organic solute, (iii) sodium-hydrogen exchange, (iv) electroneutral co-transport of a sodium, a potassium and two chloride ions, and (v) electroneutral co-transport of a sodium ion with a chloride ion. The first three mechanisms are seen in the proximal convoluted tubule, the first mechanism also in the late part of the proximal tubule, the fourth mechanism in the thick ascending limb of the loop of Henle, the fifth mechanism in the distal convoluted tubule, and the first and third mechanisms also in the distal tubule and collecting duct.

Potassium undergoes reabsorption in the proximal tubule and thick ascending limb of the loop of Henle, and secretion in the distal tubule. While the majority of filtered potassium is reabsorbed proximally, this fraction is relatively invariant, and the main physiological changes in potassium loss through the kidney are attributable to distal secretory mechanisms. One of the determinants of an increased rate of secretion of potassium distally appears to be the volume of unreabsorbed glomerular filtrate flowing through the distal tubule. Hence drugs such as thiazide diuretics, whose main effect is to decrease sodium reabsorption, can indirectly lead to increased loss of potassium as well.

The major site of action of the thiazides is the proximal part of the distal convoluted tubule, where they block the electroneutral sodium chloride co-transport mechanism (the fifth mechanism listed above). As 90% of filtered sodium has already been reabsorbed by this point, the maximal amount of sodium excretion that can be produced by thiazide diuretics is modest compared with that achieved by some other types of diuretics. Furthermore, the thiazide-induced increase in flow through tubular segments distal to the early part of the distal tubule stimulates a modest amount of potassium secretion.

Thiazides also lead to enhanced proximal reabsorption and possibly decreased distal secretion of uric acid, and hence can elevate serum uric acid levels. In addition to this, and in contrast with the loop diuretics discussed below, thiazides decrease the renal excretion of calcium ions via a direct effect on the early part of the distal tubule. Thiazides increase the excretion of magnesium ions.

Metolazone-loop diuretic combinations

Unlike other thiazide diuretics, the addition of metolazone to a loop diuretic (see below) is believed to produce a synergistic effect. This may be because metolazone has an action on proximal and distal tubules, whereas the other thiazides act only by their effect on the distal tubule. The proximal tubular effect leads to increased delivery of sodium to the loop of Henle and hence a greater effect of the loop diuretic.

Loop diuretics

These agents are also called 'high-ceiling' diuretics because the peak diuretic effect they produce is far greater than that seen with other agents. Their main site of action is the thick ascending limb of the loop of Henle, hence their more common label. The agents to be discussed under this heading include furosemide (or frusemide), ethacrynic acid and bumetanide. Unlike the thiazides, these three agents have little in common in terms of chemical structure, although both furosemide and bumetanide are sulphonamides and weak inhibitors of carbonic anhydrase.

As noted above, the loop diuretics act primarily to inhibit electrolyte reabsorption in the thick ascending limb of the loop of Henle. They act at the tubular luminal phase to inhibit the Na-K-2Cl co-transport mechanism. They also tend to produce a rapid-onset, short-lived increase in renal blood flow accompanied by an increased excretion of prostaglandins and kinins by the kidney. Parenterally administered frusemide also causes a rapid increase in venous capacitance, which occurs before the diuretic effect and results in a decrease in cardiac preload and left ventricular filling pressures. This may contribute to the early response seen in patients with pulmonary oedema.

The majority of clinical side effects experienced with loop diuretics relate to fluid and electrolyte imbalances produced by the main renal tubular actions of these agents. These actions include hyponatraemia, alkalosis, and contraction of the extracellular space.

Aldosterone antagonists

The only example of this class of drugs to be discussed here is spironolactone. This is a steroid compound which competitively antagonises the actions of mineralocorticoids such as aldosterone. Aldosterone receptors are found in a number of tissues apart from the kidney, including salivary glands and colon. The major renal effect of aldosterone is to increase sodium reabsorption in the late distal tubule and collecting duct, in exchange for secretion of potassium (or hydrogen) ions.

The aldosterone antagonists are mainly used in concert with thiazide or other diuretics in the treatment of fluid retention or hypertension. Spironolactone is frequently added to other diuretics as a means of preventing excessive potassium loss, and is used in management of primary (rare) or secondary hyperaldosteronism.

Other potassium-sparing diuretics

The two agents to be discussed under this heading are triamterene and amiloride. While these share some of the properties of spironolactone, they are not chemically related, nor are they mineralocorticoid antagonists. Both agents have some natriuretic activity of their own but are most frequently used for their ability to reduce potassium loss due to other diuretics.

The main mechanism of action appears to be inhibition of electrogenic reabsorption of sodium by cells in the distal tubule and collecting duct.

Cardiac glycosides

Cardiac glycosides have long been used as first-line therapy for controlling heart rate in patients with atrial fibrillation. There are more than 500 known cardiac glycosides. Squill was in use some 3000 years ago, and digitalis was used in Wales in the 13th century.

In 1955, Na-K ATPase inhibition was demonstrated and postulated to be its mechanism of action.

Drugs that have been used clinically include digoxin and digitoxin which both come from the foxglove plant (Digitalis), and ouabain and strophanthidin from the squill plant (Strophanthus). Ouabain was once available in Australia for intravenous use only. It was thought to have a shorter onset of action than digoxin. Digitoxin is still available in the USA but not in Australia. It has 100% oral bioavailability and a half-life of nearly one week. Its major advantage is that it is metabolised by the liver rather than being excreted unchanged by the kidneys. Hence dosage adjustment is less of an issue in patients with renal failure on this compound.

Clinical pharmacology of digoxin

Digoxin is now the only cardiac glycoside in clinical use in Australia. It can be given intravenously or orally. It can also be administered intramuscularly, but this is painful. The dosage has to be adjusted carefully in renal disease. Approximately 10% of humans have a bacterium in their gut that can metabolise digoxin. If such a patient is stable on a given dose of digoxin and is then commenced on antibiotics, which suppress this gut bacterium, it is possible that the digoxin level may rise as a result.

There are a number of clinically important drug interactions concerning digoxin. The administration of quinidine to a patient already on digoxin leads to an increase in the plasma concentration of digoxin in nearly all cases. This increase is usually of the order of 50 to 150% and begins to appear within hours. A number of other agents, particularly other antiarrhythmic drugs, produce similar but usually less dramatic increases in digoxin concentrations. These include verapamil, amiodarone, propafenone and diltiazem. In addition to these drug interactions, digitalis toxicity is in general more common in patients with low levels of potassium or magnesium.

Mechanisms of action

The mechanisms by which digitalis in general, and digoxin in particular, exert their effects are traditionally divided into 'direct' and 'indirect'. Understanding of both of these has increased significantly in recent years, although there are still a number of gaps in our knowledge.

The direct effects of digitalis are now believed to be mediated largely through two mechanisms. The first of these involves direct binding to and inhibition of the membrane bound Na-K-ATPase molecule. The second effect of digitalis is to increase the slow inward calcium current (i_{Ca}) during the action potential.

Partial inhibition by digoxin of the ATPase molecule on myocardial cells leads to an increase in intracellular sodium concentration. This causes a reduction in calcium excretion from the cell via the sodium-calcium exchange mechanism. This in turn causes an increased level of calcium within the cell and a positive inotropic effect. Furthermore, the stoichiometry of the situation is such that a very small rise in intracellular sodium concentration (approximately 1 mM) can lead to a doubling of tension development by the myocardium.

Digitalis markedly increases vagal tone and can affect sympathetic tone. Enhancement of vagal activity typically tends to cause a decrease in the sinus rate and an increase in the effective refractory period of the atrioventricular node. The main effect on ordinary atrial fibres is a shortening of their action potential duration and hence of their refactory period.

Because of their relative paucity of vagal innervation, it has traditionally been considered that the indirect, vagally mediated effects of digitalis were of little relevance to the His-Purkinje system and to ventricular myocardium, except possibly in situations of digitalis toxicity where the high sympathetic tone may play a role in provoking arrhythmias. There is emerging evidence, however, that binding of digoxin to vagal afferent fibres from ventricular myocardium may play a role in reduction of the high background sympathetic tone seen in patients with cardiac failure. Withdrawal of sympathetic tone and consequent vasodilatation and afterload reduction may well be one of the more important mechanisms of action of digitalis in cardiac failure.

Haemodynamic effects

If digoxin is given to a normal volunteer it causes both a positive inotropic effect due to drug action on the myocardium, and an increase in afterload due to the increased tone in blood vessels. A patient with cardiac failure, however, is in a different situation. As already mentioned, one of the characteristics of cardiac failure from the very early stages is a marked increase in sympathetic tone. Digoxin administration results in a withdrawal of this abnormally enhanced sympathetic tone. Thus, when a patient with cardiac failure is given digoxin, he gets the benefit of the positive inotropic effect as well as the withdrawal of sympathetic tone, which more than compensates for the direct tendency for digoxin to increase afterload. Afterload falls and the cardiac output increases.

Antiarrhythmic drugs and relevant electrophysiology

Antiarrhythmic drugs were historically classified according to the Vaughan and Williams system into 4 broad categories, called Class I, Class II, Class III and Class IV, depending on their mode of action. Class I agents are further classified into subcategories IA, IB and IC, as summarised in Table 13.2.

Table 13.2. Classification of antiarrhythmic drugs

	Drugs	**Action**
Class I	IA: quinidine, procainamide, disopyramide IB: lignocaine, mexiletine, tocainide IC: flecainide, encainide	Block fast sodium current
Class II	Beta-blockers	Block effects of catecholamines
Class III	Amiodarone, sotalol	Lengthen action potential duration
Class IV	Verapamil, diltiazem	Calcium antagonists

Clinical pharmacology of antiarrhythmic drugs
Class I Agents

Traditional antiarrhythmic drugs are generally considered as Class I agents. These have significant toxicity and act by blocking the fast inward sodium channel.

Class IA Drugs: Quinidine, procainamide, disopyramide

Quinine has been prescribed for palpitations since the 18th century. It was largely replaced for this purpose by its *d*-isomer, quinidine, after the work of Wenckebach and Frey from 1914 to 1918. The use of procainamide stems from observations by Mautz in 1936, which showed that procaine increased the threshold to electrical stimulation of ventricular muscle. Further studies led to its replacement by procainamide, which exhibited similar properties but a much longer duration of action. The antiarrhythmic properties of disopyramide were described in animals in 1962 and a clinical trial was reported in 1963.

In the clinical electrophysiology laboratory, these drugs produce very similar effects. Hence, it is not surprising that all three compounds are useful in the treatment and prophylaxis of a variety of atrial and ventricular arrhythmias, though there is a tendency to reserve procainamide for the latter.

All three have been used successfully for the reversion of, and prophylaxis against, atrial flutter and fibrillation. If administered as the sole therapy for these arrhythmias, each of these drugs may produce an acceleration of the ventricular rate. This is due, in part, to a drug-induced reduction in atrial rate, and hence reduction in repetitive concealed conduction into the A-V node. As well as this, quinidine and disopyramide, and (to a much lesser extent) procainamide, exhibit vagolytic activity, which can accelerate conduction through the A-V node. For this reason they are normally administered in conjunction with digitalis for the treatment of atrial flutter and fibrillation.

Supraventricular tachycardia of the intranodal type is most commonly and successfully treated with verapamil, which blocks the A-V nodal limb of the re-entrant circuit. The IA drugs, however, can be used with moderate success for this arrhythmia. They can also be quite useful in supraventricular tachycardias caused by an accessory atrioventricular connection (as seen in Wolff-Parkinson-White syndrome). In these cases, the drugs act by slowing conduction in part of the circuit to the point of block.

Class IA drugs are effective in most cases in suppressing ventricular ectopic beats by their effect on automaticity. Lignocaine and mexiletine have largely replaced these drugs for treatment of ventricular tachycardia or fibrillation in association with acute myocardial infarction. All three agents, however, may be useful in the difficult and increasingly recognised clinical problem of chronic, recurrent ventricular tachycardia or fibrillation. In this condition, choice of therapy may be best guided by clinical electrophysiological studies in which programmed stimulation is used in an attempt to provoke the arrhythmia.

Quinidine is usually administered orally. In Australia, it is usually prescribed as a long-acting preparation (for example, Kinidin Durules, 2–4 every 12 hours). This produces reasonably constant blood levels for about 12 hours, after which there is a fairly rapid decline. As with all antiarrhythmic therapy, it is advisable where possible to adjust dosage according to serum drug levels to ensure that these are in the therapeutic range. The cardiovascular side effects of quinidine include hypotension, which may (particularly at toxic concentrations) be partly due to its known negative inotropic effects but is also attributable to vasodilation produced by the alpha-adrenergic blocking action of the drug. In addition, therapeutic concentrations of quinidine occasionally may produce a potentially lethal ventricular tachycardia ('*torsade de pointes*') or fibrillation, usually in association with marked Q–T interval prolongation.

Procainamide may be administered both by oral and intravenous routes. The cardiovascular side effects of procainamide are very similar to those of quinidine except that the drug has no alpha-adrenergic blocking activity.

Disopyramide may also be administered by the intravenous route. It shares a moderate negative inotropic effect with quinidine and procainamide, though this may be masked to some extent by a tendency to produce peripheral vasoconstriction. Nevertheless, this effect is capable of precipitating overt cardiac failure in patients with pre-existing depression of ventricular function. Widening of the QRS complex, prolongation of the Q–T interval and drug-induced ventricular tachyarrhythmias have all been reported as occasional side effects.

IB Drugs: Lignocaine, mexiletine, tocainide

Lignocaine is the oldest and best known of this group (it was synthesised in 1946). It has achieved widespread acceptance as first line pharmacological therapy for serious ventricular arrhythmias in acute myocardial infarction. It is sometimes of value in the treatment of supraventricular arrhythmias, but these are usually best managed with other drugs.

Because of extensive first-pass metabolism in the liver, lignocaine must be administered parenterally.

Routine use of lignocaine in acute ventricular arrhythmias has come under question in recent years for two reasons. (i) A number of animal studies have suggested that lignocaine may increase the electrical defibrillation threshold significantly. (ii) Of some concern are two studies using meta-analysis, which have suggested a significant increase in fatal bradyarrhythmias in patients with acute myocardial infarction treated with prophylactic lignocaine. Precipitation of ventricular tachyarrhythmias with or without Q–T prolongation occurs rarely if at all with lignocaine.

Central nervous system side effects are not uncommon with lignocaine. These include paraesthesiae (often perioral), mental changes, tremor, convulsions and coma.

Mexiletine and tocainide are chemically very similar to lignocaine. They share the advantages of being effective when given by mouth. As with lignocaine, they are both most useful in the treatment of ventricular arrhythmias, and a patient who responds well to parenterally administered lignocaine will frequently also respond to oral therapy with mexiletine or tocainide. The side effects of these drugs are similar to those listed for lignocaine. In addition, gastrointestinal symptoms, especially nausea, are a common complaint. Since mexiletine is less expensive and more readily available than tocainide, it would seem to be the drug of choice when oral therapy is required.

IC Drugs: Flecainide, encainide, lorcainide, propafenone

These drugs, of which only flecainide is freely available in Australia, are discussed briefly. There are a number of studies indicating that all three are very effective in suppressing both supraventricular and ventricular arrhythmias. It should be noted, however, that they also have considerable negative inotropic properties and tend to prolong intracardiac conduction times, even in therapeutic concentrations. Arrhythmogenesis has been reported for encainide and flecainide, and led to their withdrawal from the CAST study, a large American study of antiarrhythmic drug therapy in 1991.

Class II agents

Class II antiarrhythmic agents include the generally safe antisympathomimetic drugs, particularly the beta-adrenoceptor blockers. Beta-blocking agents are often effective both in reversion of, and in prophylaxis against, supraventricular tachycardia, where they probably act largely by prolonging refractoriness and slowing conduction in the AV node. Their role in this arrhythmia (particularly for acute therapy) has, however, been largely overshadowed by verapamil. In atrial fibrillation and flutter (especially if due to thyrotoxicosis), beta-blocking agents can be useful in slowing the ventricular response by their effect on the AV node, but they are generally of little use in restoring sinus rhythm. An exception to this is sotalol, which is discussed with the Class III drugs.

Beta-blocking agents also have value in the therapy of ventricular tachyarrhythmias, though they have not generally been used as first-line drugs for this indication in the past. They are of particular use in arrhythmias caused by increased circulating catecholamines (anxiety, exercise, phaeochromocytoma), and arrhythmias of the congenital long Q–T inter-val syndrome. Some recent studies have also shown a reduction in ventricular arrhythmias in acute myocardial infarction after the early intravenous administration of beta-blocking drugs.

Class III agents

The best known drug of this class of antiarrhythmics is amiodarone. It was first used in France in 1962 as a vascular smooth-muscle relaxant, and has been widely used in Europe and South America as an antiarrhythmic agent for well over a decade. It came into use in the United States and Australia in the 1980s. Apart from its marked ability to prolong the duration of the cardiac action potential (Class III activity), amiodarone is also a smooth-muscle relaxant, a non-competitive antiadrenergic agent, and demonstrates some degree of Class I and IV activity, at least *in vitro*.

Whatever its basic mechanism (or mechanisms) of action, it is a very useful antiar-rhythmic agent with demonstrated effectiveness in the therapy and prophylaxis of most types of arrhythmia. It is particularly effective in the treatment of atrial fibrillation, su-praventricular arrhythmias associated with Wolff-Parkinson-White syndrome, ventricular arrhythmias complicating hypertrophic cardiomyopathy (which respond poorly to beta-blocking agents or calcium antagonists) and refractory, recurrent ventricular tachycardia and fibrillation. In the latter life-threatening situation, amiodarone has proved effective in large numbers of patients whose condition had failed to respond to a series of other estab-lished and experimental drugs.

As often happens in medicine, such benefits come at a price. Amiodarone is expen-sive and its clinical use is complicated by its very unusual pharmacokinetics and unwanted side effects.

The administration of amiodarone (normally by mouth) is complicated by a vari-able bioavailability (20–80%), a huge volume of distribution (5000 litres) and a terminal half-life of elimination which is usually 35–40 days, but may exceed 100 days. The major metabolite accumulates in high concentration in plasma and tissues, and possesses very similar electrophysiological properties to amiodarone. Dosage regimens vary from clini-cian to clinician, but most recommend a loading dose of 600–2000 mg/day for 1–8 weeks, followed by reduction to a maintenance dose, usually of the order of 200–400 mg/day. Many of the side effects are dose-dependent and each patient should receive the minimum effective dose.

The cardiovascular side effects can include hypotension (usually a problem only with intravenous use), bradycardia (which may be aggravated by concomitant therapy with beta-blocking drugs or verapamil), and Q–T interval prolongation (normally thera-peutic, but occasionally excessive and rarely associated with ventricular tachycardias). Non-cardiac effects include photosensitivity, disturbances of sleep, resting tremor, thyro-toxicosis and hypothyroidism, and pulmonary alveolitis (sometimes fatal). The interaction between amiodarone and the thyroid is complex and has been well described. While thy-roid function should be assessed before the start of amiodarone therapy, overt thyroid disease develops in less than 2% of patients. One of the best known, but least important, side effects of amiodarone therapy is the development of corneal microdeposits, which can be seen in 98% of patients receiving long-term treatment. These deposits rarely pro-duce symptoms; blurred and halo vision occurs in 1 to 2% of cases and diminishes after reduction of the dose. Amiodarone may interact with other drugs. Its additive effects with beta-blocking agents and verapamil, and its ability to elevate serum digoxin levels, have already been noted. In addition, potentiation of the effects of warfarin may occur, which usually necessitates reduction of the anticoagulant dose by about half.

Sotalol is a non-cardioselective beta-blocking agent with marked Class III activity. Unlike other beta-blocking agents the prolongation of the duration of the action potential is apparent at once (within minutes, if administered intravenously), and this drug is showing promise in clinical trials in the treatment of supraventricular and ventricular arrhythmias. The oral bioavailability of sotalol is about 60%, and there is no significant hepatic first-pass metabolism. Sotalol can produce any of the characteristic side effects associated with beta-blockers, and in addition has been reported to cause polymorphic ventricular tachycardia ('torsade de pointes') associated with lengthening of the Q–T interval. This side effect, which may be fatal is probably more common in the presence of high sotalol concentrations, potassium depletion or the co-administration of other drugs known to prolong the Q–T interval.

Class IV agents

The Class IV antiarrhythmic agents include the well known calcium channel blockers verapamil and diltiagen. Verapamil is the prototype for this class of drug. It has been in clinical use since 1966, and has become the drug of first choice for short-term therapy of supraventricular tachycardia, in which it acts by blocking the slow conducting (AV nodal) limb of the re-entrant circuit. The usual dosage is 5–10 mg administered intravenously over 5–10 minutes, with careful monitoring of the ECG and blood pressure. In atrial fibrillation or flutter, verapamil usually slows the ventricular response, but is unlikely to induce reversion to sinus rhythm. Long-term oral therapy with verapamil can be useful in prophylaxis against recurrent supraventricular tachycardias, but can be complicated by the pharmacokinetics of the drug. Verapamil is not generally employed for treatment of recurrent ventricular tachyarrhythmias. Some studies have demonstrated a good response to verapamil in a small subgroup of patients with recurrent ventricular tachycardia.

Cardiac depression is the most serious side effect of verapamil. It is rarely a problem in patients with normal left ventricular function, but can be quite severe in already diseased or beta-blocked hearts, especially when verapamil is administered intravenously. Non-cardiac side effects are occasionally a problem. These include tiredness, constipation, pruritus, headache and vertigo. Constipation in particular can be very troublesome, especially to elderly patients.

Because of their additive effects on the AV node and on myocardial contractility, the combination of verapamil and beta-blocking agents is potentially dangerous. Recent experience suggests that they can be safely administered together in many patients, but the initiation of such therapy is best carried out under careful supervision. Similarly, the combined administration of digoxin and verapamil can be very useful, especially in atrial fibrillation, but caution must be exercised both because of their additive effects on AV conduction and because verapamil tends to elevate serum levels of digoxin.

Anti-platelet agents in cardiology

These drugs are explained in Chapter 14.

Antithrombotic agents

Heparin

Heparin was first isolated from the canine liver by a medical student in 1916 and has been in regular clinical use for over 50 years. Structurally it is a mixture of sulfated glycosaminoglycans, ranging in molecular weight from less than 5000 to more than 30 000 with an average of 12 000 to 15 000, depending on the source. Only about one third of this heparin mixture has significant anticoagulant effect.

Heparin exerts most of its anticoagulant effect by binding to and greatly increasing the activity of an $alpha_2$-globulin called antithrombin III. Antithrombin-III normally complexes with and inactivates a number of activated clotting factors, particularly thrombin and Factor Xa. When heparin binds to antithrombin III it produces a conformational change that dramatically increases the affinity of antithrombin III for thrombin, factor Xa and other protease enzymes of the coagulation cascade. This eventually leads to a dose-dependent prolongation of blood clotting which can be monitored with assays such as the activated partial thromboplastin time (APTT) and the thrombin time (TT). Heparin has other effects, including some inhibition of platelet function, increased permeability of vessel walls and inhibition of proliferation of vascular smooth muscle, but this presentation concentrates on the antithrombotic actions of this agent.

While thrombin is more sensitive to inhibition by the heparin-antithrombin-III complex than is factor Xa, it has recently become recognised that the low molecular weight components of the heparin mixture (those with fewer saccharide residues) are unable to bind to thrombin and antithrombin-III simultaneously, and thus selectively inhibit factor Xa activity. This has led to the marketing and promotion of specific low molecular weight fractions of heparin for antithrombotic prophylaxis, the aim being to inhibit factor Xa and hence intravascular coagulation, without inhibiting thrombin activation and seriously impairing normal haemostasis. In this way it may prove possible to separate the beneficial actions and the bleeding complications of heparin, and further enhance the clinical value of this compound.

Heparin is poorly absorbed orally, and must be administered by intravenous or subcutaneous injection. Since there is no satisfactory assay for circulating heparin, the dosage is normally adjusted according to the APPT or TT, as noted above. The dose response curve for heparin is not linear; rather, the anticoagulant response increases disproportionately in intensity and duration as the dose increases. The apparent biological half-life of intravenous heparin is of the order of 30–60 minutes, increasing somewhat with dosage. Heparin binds initially to saturable sites on endothelial cells. Heparin is eliminated by mechanisms that are still unclear, but there are reports of reduced heparin requirements in patients with renal failure.

It has been confirmed that fibrin binds to thrombin and protects it from inactivation by the heparin-antithrombin-III complex. The result of this is that about 20 times more heparin is needed to inactivate fibrin-bound thrombin than to inactivate prothrombin. This does not apply to a number of more recently introduced thrombin inhibitors such as hirudin (see below). This effect explains the observation that preventing extension of established venous thrombosis requires higher concentrations of heparin than does preventing its formation, as well as the relative inefficacy of heparin in inhibiting thrombin activity after successful coronary thrombolysis.

The most common and feared side effect of heparin is bleeding. With well monitored administration intravenously or subcutaneously the incidence of major bleeding appears to range from about 4–6%. This can be increased by concomitant use of aspirin, co-existent alcoholic liver disease or other major hepatic dysfunction and possibly renal failure. Thrombocytopenia is also a well-recognised and usually asymptomatic complication of heparin therapy, with an incidence ranging from 2% or less, to over 20%. In a much smaller number of patients (probably well under 1% of those given heparin), thrombocytopenia is associated with arterial or venous thrombosis (this combination is sometimes known as 'HITTS': Heparin Induced Thrombocytopenia and Thrombosis). Venous thrombosis in particular may also result from heparin resistance caused by the neutralising effect of heparin-induced release of platelet factor 4. In patients with persistent heparin-induced thrombocytopenia who require continuing antithrombotic therapy, low molecular weight heparin may have cross-reactivity with standard heparin, and the use of heparinoid appears to be a more successful alternative. Less common side effects of heparin in long-term use include various allergic reactions, alopecia and osteoporosis.

Warfarin (coumadin)

Dishydroxycoumarin (dicumarol) was identified in 1939 as the causative agent for the haemorrhagic disorder described in cattle that ingested spoiled sweet clover. A few years later a synthetic congener named warfarin was developed. In the 1950s, warfarin and related compounds became widespread therapy for the prevention and treatment of thromboembolic disease. The chemistry and pharmacology of these agents is well described in the literature and are only outlined here. In the remainder of this section the term warfarin is be used, but most of what is presented applies equally to the other coumadin derivatives.

Warfarin is an antagonist of Vitamin K. The coagulation factors II, VII, IX and X and the anticoagulant proteins C and S require Vitamin C as a co-factor for their activation. All of these factors, except possibly protein S, are synthesised mainly in the liver. Therapeutic doses of warfarin decrease both the amount and activity of each of the Vitamin K-dependent coagulation factors. Warfarin has no direct effect on the activity of any fully activated coagulation factors already present in the blood, and hence the time required for the effects of warfarin to manifest depends on individual rates of clearance of each of the factors. Factor VII and protein C have half-lives of approximately 6–8 hours. The half-lives of factors IV, X and II are approximately 24, 36 and 54 hours respectively, and the half-life of protein S is approximately 30 hours. Thus the effects of the reduction in factor VII and protein C are manifested long before effects on other coagulation factors. Because factor VII is of limited relevance to intravascular coagulation, patients in the first 24 hours or so after the introduction of warfarin therapy may manifest a 'hypercoaguable' state secondary to the reduction in protein C. For this reason, and also because of the long half-lives of the other vitamin K-dependent clotting factors that are more important than factor VII in intravascular coagulation, concomitant heparin therapy should be continued for several days after the introduction of warfarin.

Warfarin is well absorbed orally, although food can reduce this to some extent. It freely crosses the placenta. Warfarin is transformed into inactive metabolites by the liver and kidneys and eliminated with a half-life ranging from 20–60 hours. There are large numbers of potentially important interactions between warfarin and other ingested substances, including many drugs. These are well covered in standard textbooks. The major toxic complication of warfarin is, of course, bleeding. If necessary, the effects of warfarin can be reversed with Vitamin K or by replacing clotting factors exogenously, using fresh frozen plasma or transfusions of fresh whole blood. Warfarin should not be used during pregnancy because of its teratogenic effects on the foetus and risk of maternal bleeding. Other occasional reactions to warfarin include rashes, itching, fever and gastrointestinal upsets.

Regular monitoring is an important part of therapy with warfarin. Traditionally this was done using the prothrombin time or its inverse, the prothombin index. Prolongation of prothrombin time relative to a controlled sample of plasma occurs when any of factors V, II, VII or X are decreased significantly. Many countries have introduced the International Normalised Ratio (INR) for reporting and standardising warfarin effect. This is based on the ratio of the patient prothrombin time to a controlled prothrombin time that would have been obtained using a standard World Health Organization technique.

Recommendations for the ideal therapeutic level of the prothrombin time or INR vary according to indication.

Thrombolytic agents

Widespread use of thrombolytic agents has revolutionised the management of acute myocardial infarction in the past decade. The following is only a very brief outline of the biochemistry and pharmacology of some of the more important of these new agents.

Plasmin is a serine protease (790 amino acids), which breaks the arginine-lysine bonds found in many clotting-cascade proteins, including fibrin. 'Specificity' for fibrin is only due to the facts that plasminogen binds selectively to partially lysed fibrin, and plasminogen is more readily converted to plasmin when already bound to fibrin. Inactive plasminogen is converted to plasmin by a number of activators, including tPA, urokinase and streptokinase-plasminogen complex. There are a number of endogenous plasmin inhibitors: alpha$_2$-antiplasmin, alpha$_2$-macroglobulin, alpha$_1$-antitrypsin, C$_1$-esterase inhibitor and antithrombin III. Extensive activation of circulating plasminogen to plasmin (for example by streptokinase) results in its mopping up of all available alpha$_2$-antiplasmin, the most important of the endogenous inhibitors. Since there is more plasminogen than alpha 2-antiplasmin, this eventually produces a systemic lytic state. This is seen with streptokinase and urokinase and high doses of tPA, and produces depletion of plasminogen and fibrinogen. Generally fibrinogen and fibrin degradation products are indistinguishable, but the 'D-D dimer' fragment is relatively specific for fibrin degradation, and has been used to monitor successful lysis of fibrin.

Tissue plasminogen activator (tPA) is a 527 amino acid glycoprotein made by many cell types, including endothelial cells, liver and myocardium. It binds to fibrin as well as plasminogen (hence 'clot-selectivity'). When given pharmacologically, any tPA that does not quickly bind to fibrin tends to bind to an inactivator (PAI-1) and circulate in blood in this inactive form. tPA has a redistribution half-life of 3–6 minutes and a beta half-life of 20–40 minutes.

Urokinase, another endogenous plasminogen activator (411 amino acids) is not fibrin specific. It also activates circulating plasminogen, producing a systemic lytic state. Its redistribution half-life is eight minutes and its beta half-life 48 minutes. tPA and urokinase activate plasminogen by different mechanisms, hence there is a potential for synergistic effects of the two agents.

Streptokinase (415 amino acids) comes from beta-haemolytic Streptococcus. It is not an enzyme, unlike urokinase and tPA which are serine proteases. It forms a one-to-one complex with plasminogen, and this new substance (streptokinase-plasminogen complex) is able to activate plasminogen to plasmin. It is not fibrin specific, and produces a systemic lytic state, with raised levels of fibrin and fibrinogen degradation products and reduced fibrinogen levels. Many individuals who have not been given streptokinase therapeutically already have antibodies to this substance from prior exposure to Streptococci. Streptokinase has a half-life of only 30–90 minutes, but the half-life of the streptokinase-plasminogen complex is much longer because it is resistant to alpha$_2$-antiplasmin (see below).

The GISSI-II, International Streptokinase/tPA, and ISIS-III trials[1] showed no significant differences between tPA, APSAC and streptokinase in terms of mortality reduction. These studies, however, were heavily criticised on the grounds that the standard heparin regimen was subcutaneous heparin averaging about 25 000 units per day. There is considerable evidence that tPA in particular (because of its short half-life and other factors), requires intravenous heparin as adjuvant therapy to maximise its ability to open and maintain patency of infarct-related arteries.

This controversy eventually led to the GUSTO (Global Utilisation of Streptokinase and tPA for Occluded Arteries) Trial.[2] There were four arms to this study, including standard streptokinase therapy with subcutaneous heparin, streptokinase therapy with intravenous heparin, a combination of streptokinase and tPA in slightly reduced doses with intravenous heparin, and finally a 'front-loaded' tPA regimen in which the tPA was given more rapidly than had traditionally been the case, and in concert with high dose intravenous heparin. Briefly, the first three regimens were equivalent in terms of their effects on mortality, although the combination therapy led to slightly more bleeding. The final (front-loaded tPA plus IV heparin) arm of the study gave a statistically significant further reduction in mortality compared to the other three regimens (6.3% total mortality at 30 days versus 7.0 to 7.4%). The benefit was most marked in those under 75 years of age having an anterior myocardial infarct.

As result of the GUSTO results it appears that tPA and intravenous heparin became 'standard therapy' for acute myocardial infarction, at least in patients under 75 who present within six hours of the onset of their pain.

Urokinase has been less extensively trialled than streptokinase and tPA, and is considerably more expensive than streptokinase. There is no reason to suspect that it is any more effective.

Two other major indications for use of tPA rather than streptokinase exist. These are where the patient is known or suspected to be allergic to streptokinase, and where the patient has had streptokinase more than three to five days previously and less than 12 months previously. This is not only because of the risk of allergic reactions, but also because these patients have been shown to have persistent streptokinase antibodies which would be expected to reduce the efficacy of streptokinase.

Theoretically tPA, being fibrin-specific, should produce less bleeding than streptokinase. This has not been borne out by the large-scale trials, and in fact there has been a suggestion that the opposite is the case, although the difference is only marginal. There is little doubt that tPA is better than streptokinase at producing rapid opening of the acutely occluded coronary artery. The problem appears to be that, because of its short half-life, reocclusion is more frequent than with streptokinase. Pooling the results of patency trials with streptokinase and tPA suggests that the percentage of patent infarct-related arteries at 90 minutes is 45% for streptokinase and 76% for tPA. However, at 24 hours the figures are both about 80 to 85%, and at three weeks about 75% in both groups.

Recent work has revolved around modified forms of tPA, one of which, rPA, is now available in Australia. Its efficacy is very similar to that of tPA but is given as a double bolus rather than as an infusion which may be convenient. It remains to be seen how many hospitals switch over to use of rPA. A number of other modified tPAs are being evaluated in clinical trials and several more may appear in the market in the next few years. It is also possible that combinations of the new antiplatelet agents, the IIb/IIIa antagonists (such as ReoPro, Eli Lilly) may have a use in acute myocardial infarction combined with lower doses of thrombolytic. These protocols are currently under investigation.

As a final point on the cost benefit analysis for thrombolytic therapy, it has been calculated that the risk of death or serious bleeding directly related to thrombolytic therapy is of the order of three to four per thousand patients, compared with approximately 50 lives saved per thousand patients given thrombolytic therapy. On the face of it there seems little doubt that the odds are in favour of thrombolytic therapy.

References

1.   Gruppo Italiano per lo Studio della Sopravvienza nell'Infarcto Miocardico: GISSI-2: A factorial randomised trial of alteplase versus streptokinase and heparin versus no heparin among 12,490 patients with acute myocardial infarction. *Lancet* 1990; **336**:65–71.
2.   The GUSTO Investigators. An international randomized trial comparing four thrombolytic strategies for acute myocardial infarction. *N Engl J Med* 1993; **329**:673–82.

Further reading

Goodman LS, Gilman A, Hardman JG, Limbird LE. *Goodman and Gillman's The pharmacological basis of therapeutics*, 9th ed. New York: Mcgraw Hill 1996.

Chapter 14

Antiplatelet and anticoagulant therapy in interventional cardiology

Harry C. Lowe and Antonio Colombo

The patient is given aspirin (1.0 g per day) for three days, starting the day before the procedure. Heparin and low molecular weight dextran are administered during dilatation; warfarin is started after the procedure and is continued until the follow-up study six to nine months later.

Andreas R Gruntzig, 12 July 1979[1]

Cardiovascular disease accounted for 41% of all deaths in Australia in 1997, costing an estimated $3.7 billion. A large proportion of these deaths was due to coronary disease, and the largest single cause of death was myocardial infarction, accounting for 29 000 deaths.[2] Use of therapeutic coronary intervention, by coronary angioplasty and, more recently, coronary stenting, has grown rapidly in the treatment of symptomatic coronary disease.[3] This rapid increase has in part been made possible by improvements in antiplatelet and anticoagulant therapy.

Tables 14.1 and 14.2 provide details of the various trials mentioned in this chapter.

Table 14.1. Acronyms for trials

CACHET	Comparison of Abciximab Complications with Hirulog (and back-up Abciximab) Events Trial[62]
CAPTURE	Chimeric 7E3 antiplatelet in unstable angina refractory to standard treatment[38]
EPIC	Evaluation of c7E3 for prevention of ischaemic complications[72]
EPILOG	Evaluation of PTCA to improve long-term outcome by c7E3 GP IIb/IIIA receptor blockade[30]
EPISTENT	Randomised placebo-controlled and balloon angioplasty controlled trial to assess safety of coronary stenting with the use of platelet glycoprotein-IIb/IIIa blockade[93]
GUSTO	Global use of strategies to open occluded arteries[71]
HELVETICA	Hirudin in a European trial versus heparin in the prevention of restenosis after PTCA[70]
IMPACT II	Randomised placebo-controlled trial of effect of eptafibatide on complications of percutaneous coronary intervention[77]
ISAR	Intracoronary stenting and antithrombotic regimen[20]
PRISM PLUS	Platelet receptor inhibition in ischaemic syndrome management in patients limited by unstable angina symptoms and signs[80]
PURSUIT	Platelet glycoprotein IIb/IIIa in unstable angina; suppression using integrelin therapy[78]
RAPPORT	Reopro in acute MI Primary PTCA organisation trial[76]
RESTORE	Randomized efficacy study of tirofiban for outcomes and restenosis[79]
STARS	Stent antithrombotic regimen study[19]

Table 14.2. GP IIb/IIIa receptor antagonist trials in percutaneous intervention. 30-day outcome (death and non-fatal MI)

Trial	Patient No	Indication	Drug	Placebo (%)	IIb/IIIa (%)	Risk Redn (%)	Ref
CAPTURE	1252	PTCA	Abciximab	9.0	4.8	47.1	(38)
EPIC	2099	PTCA	Abciximab	10.1	7.0	30.6	(72)
EPILOG	2792	PTCA	Abciximab	9.1	4.0	56.0	(30)
EPISTENT	1603	STENT	Abciximab	10.8	5.3	51.0	(93)
IMPACT II	4010	PTCA	Eptifibatide	8.4	7.1	15.4	(77)
RESTORE	2139	PTCA	Tirofiban	6.3	5.1	19.3	(79)

Rationale for drug use in coronary intervention

Coronary balloon angioplasty, by its very nature, causes atherosclerotic plaque rupture, exposure of the subendothelium to flowing blood, platelet adherence and aggregation, thrombin formation and the generation of fibrin.[4] The stainless steel coronary stent adds a potent thrombogenic stimulus to this already prothrombotic environment.[5] For this reason, the advances in coronary stenting described in Chapter 21 have relied heavily on recent improvements in drug strategies to overcome this inherent tendency to thrombosis.

Drug strategies have focused on two main pathways. First, the central role of thrombin in fibrin production and platelet activation has lead to the development of agents directed at reducing thrombin generation. These include antithrombin III-dependent inhibitors (heparin and its derivatives), the direct thrombin inhibitors (hirudin, bivalirudin and others) and the indirect thrombin inhibitor warfarin. Second, in part because of a realisation of the limited clinical effects of antithrombin agents, there has been increased attention on the central role of the platelet, and development of a number of antiplatelet agents. Here individual agents are discussed, and trial data assessing their use in coronary intervention is assessed. Warfarin and Low Molecular Weight Heparins (LMWHs) are the subject of excellent reviews elsewhere[6,7] and are discussed only briefly.

Aspirin

Aspirin was first tested clinically for a variety of rheumatic conditions in 1899.[8] Its use in cardiovascular disease was described more than 40 years ago, demonstrating a protective effect in acute myocardial infarction,[9] later found to be due to an inhibitory effect on platelets.[10] Aspirin inhibits platelet thromboxane A2 and prostaglandin I2 synthesis by the irreversible acetylation of cyclo-oxygenase.[11] This occurs rapidly, within approximately 30 minutes, and lasts for the lifetime of the platelet, around 10 days. The effect is dose-dependent from 5 mg to 100 mg, with 100 mg causing almost complete inhibition of thromboxane A2.[11] Aspirin has a number of disadvantages, however. It is a relatively weak antiplatelet agent; it has no effect on thromboxane A2 independent pathways; it does not alter platelet adhesion or secretion and its effects are variable between individuals (reviewed in 12). Aspirin causes a dose-dependent risk of major upper gastrointestinal tract bleeding of up to threefold in doses up to 325 mg.[13] The risk is not eliminated by doses less than 100 mg or by coated formulations, but is increased further in doses greater than 325 mg.[11,13] Aspirin also causes dose-dependent increases in nausea, epigastric pain and intracranial haemorrhage, and a non-dose-dependent increase in constipation.[11]

Thienopyridine derivatives (ticlopidine, clopidogrel)

Ticlopidine and clopidogrel are two structurally closely related thienopyridine derivatives.[14] Clopidogrel differs from ticlopidine only by the addition of a carboxymethyl group. Both drugs are inactive *in vitro*, but active orally following hepatic metabolism to one or more metabolically active forms. Excretion is principally renal.[15] The mechanism of action *in vivo* is not completely clear, but *in vitro* studies suggest both ticlopidine and clopidogrel inhibit binding of ADP to low affinity puringenic type two receptors on the platelet, preventing activation of the GP IIb/IIIa receptor and consequent platelet activation.[16] Neither agent promotes platelet conformational change or calcium influx, suggesting the type 1 ADP receptor is not activated and neither agent affects the cyclo-oxygenase pathway, providing a mechanism of action independent from aspirin.[16] Like aspirin, ticlopidine and clopidogrel provide platelet inhibition that is irreversible, and after stopping therapy an effect is present for 7–10 days, equivalent to the lifespan of the platelet. Inhibition is dose-dependent; 20–30% platelet inhibition is achieved in 2–3 days of treatment with 500 mg/day ticlopidine or 75 mg/day clopidogrel.[16,17] The reason for this delay in effect is not known.

Ticlopidine and clopidogrel share a number of side effects. In general, however, side effects occur less frequently with clopidogrel therapy, such that its side-effect profile is similar to that of aspirin.[14,16] Neutropenia (neutrophil count <1200/ml) occurs in 2.4% of patients receiving ticlopidine chronically, and is severe (neutrophil count <450/ml) in 0.9%.[18] It occurs more frequently in elderly females and is associated with a risk of overwhelming infection that can be fatal.[16] It occurs less often in short-term treatment. In two trials of ticlopidine given for 1 month after stenting, the rates of neutropenia were 0.5% and 0.2%, which did not differ significantly from controls (0%).[19,20] Neutropenia is uncommon with clopidogrel. In a trial of 19,185 patients given either clopidogrel or aspirin chronically, severe neutropenia occurred in 0.1%, which did not differ significantly from aspirin (0.17%).[21] Similarly, given acutely for one month after stenting, in addition to aspirin, the incidence of neutropenia was 0% for clopidogrel compared to 0.3% for ticlopidine.[22] Thrombotic thrombocytopenic purpura may occur with long-term ticlopidine treatment, but is very rare in short-term dosing.[23,24] Other side effects shared by the two agents are gastrointestinal (diarrhoea, nausea and dyspepsia) and dermatological (rash, urticaria).[18,25]

IIb/IIIa receptor antagonists

Over the last decade a new class of compound, the platelet IIb/IIIa receptor antagonists, has been introduced. This has resulted from recognition of the importance of the platelet IIb/IIIa receptor in fibrinogen binding to platelets, and use of recombinant technology in designing antagonists.[26,27] The prototype IIb/IIIa receptor antagonist, abciximab (Repro®, Eli Lily & Co.), is a chimeric humanised Fab fragment of a monoclonal antibody to the IIb/IIIa $\alpha_{IIb}\beta_3$) receptor. It also binds with equal affinity to the vitronectin $\alpha_v\beta_3$ receptor, which is present on vascular endothelial and smooth muscle cells, as well as the platelet, and shares the same β_3 sub-unit as the GP IIb/IIIa receptor.[28]

There are two other types of IIb/IIIa antagonists. The first, the peptide eptifibatide, is a synthetic analogue of barbourin, a naturally occuring disintegrin from the venom of the rattlesnake *Sistrurus barbouri*.[29] The second is a group of smaller peptides having the Arg-Gly-Asp (RGD) sequence in common. These include tirofiban, lamifiban and xemilofiban. Despite the diverse structure and methods of synthesis, these agents all bind resting and activated platelets.

Abciximab is given as a bolus (0.25 mg/kg) followed by a 12-hour infusion (0.125 mg/kg/min).[30] Abciximab has a high affinity for the GP IIb/IIIa receptor, a rapid onset of action and provides greater than 80% receptor blockade after bolus administration.[31] Platelet function as assessed by standard means[32] returns to normal within 24–36 hours of treatment with a bolus and 12 hour infusion.[33,34] However, flow cytometric analyses have shown that at 8 and 15 days after treatment, abciximab still provides 29% and 13% receptor blockade.[35] This suggests a longer-term effect on platelets not detected by standard means.

Thrombocytopenia occurs with the IIb/IIIa antagonists. In some cases this appears clinically similar to, and is difficult to distinguish from, heparin-induced thrombocytopenia.[36] In some cases it appears to be a particular effect of abciximab, with an acute (<24 hours after drug initiation) and marked fall in platelet count (to <20 x 10⁹ platelets/ml). This occurs in between 0.3% and 0.79% of patients[37,38] and responds to cessation of all antiplatelet and anticoagulant therapy and platelet infusion, without major complication.[37,39] The pathogenesis is unclear, although it may be related to the generation of human anti chimeric antibodies (HACA), which occurs in up to 6% of abciximab-treated patients.[30]

Other antiplatelet agents

Agents are under development that block various other pathways in the cascade of platelet activation. These include antibodies to von Willebrand Factor (vWF), glycoprotein Ib/IX, inhibitors of vWF binding to Ib/IX, ridogrel and cilostazol.[12,40,41]

Antithrombotics

Unfractionated heparin

Heparin was first isolated in 1916, its name reflecting its original isolation from the liver.[42] It contains a unique pentasaccharide sequence that confers the ability to reversibly bind to the lysine residues on antithrombin III.[43,44] This binding induces a conformational change on the arginine-reactive centre of antithrombin III, which then inhibits the serine active site of thrombin and other enzymes.[45] Unfractionated heparin refers to the variability of the heparin molecule. The mean molecular weights are 15 000, but with variation from 3000 to 30 000 Daltons. Only one-third of these molecules have anticoagulant effect at therapeutic doses.[45,46] The pharmacokinetics of heparin are incompletely understood and complicated by the fact that there is no useful heparin assay. In therapeutic doses the dose response is also variable and non-linear.[45,47] Practically, this means that heparin has a narrow therapeutic window, and dosing has to be carefully monitored by measures of biologic activity, such as the activated clotting time (ACT) or activated partial thromboplastin time (APTT). The half-life following intravenous injection increases with increasing dose, from 30 minutes for a 25 unit/kg bolus to 152 minutes for a 400 unit/kg bolus.[45,48] The mechanisms of metabolism and elimination are unclear.[45] Heparin also has effects other than as an anticoagulant, including inhibition of vascular smooth muscle cell proliferation[49] and increasing vessel permeability.[50]

Low molecular weight heparin

The low molecular weight heparins (LMWHs) constitute the group of heparin molecules between 4000 and 5500 Daltons, and include three formulations: enoxaparin, dalteparin and tinzaparin.[6] LMWHs act mainly to inhibit activated clotting factors, and they have less effect on platelet aggregation and vessel permeability than heparin. These effects suggest LMWHs are likely to be more antithrombotic but less haemorrhagic than unfractionated heparin.[6,51] In addition, LMWHs do not bind to endothelium or to plasma proteins to any degree and show good bioavailabilty following subcutaneous injection. This means they are easier to administer and do not require monitoring, making their clinical use much simpler.[6,51]

Direct thrombin inhibitors

Direct thrombin inhibitors inactivate both free and fibrin bound thrombin.[52] There are two types: (i) the specific thrombin inhibitors hirudin (desirudin) and bivalirudin (hirulog) and (ii) the active site inhibitors including argatroban, efegatran and inogatran. The former bind to two sites on thrombin, the substrate recognition site and the active site, which increases specificity for thrombin. The latter bind only to the active site, which is similar to a number of other serine proteases, so reducing specificity.[53-55]

Hirudin was derived originally from the salivary glands of the medicinal leech *Hirudo medicinalis*, and is now synthesised in a recombinant form. It is a 65 amino acid polypeptide.[53] Bivalirudin (hirulog) is a synthetic 20 amino acid molecule; an active portion is bound to a 12 amino acid sequence analogous to the carboxyterminal portion of hirudin.[54] The direct thrombin inhibitors do not bind plasma proteins, producing a more predictable anticoagulant response.[56] Monitoring of effect is still required for hirudin despite this, since the therapeutic window for this agent is narrow.[5] However, bivalirudin is safe across a range of weight-adjusted doses, so may not require monitoring.[58] Bivalirudin may also offer the advantage over hirudin of activation of the anticoagulant protein C.[59]

The active site thrombin inhibitors include argatroban, efegatran and inogatran. Inogatran is a synthetic low molecular weight peptide which, like the other two agents, showed promising antithrombotic effects in a number of animal models.[60,61]

Treatment following coronary angioplasty

Aspirin was used with heparin, dextran and warfarin in the very first cases of angioplasty in the late 1970s.[1] It has since been used alone as standard antiplatelet therapy following angioplasty,[62] and has been demonstrated to reduce the incidence of periprocedural abrupt vessel closure and myocardial infarction.[63]

In the 1980s *ticlopidine* was also shown, in combination with aspirin, to reduce ischaemic complications related to angioplasty.[64] Given that this combination has recently demonstrated increased platelet inhibition compared with aspirin alone in patients undergoing angioplasty without stenting, and that many patients are now pre-treated with ticlopidine prior to intervention, use of the combination of aspirin and ticlopidine for angioplasty has been recently re-examined.[65]

Heparin has been used routinely to provide periprocedural anticoagulation for angioplasty for more than a decade. It has not, however, been the subject of randomised trials for this indication, but experimental animal data and its efficacy in reducing thrombotic complications in the setting of unstable angina suggest these trials will not be undertaken.[66,67] The principal modification to heparin therapy has been a trend toward lower weight-adjusted doses. Following the introduction of IIb/IIIa receptor antagonists in combination with heparin, the EPILOG trial demonstrated equal efficacy and reduced bleeding complications with a weight-adjusted heparin dose of 70 µg/kg, aiming for an ACT of >200 seconds, compared to a standard heparin dose of 100 µg/kg.[30]

The thrombin inhibitors *bivalirudin* and *hirudin* have both been used as alternatives to heparin in coronary angioplasty. Bivalirudin was found to be at least equivalent to heparin in an early dose ranging study.[68] Subsequently, in 4098 patients with unstable angina and post infarct angina, bivalirudin was compared with heparin.[69] Although there was no benefit for bivalirudin overall, in the sub-group with unstable angina, the endpoint of death, myocardial infarction (MI) or urgent revascularisation was significantly reduced compared with those treated with heparin (4% v 10%. P=0.003).[69] Of note also in this trial, the bivalirudin group had a low (3.7% incidence of >3g/dl Hb loss) rate of bleeding, even when the ACT was >350.[69]

Hirudin has also been compared to heparin following angioplasty for unstable angina in 1141 patients who received either heparin or one of two hirudin regimens. Although a benefit for hirudin was seen at 96 hours, this did not extend to 6 months.[70] A similar finding was observed in the GUSTO IIb study, with hirudin being no more effective than heparin at 30 days. In the GUSTO study 12 142 patients with acute coronary syndromes were randomised to hirudin or heparin, and 22–23% underwent coronary angioplasty (PTCA).[71]

Abciximab was the first IIb/IIIa receptor antagonist to be evaluated by a large-scale clinical trial. This was in the EPIC trial, with 2099 patients undergoing high-risk angioplasty or directional atherectomy.[72] Patients received aspirin and 10 000 to 12 000 units of heparin, aiming for an ACT of 300–350 and maintained as an infusion for at least 12 hours. In addition, they received abciximab as a bolus (0.25 mg/kg), a bolus plus 12-hour infusion (10 µg/min), or placebo. The 30 day endpoint of death, MI or urgent revascularisation occurred in 11.4%, 8.3% and 12.8% respectively, a significant reduction for the bolus and infusion group (p=0.008). An improvement in outcome was observed also at 6 months and 3 years.[73] Subsequent sub-group analyses demonstrating benefit in patients with acute MI[74] and unstable angina[75] provided the rationale for two further trials in these patient sub-groups.[38,76]

The RAPPORT trial examined 483 patients undergoing primary angioplasty for acute MI. They were randomised to either abciximab bolus and 0.125 µg/kg/min infusion or placebo. All patients received aspirin and 100 µg/kg heparin bolus to maintain an ACT greater than 300 secs. Of the 483 enrolled patients, abciximab significantly reduced the incidence of death, reinfarction or urgent target vessel revascularisation compared to placebo at 7 days, (3.3% v 9.9% p=0.003), 30 days (5.8% v 11.2% p=0.03) and 6 months (17.8% v 11.6% p=0.05).[76]

A similar, though less robust, effect was seen in the CAPTURE study of 1265 patients undergoing angioplasty in the context of refractory unstable angina.[38] Patients received placebo or an abciximab bolus and weight-adjusted infusion from 18–24 hours prior to angioplasty until one hour afterwards. The 30-day combined endpoint of death or MI was reduced (4.8% v 9.0% p=0.003), but no benefit was demonstrable at 6 months.[38]

These latter two studies used modified heparin and abciximab doses, both derived from a follow-up study to the EPIC trial, the EPILOG study, which randomised patients undergoing angioplasty to placebo or abciximab with low-dose or standard-dose heparin.[30] Patients with acute myocardial infarction or electrocardiogram changes of unstable angina within the previous 24 hours were excluded. Heparin was given weight adjusted either to 70 µg/kg (low dose), or 100 µg/kg (standard dose). The abciximab infusion dose was also weight adjusted to 0.125 µg/kg/min to a maximum of 10 µg/min. A benefit in the 30-day combined endpoint of death, MI and urgent revascularisation was observed for abciximab and low-dose heparin (5.2%) and abciximab and standard-dose heparin (5.4%) v placebo (11.7%) (p<0.001).[30]

Eptifibatide was studied in 4010 patients undergoing coronary intervention in the IMPACT II trial.[77] More than 90% of the patients were treated by angioplasty alone. Patients were randomised to low-dose eptifibatide (135 µg/kg bolus plus 0.5 µg/kg/min infusion), high dose eptifibatide (the same bolus dose plus 0.75 µg/kg/min infusion) or placebo. There was a decrease of borderline significance in the 30 day combined endpoint of death, MI, and revascularisation for eptifibatide, which was less marked in the high-dose group. There was no difference in outcomes at 6 months.[77] Discussion followed this trial, however, suggesting that the eptifibatide dose used was too low. A subsequent trial used a higher eptifibatide dose of 180 μg/kg bolus followed by a 2.0 μg/kg/min infusion for patients with acute coronary syndromes;[78] 23.3% of the eptifibatide group and 24.8% of the placebo group underwent percutaneous revascularisation or coronary bypass surgery (CABG). There was a small but significant reduction in death or non-fatal MI (14.2% v 15.7%; p=0.004), suggesting the larger dose may be more effective.[78]

Tirofiban was trialled in 2139 patients with acute coronary syndromes undergoing percutaneous revascularisation.[79] More then 90% were treated with angioplasty alone. Patients received either placebo or tirofiban (10 μg/kg bolus followed by a 36-hour infusion of 0.15 μg/kg/min). At 30 days, the combined endpoint of death, MI, revascularisation or need for non-elective stenting during the procedure was not significantly different in the tirofiban and placebo groups (10% v 12.2%; p=0.16), although there was a difference at 7 days (7.6% v 10.4%; p=0.022). Evidence supporting use of tirofiban in patients undergoing angioplasty also comes from the PRISM PLUS trial.[80] This examined use of tirofiban, tirofiban and heparin, and heparin alone in patients with unstable angina. By sub-group analysis, 475 of the study group of 1570 underwent PTCA at 2–4 days after the 48-hour study drug infusion, although this was not randomised. Death or myocardial infarction occurred in 5.9% of the tirofiban and heparin group v 10.2% of the heparin alone group (RR 0.56 95%, CI 0.29 to 1.09).

Overall, there is compelling evidence for the use of aspirin and heparin following angioplasty. There is strong evidence for the use of abciximab, particularly in high-risk patients, and less evidence supporting use of the other agents.

Treatment following coronary stenting

The early experience of coronary stenting has been well documented[14, 81] and was associated with high rates of stent thrombosis—ranging from 6% to 20% despite heavy antithrombotic regimens including aspirin, dipyridamole, dextran, heparin and warfarin. These early studies also reported excessive bleeding.[81,83]

Intravascular ultrasound (IVUS) was pivotal in demonstrating that many stents with satisfactory angiographic appearance were underdeployed.[84] This provided a reason for the initially high rates of stent thrombosis, and a rationale for proceeding to high-pressure balloon inflation to ensure optimal stent deployment, following this with a simplified antiplatelet regimen without anticoagulation. A number of the initial registries used only aspirin and ticlopidine, with or without heparin, and reported stent thrombosis rates of 0–1.4% and bleeding rates of 0–2.2%.[84,85] Two subsequent randomised but not blinded trials, ISAR and STARS, confirmed the registry findings.[19,20] In the ISAR trial, the aspirin and ticlopidine group had a 1.6% combined cardiac endpoint compared with 6.2% (p<0.01) for the phenprocoumon group, and no incidence of stent thrombosis compared with 5.0% (p<0.01).[20] The STARS trial demonstrated a similar improvement of 0.5% v 2.7% (p=0.07) in a combined cardiac endpoint for aspirin and ticlopidine versus warfarin.[19] The STARS study included a group randomised to aspirin alone. This group had a combined endpoint of 3.6%, higher than the warfarin group.[19]

Whether ticlopidine is required in addition to aspirin for all sub-sets of stented patients is not known. Initially, a number of non-randomised registries with small patient numbers suggested aspirin alone in selected patients was associated with a low rate of complications,[86,87] proposing the hypothesis that aspirin alone may be sufficient in low-risk patients.[88] This question has been largely bypassed by the advent of clopidogrel. Clopidogrel has fewer side effects than ticlopidine, and recent data suggest these two agents are equally effective when used in combination with aspirin following stent implantation. In a recent non-randomised study, there was no difference in the rates of subacute thrombosis or major cardiac events (1.5% v 1.4% and 3.1% v 2.4%, p=NS respectively for ticlopidine versus clopidogrel, both for one month) whereas the clopidogrel group had a significantly lower rate of side effects (neutropenia, diarrhoea and rash) compared to ticlopidine (10.6% v 5.3%; p=0.006).[22] A subsequent single-centre observational study of 500 patients compared aspirin and clopidogrel (300 mg loading dose and 75 mg/day for two weeks) with aspirin and ticlopidine (500 mg loading dose and 250 mg bd for two weeks) and found no difference in 30-day event rates (0.8% v 1.6%; p=NS) and no incidence of neutropenia or thrombotic thrombocytopenic purpura (TTP).[89] This study was not randomised or powered to detect equivalence and since similar results were obtained in another registry giving clopidogrel or ticlopidine for 2–4 weeks, without a loading dose,[90] the issues of optimal agent, duration of therapy, and need for a loading dose, remain unanswered. The ongoing CREDO trial may answer these questions,[91] but with new agents such as cilostazol already undergoing preliminary testing,[41] this field is likely to continue to change rapidly. At present, aspirin with clopidogrel given as a loading dose of 150–300 mg, followed by 75 mg/day for 2–4 weeks, is commonly accepted practice.

Stents also have the potential for providing local drug delivery by means of stent coatings. A heparin-coated stent has been tested clinically in the Benestent II trial of 827 patients, who received either angioplasty, or a heparin-coated stent and ticlopidine for one month. The combined endpoint at 6 months of death, MI, repeat PTCA or CABG was reduced in the stent group compared with angioplasty (12.8% v 19.3%; p=0.016) with a similar effect observed at 12 months.[92]

The benefits observed with IIb/IIIa receptor antagonists with angioplasty and the more prothrombotic environment in the context of stenting provided the rationale for use of these agents in stenting. The principal source of data comes from the EPISTENT trial, which compared stent alone v abciximab and PTCA v abciximab and stent in a total of 2,399 patients. The two stent groups also received ticlopidine. The 30 day combined endpoints of death, MI or urgent revascularisation were 10.8%, 6.9% and 5.3% (p<0.001) respectively; significantly lower for the stent alone group.[93] Major bleeding was increased non-significantly in the stent alone group. An additional finding from EPISTENT was the similar outcomes of PTCA with abciximab compared to stent alone. Some data are also available from an analysis of the EPILOG trial.[30,94] Unplanned stenting was significantly less in the abciximab group compared to placebo (9.1% v 14.7% p<0.01). Interestingly, this benefit was more pronounced for those with eccentric complex lesions, compared to concentric straightforward lesions.[94]

Oral GP IIb/IIIa antagonists are theoretically attractive in their potential to provide longer term platelet inhibition following revascularisation, but their place has yet to be defined.[95] The oral agent xemilofiban in doses greater than 10 mg showed >50% inhibition of aggregation in response to ADP and collagen when given alongside abciximab in stented patients, with an effect present out to 2 weeks.[96] Xemilofiban was also given to 23 patients with unstable angina undergoing angioplasty; rapid and sustained platelet inhibition was demonstrated, but was associated with excessive bleeding.[97] However, a recently completed study in 7232 patients randomised to one of two xemilofiban doses or placebo suggested no benefit.[98]

Despite a large number of clinical trials, the optimal antiplatelet and antithrombotic regimen post stenting remains unclear. Evidence suggests that abciximab reduces ischaemic complications. The evidence for the other IIb/IIIa receptor antagonists is less compelling. The optimal combination of IIb/IIIa antagonist, aspirin, and clopidogrel or ticlopidine, and the treatment duration are also unclear. Common clinical practice, in part because of cost concerns, has reserved the use of the IIb/IIIa antagonists for rescue rather than prophylactic use, and favours clopidogrel over ticlopidine in addition to aspirin.

Future prospects

The pace of change in antiplatelet and anticoagulant therapies in the last decade has been rapid, with a number of factors influencing future improvements. Significantly, the endpoints of stent thrombosis and cardiovascular morbidity have become low in the more recent trials. At one month, stent thrombosis is 0.5–1.4%, mortality 0–0.9% and any major adverse cardiac event 2.3–2.4%.[19,20] Thus any new drug therapy is likely to need randomised trials involving large numbers of patients, to demonstrate an improvement in efficacy over standard therapy.[99] Partly in recognition of this and partly in response to questions over the cost of new agents, a number of the latest trials are aimed at demonstrating equivalence of effect with fewer side effects and/or lower cost. An example is the upcoming CACHET trial of bivalirudin with abciximab backup compared with abciximab and weight-adjusted heparin for angioplasty and stenting, aimed at exploiting the low incidence of bleeding and favourable short-term outcome with bivalirudin, and this may provide some answers as to which particular groups of patients are likely to benefit from abciximab.[62] A large number of potential new agents are becoming available, and it seems likely that many will be tested in a similar way.[99]

A number of other developments may influence new therapies. The recognition of certain patient sub-sets at particular risk of thrombosis through genetic,[100] clinical or other variables will mean therapies may be able to be specifically targeted. Technological advances such as molecular biological techniques have already contributed to development of the IIb/IIIa receptor antagonists and thrombin inhibitors.[26] These techniques are now being extended to examine the pathways of gene expression that precede events at the cell surface, and may provide the next avenue of therapeutic potential.[101]

References

1. Gruntzig AR, Senning A, Siegenthaler WE. Nonoperative dilatation of coronary-artery stenosis. *N Engl J Med* 1979; **301**:61–8.
2. Australian Institute of Health and Welfare. *Heart, stroke and vascular diseases, Australian facts 1999*. Australian Institute of Health and Welfare and Heart Foundation of Australia.
3. Lane DM. Dramatic increase in the use of coronary stents. *Am J Cardiol* 1999; **84**:1141.
4. Badimon L, Badimon JJ, Fuster V. Pathogenesis of Thrombosis. In Fuster V, Verstrate M (eds). *Thrombosis in cardiovascular disorders*. Philadelphia: WB Saunders 1992, 17–39.
5. Serruys PW, Strauss BH, Beatt KJ *et al*. Angiographic follow-up after placement of a self-expanding coronary artery stent. *N Engl J Med* 1991; **3214**:13–17.
6. Turpie AGC, successors to heparin: new antithrombotic agents. *Am Heart J* 1997; **134**:S71–S77.
7. Tcheng JE, Kong DF. Vale, warfarin: a stentorian farewell. *Am Heart J* 1999; **138**:602–4.
8. Rainsford KD. *Aspirin and the salicylates*. London: Butterworth 1984
9. Craven LL. Experiences with aspirin (acetylsalicyclic acid) in the nonspecific prophylaxis of coronary thrombosis. *Mississippi Valley Med J* 1953; **75**:38–40.
10. Weiss HJ and Aledort LM. Impaired platelet-connective tissue reaction in man after aspirin ingestion. *Lancet* 1967; **2**:495–97.
11. Patrono C. Aspirin as an antiplatelet drug. *N Engl J Med* 1994; **330**:1287–93.
12. Theroux P. Antiplatelet therapy: do the new platelet inhibitors add significantly to the clinical benefits of aspirin ? *Am Heart J* 1997; **134**:S62–S70.

13.   Kelly JP, Kaufman DW, Jurgelon JM *et al*. Risk of aspirin-associated major upper-gastrointestinal bleeding with enteric-coated or buffered product. *Lancet* 1996; **348**:1413–16.

14.   Sharis PJ, Cannon CP, Loscalzo J. The antiplatelet effects of ticlopidine and clopidogrel. *Ann Intern Medicine* 1998; **129**:394–405.

15.   Verstraete M, Zoldhelyi P. Novel antithrombotic drugs in development. *Drugs* 1995; **49**:856–84.

16.   Herbert JM, Frehel D, Vallee E *et al*. Clopidogrel, a novel antiplatelet and antithrombotic agent. *Cardiovasc Drug Rev* 1993; **11**:180–98.

17.   Coukell AJ, Markham A. Clopidogrel. *Drugs* 1997; **54**:745–50.

18.   Hass WK, Easton JD, Adams HP Jr *et al*. A randomised trial comparing ticlopidine with aspirin for the prevention of stroke in high risk patients. Ticlopidine Aspirin Stroke Study Group. *N Engl J Med* 1989; **321**:501–7.

19.   Leon MB, Baim DS, Popma JJ *et al*. A clinical trial comparing three antithrombotic-drug regimens after coronary-artery stenting. Stent Anticoagulation Restenosis Study Investigators. *N Engl J Med* 1998; **339**:1665–71.

20.   Schomig A, Neuman FJ, Kastrati A *et al*. A randomised comparison of antiplatelet and anticoagulant therapy after the placement of coronary-artery stents. *N Engl J Med* 1996; **334**:1084–9.

21.   CAPRIE steering committee. A randomised, blinded, trial of clopidogrel versus aspirin in patients at risk for ischaemic events (CAPRIE). *Lancet* 1996; **348**:1329–1339.

22.   Moussa I, Oetgen M, Roubin G *et al*. Effectiveness of clopidogrel and aspirin versus ticlopidine and aspirin in preventing stent thrombosis after coronary stent implantation. *Circulation* 1999; **99**:2364–66.

23.   Muszkat M, Shapira MY, Sviri S *et al*. Ticlopidine-induced thrombotic thrombocytopenic purpura. *Pharmacotherapy* 1998; **18**:1352–5.

24.   Bennett CL, Weinberg PD, Rozenberg-Ben-Dror K *et al*. Thrombotic thrombocytopenic purpura associated with ticlopidine. A review of 60 cases. *Ann Intern Med* 1998; **128**:541–4.

25.   Molony BA. An analysis of the side effects of ticlopidine. In Haas SK and Easton. JD (eds) *Ticlopidine, platelets and vascular disease*. New York: Spinger-Verlag 1993, 117–39.

26.   Topol EJ, Byzova TV, Plow EF, Platelet GPIIb-IIIa blockers. *Lancet* 1999; **353**:227–31.

27.   Lefkovitz J, Plow EF, Topol EJ. Platelet Glycoprotein IIb/IIIa receptors in cardiovascular disease. *N Engl J Med* 1995; **332**:1553–9.

28.   Nakada MT, Jordan RE, Knight. DM., Abciximab (reopro, chimeric 7E3 Fab) cross reactivity with AvB3 integrin receptors: a potential mechanism for the prevention of restenosis. *J Am Coll Cardiol* 1997; **29**:243A.

29.   Scarborough RM. Development of eptifibatide. *Am Heart J* 1999; **138**:1093–104.

30.   EPILOG investigators. Platelet glycoprotein IIb/IIIa receptor blockade and low-dose heparin during percutaneous coronary revascularisation. *N Engl J Med* 1997; **336**:1689–96.

31.   Coller BS, Scudder LE, Beer J *et al*. Monoclonal antibodies to platelet glycoprotein IIb/IIIa as antithrombotic agents. *Ann N Y Acad Sc* 1991; **614**:193–213.

32.   Born GVR, Aggregation of blood platelets by adenosine diphosphate and its reversal. *Nature* 1969; **194**:927–29.

33.   Tcheng JE, Ellis SG, George BS *et al*. Pharmacodynamics of chimeric glycoprotein IIb/IIIa integrin anti-platelet antibody Fab 7E3 in high-risk coronary angioplasty. *Circulation* 1994; **90**:1757–64.

34.   Mascelli MA, Worley S, Veriabo NJ *et al*. Rapid assessment of platelet function with a modified whole-blood aggregometer in percutaneous transluminal angioplasty patients receiving anti-GP IIb/IIIa therapy. *Circulation* 1997. **96**:3860–3866.

35.   Mascelli MA, Lance ET, Damaraju L *et al*. Pharmacodynamic profile of short-term abciximab treatment demonstrates prolonged platelet inhibition with gradual recovery from GP IIb/IIIa receptor blockade. *Circulation* 1998; **97**:1680–88.

36.   Madan M, Berkowitz SD, and Tcheng JE. Glycoprotein IIb/IIIa integrin blockade. *Circulation* 1998; **98**:2629–35.

37.   Berkowitz SD, Harrington RA, Rund MM, Tcheng JE. Acute profound thrombocytopenia after c&E3 Fab (abciximab) therapy. *Circulation* 1997; **95**:809–13.

38.   CAPTURE and investigators. Randomised placebo-controlled trial of abciximab before and

during coronary intervention in refractory unstable angina:the CAPTURE study. *Lancet* 1999; **349**:1429–35.

39. Berkowitz SD, Harrington RA, Rund MM *et al*. Acute profound thrombocytopenia after c7E3 Fab (abciximab) therapy (letter). *Circulation* 1997; **96**:3810.

40. Weitz JI, Califf RM, Ginsberg JS *et al*. New Antithombotics. *Chest* 1995; **108** (suppl 4):471S–85S.

41. Yoon Y, Shim W, Lee D *et al*. Usefulness of cilostazol versus ticlopidine in coronary artery stenting. *Am J Cardiol* 1999; **84**:1375–80.

42. McLean J. The thromboplastic action of cephalin. *Am J Physiol* 1916; **41**:250–7.

43. Rosenberg RD, Lam L. Correlation between structure and function of heparin. *Proc Nat Acad Sci* 1979; **76**:1218–22.

44. Choay J, Petitou M, Lormeau JC *et al*. Structure-activity relationship in heparin: a synthetic pentasaccharide with high affinity for anti-thrombin III and eliciting high anti-factor Xa activity. Biophysical Research Communications 1983; **116**:492-9.

45. Hirsh J. Heparin. *N Engl J Med* 1991; **324**:1565–74.

46. Andersson LO, Barrowcliffe TW, Holmer E *et al*. Anticoagulant properties of heparin fractionated by affinity chromatography on matrix-bound antithrombin III adn by gel filtration. *Thrombosis Res* 1976; **9**:575–83.

47. de Swart CAM, Hijmeyer B, Roelofs JMM *et al*. Kinetics of intravenously administered heparin in normal humans. *Blood* 1982; **47**:385–417.

48. Bjornsson TO, Wolfram BS, and Kitchell BB. Heparin kinetics determined by three assay methods. *Clin Pharm Ther* 1982; **31**:104–13.

49. Clowes AW, Karnovsky MJ. Supression by heparin of smooth muscle cell proliferation in injured arteries. *Nature* 1977; **265**:625–6.

50. Blajchman MA, Young E, Ofusu FA. Effects of unfractionated heparin, dermatan sulfate and low molecular weight heparin on vessel wall permeability in rabbits. *Ann N Y Acad Sci* 1989; **556**:245–54.

51. Hirsh J, Levine MN. Low-molecular weight heparin. *Blood* 1992; **79**:1–17.

52. Weitz JI, Huboda M, Massel D *et al*. Clot-bound thrombin is protected from inhibition by heparin-antithrombin III but is susceptible to inactivation by antithrombin III-dependent inhibitors. *J Clin Invest* 1990; *86*:385–91.

53. Stone SR, Hofsteenge J. Kinetics of inhibition of thrombin by hirudin. *Biochemistry* 1986; **25**:4622–28.

54. Maraganore JM, Bourdon P, Jablonski J *et al*. Design and characterisation of the hirulogs: a novel class of bivalent peptide inhibitors of thrombin. *Biochemistry* 1990; **29**:7095–101.

55. Hirsh J, Weitz JI. New Antithrombotic Agents. *Lancet* 1999; **353**:1431–36.

56. Marbet GA, Verstraete M, Kienast J *et al*. Clinical pharmacology of intravenously administered recombinant desulfatohirudin (CGP 39393) in healthy volunteers. *J Cardiovasc Pharmacol* 1993; **22**:364–72.

57. GUSTO investigators. Randomized trial of intravenous heparin versus recombinant hirudin for acute coronary syndromes. *Circulation* 1994; **90**:1631–37.

58. Bittl JA. comparative safety profiles of hirulog and heparin in patients undergoing coronary angioplasty. *Am Heart J* 1995; **130**:658–65.

59. Bates SM and Weitz JI. Direct thrombin inhibitors for treatment of arterial thrombosis: potential differences between bivalirudin and hirudin. *Am J Cardiol* 1998; **82**:12P–18P.

60. Uriuda Y, Wang Q-D, Grip L *et al*. Antithrombotic activity of inogatran, a new low-molecular weight inhibitor of thrombin, in a closed chest porcine model of coronary artery thrombosis. *Cardiovasc Res* 1996; **32**:320–7.

61. Gustavsson D, Elg M, Lenfors S *et al*. Effects of inogatran, a new low molecular weight thrombin inhibitor, in rat models of venous thrombosis, thrombolysis and bleeding time. *Blood Coag Fibrinol* 1996; **7**:69–79.

62. Topol EJ. Evolution of improved antithrombotic and antiplatelet agents: genesis of the comparison of abciximab complications with hirulog (and back-up abcixiamb) events trial (Cachet). *Am J Cardiol* 1998; **82**:63P–68P.

63. Schwartz L, Bourassa MG, Lesperance J *et al*. Aspirin and dipyridamole in the prevention of

restenosis after percutaneous transluminal coronary angioplasty. *N Engl J Med* 1988; **318**:1714.19.

64.   White CW, Chaitman B, Lassar TA *et al*. Antiplatelet agents are effective in reducing the immediate complications of PTCA: results from the ticlopidine multicenter trial. *Circulation* 1987; **76** (suppl):IV–400A.

65.   van de Loo A, Nauck M, Noory E *et al*. Enhancement of platelet inhibition of ticlopidine plus aspirin vs aspirin alone given prior to elective PTCA. *Eu Heart J* 1998; **19**:96–102.

66.   Lukas MA, Deutsch E, WK. Beneficial effect of heparin therapy on PTCA outcome in unstable angina. *J Am Coll Cardiol* 1988; **11** (suppl):132A.

67.   Heras M, Chesebro JH, Penny WJ *et al*. Importance of adequate heparin dosage in arterial angioplasty in a porcine model. *Circulation* 1988; **78**:654–60.

68.   Topol EJ, Bonan R, Jewitt D *et al*. Use of a direct antithrombin, hirulog, in place of heparin during coronary angioplasty. *Circulation* 1993; **87**:1622–29.

69.   Bittl JA, Strony J, Brinker HA *et al*. Treatment with bivalirudin (hirulog) as compared to heparin during coronary angioplasty for unstable or postinfarct angina. *N Engl J Med* 1995; **333**:764–69.

70.   Serruys PW, Herrman J-PR, Simon R *et al*. A comparison of hirudin with heparin in the prevention of restenosis after coronary angioplasty. *N Engl J Med* 1995; **333**:757–63.

71.   GUSTO IIb investigators. A comparison of recombinant hirudin with heparin for the treatment of acute coronary syndromes. *N Engl J Med* 1996; **335**:775–82.

72.   EPIC investigators. Use of a monoclonal antibody directed against the platelet glycoprotein IIb/IIIa integrin platelet antibody Fab 7E3 in high-risk coronary angioplasty. *N Engl J Med* 1994; **330**:956–61.

73.   Topol EJ, Ferguson JJ, Weisman HF *et al*. Long term protection from myocardial ischaemic events in a randomised trial of brief integrin b3 blockade with percutaneous intervention. *J Am Med Assoc* 1997; **278**:479–84.

74.   Lefkovitz J, Ivanhoe RJ, Califf RM *et al*. Effects of platelet glycoprotein IIb/IIIa receptor blockade by a chimeric monoclonal antibody (abciximab) on acute and six-month outcomes after percutaneous transluminal coronary angioplasty for acute myocardial infaction. *Am J Cardiol* 1996; **77**:1045–51.

75.   Lincoff AM, Califf RM, Anderson KM *et al*. Evidence for prevention of death and myocardial infarction with platelet membrane glycoprotein IIb/IIIa blockade by abciximab (c7E3 Fab) among patients with unstable angina undergoing percutaneous coronary revascularisation. *J Am Coll Cardiol* 1997; **30**:149–56.

76.   Brener SJ, Barr LA, Burchenal JEB *et al*. Randomised, placebo-controlled trial of platelet glycoprotein IIb/IIIa blockade with primary angioplasty for acute myocardial infarction. *Circulation* 1998; **98**:734–41.

77.   IMPACT II investigators. Randomised placebo-controlled trial of effect of eptafibatide on complications of percutaneous coronary intervention: IMPACT II. *Lancet* 1997; **349**:1422–28.

78.   PURSUIT, trial investigators. Inhibition of platelet glycoprotein IIb/IIIa with eptifibatide in patients with acute coronary syndromes. *N Engl J Med* 1998; **339**:436–43.

79.   Gibson CM, Goel M, Cohen DJ *et al*. Six-month angiographic and clinical follow-up of patients prospectively randomized to receive either tirofiban or placebo during angioplasty in the RESTORE trial. Randomized Efficacy Study of Tirofiban for Outcomes and Restenosis. *J Am Coll Cardiol* 1998; **32**:28–34.

80.   PRISM-PLUS study investigators. Inhibition of the platelet glycoprotein IIb/IIa receptor with tirofiban in unstable angina and non-Q wave myocardial infarction. *N Engl J Med* 1998; **338**:1488–97.

81.   Eeckout E, Kappenberger L, Goy JL. Stents for intracoronary placement: current concepts and future directions. *J Am Coll Cardiol* 1996; **27**:757–65.

82.   Sigwart U, Puel J, Mirkovitch *et al*. Intravascular stents to prevent occlusion and restenosis after angioplasty. *N Engl J Med* 1987; **613**:701–6.

83.   Mak KH, Belli G, Ellis SG *et al*. Subacute stent thrombosis: evolving issues and current concepts. *J Am Coll Cardiol* 1996; **27**:494–503.

84.   Colombo A, Hall P, Nakamura S *et al*. Intracoronary stenting without anticoagulation accomplished with intravascular ultrasound guidance. *Circulation* 1995; **91**:1676–88.

85.   Karrilon GJ, Morice MC, Benveniste E *et al*. Intracoronary stent implantation without ultrasound

guidance and with replacement of conventional anticoagulation by antiplatelet therapy. 30 day clinical outcome of the French Multicenter Registry. *Circulation* 1996; **94**:1519–27.

86. Albeiro R, Hall P, Itoh A *et al.* Results of a consecutive series of patients receiving only antiplatelet therapy after optimized stent implantation. Comparison of aspirin alone versus combined ticlopidine and aspirin therapy. *Circulation*; **95**:1145–56.

87. Roy PR, Lowe HC, Walker BW *et al.* Intracoronary stenting without intravascular ultrasound guidance followed by antiplatelet therapy with aspirin alone in selected patients. *Am J Cardiol* 1996; **77**:1105–7.

88. Lowe HC, Baron D, Roy PR. Combined Ticlopidine and Aspirin Versus Aspirin Therapy Alone After Stent Implantation. *Circulation* (letter) 1996; **74**:2993.

89. Berger PB, Bell MR, Rihal CS *et al.* Clopidogrel versus ticlopidine after intracoronary stent placement. *J Am Coll Cardiol* 1999; **34**:1891–4.

90. Mishkel GJ, Aguirre FV, Ligon RW *et al.* Clopidogrel as adjunctive therapy during coronary stenting. *J Am Coll Cardiol* 1999; **34**:1884–90.

91. Klein LW and Calvin JE. Use of clopidrogel in coronary stenting: what was the question? *J Am Coll Cardiol* 1999; **34**:1895–98.

92. Serruys PW, van Hout B, Bonnier H *et al.* Randomised comparison of implantation of heparin-coated stents with balloon angioplasty in selected patients with coronary artery disease (Benestent II). *Lancet* 1998; **352**:673–81.

93. EPISTENT investigators. Randomised placebo-controlled and balloon angioplasty controlled trial to assess safety of coronary stenting with the use of platelet glycoprotein-IIb/IIIa blockade. *Lancet* 1998; **352**:87–92.

94. Dangas G, Colombo A. Platetet glycoprotein IIb/IIIa antagonists in percutaneous coronary revascularisation. *Am Heart J* 1999; **138**:S16–23.

95. Ferguson JJ and Lau TK. New antiplatelet agents for acute coronary syndromes. *Am Heart J* 1998; **135**:S194–S200.

96. Kereiakes DJ, Kleiman N, Ferguson JJ *et al.* Sustained platelet glycoprotein IIb/IIIa blockade with oral xemilofiban in 170 patients after coronary stent deployment. *Circulation* 1997; **96**:1117–21.

97. Simpendorfer C, Kottke-Marchant K, Topol EJ. First experience with chronic platelet GP IIa/IIIb receptor blockade: a pilot study of xemilofiban, an orally active antagonist in unstable angina patients eligible for PTCA. *J Am Coll Cardiol* 1996; **27**:242A.

98. Ferguson JJ. Meeting Highlights. *Circulation* 1999; **100**:570–5.

99. Califf RM. A perspective on the regulation of the evaluation of new antithrombotic drugs. *Am J Cardiol* 1998; **82**:25P–35P.

100. Walter DH, Schachinger V *et al.* Platelet glycoprotein IIIa polymorphisms and risk of coronary stent thrombosis. *Lancet* 1997; **350**:1217–19.

101. Topol EJ, Serruys PW. Frontiers in interventional cardiology. *Circulation* 1998; **98**:1802–20.

Chapter 15

The Electrocardiogram in Ischaemic Heart Disease

Geoffrey S. Oldfield

Electrical activation of the heart

Anatomy

The electrical system of the heart consists of specialised muscle fibres. To the naked eye, these are unrecognisable from contractile muscle and require histochemical techniques to be recognised. The components of this system are the sino-atrial (SA) node, the internodal pathways, the atrio-ventricular (AV) node, the Bundle of His and the Purkinje system (Fig 15.1). It is interesting that the discovery of the various parts of the pathway was in reverse order of activation, commencing with Purkinje in 1845 and finishing with Keith & Flack discovering the sinus node in 1907.

The SA node is the primary cardiac pacemaker and is found high in the right atrium, just anterolateral to its connection with the superior vena cava (SVC). It is approximately 25 mm in length and is richly supplied with autonomic nerve fibres and blood vessels. It is connected to the AV node by three internodal tracts—the anterior, middle and posterior internodal tracts. The anterior tract passes anteriorly and to the left of the superior vena cava, entering the anterior inter-atrial band, and then splits into two parts, the first passing to the left atrium (Bachmans' Bundle), the second descending anteriorly in the inter-atrial

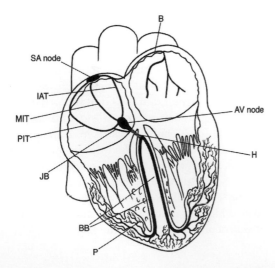

Figure 15.1. The electrical system of the heart. B = Bachman's bundle of the anterior internodal tract, IAT = interatrial bundle of anterior internodal tract, MIT = middle internodal tract, PIT = posterior internodal tract, JB = James' bypass fibres, H = common bundle of His, BB = bundle branches, P = Purkinje network.

septum to the AV node. The middle internodal tract runs in the inter-atrial septum to the AV node, whilst the posterior internodal tract terminates with most of its fibres bypassing the proximal and middle portions of the AV node to enter the distal portion (James' By-pass Tract). The AV node is approximately 6 x 3 x 2 mm in size and lies in the right atrium, on the right side of the inter-atrial septum, in front of the opening of the coronary sinus above the attachment of the septal cusp of the tricuspid valve. The distal 'tail' of the AV node is contiguous with the Bundle of His, which is approximately 20 x 3 mm. It bifurcates early into 'branching' and 'penetrating' segments. The branching segments arise immediately distal to the AV node in the proximal His Bundle. It branches proximally to form the posterior fibres of the left bundle branch, then divides to form the anterior fibres of the left bundle branch and the right bundle branch.

The 'penetrating' branch runs through the central fibrous structure and has no contact with myocardium. The right main bundle runs down the right side of the interventricular septum towards the apex. Initially it lies deep in the endocardium and has only a few branches, but on reaching the moderator band its free edge runs inwards to the base of the anterior papillary muscle of the right ventricle, where it branches to supply the whole of the right ventricular endocardium. The left main His Bundle emerges on the left side of the interventricular septum (IVS), just below the non-coronary cusp of the aortic valve and passes down the septum, sending branches into the septum until about a third of the way down the IVS. Here it breaks into posterior and anterior branches that pass the postero-medial and antero-lateral papillary muscles, where it branches to form the complex Purkinje network of fibres supplying the left ventricular endocardium.

Mode of activation of myocardium

The normal impulse originates in the SA node and passes longitudinally through the atria as a 'wavefront', initially activating the right atrium in a rightwards and anterior direction. This is followed by activation of the left atrium, in a left and posterior direction. The 'wavefront' is rapid, travelling longitudinally and contiguously at approximately 1000 mm/ second throughout the atrial muscle.

The impulse arrives at the AV node via the specialised internodal pathway, where it is delayed due to decremented conduction. The earliest sub-endocardial depolarisation is detected simultaneously on the left central side of the interventricular septum, and on the high anterior and infero-apico-septal regions. The wave of depolarisation then spreads transversely from endocardium to epicardium through the thickness of the left and right ventricular walls. The epicardial depolarisation is detected first on the right antero-apical region, followed by the anterior and posterior para-septal regions of the left ventricle. The lateral wall and basal septum are activated last. The Purkinje system extends to varying depths into the sub-endocardial layer in each individual, penetrating 3–4 mm into the free ventricular walls from the endocardium. Activation of the sub-endocardial layer (which is electrically silent) is not recorded on the surface electrocardiogram (ECG). It was originally theorised by Sodi-Pallares[1-4] that the island of Purkinje tissue acted as a 'closed polarised island' where activation from the many Purkinje fibres spreads outwards in a 'spherical' manner through the myocardium. It was not until activation reached the endocardium that the 'closed islands' opened and net activation began to spread to the epicardium so a positive potential would be recorded (Fig. 15.2). Sodi-Pallares referred to the (electrically silent) Purkinje ridge sub-endocardial layer as the 'electrical sub-endocardial surface'. The thickness or depth of this sub-endocardial layer is highly variable. Durrer[5] and others subsequently showed the complete sequence of ventricular activation of the heart.

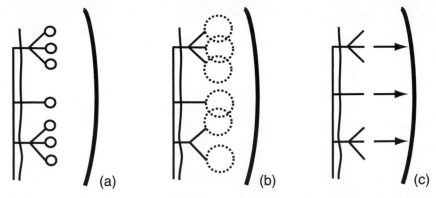

Figure 15.2. *Diagrammatic representation of Sodi-Pallares' 'electrical endocardial surface' concept. Electrical activation arrives at the endocardial surface via the Purkinje fibres. At first, activation is restricted to closed polarized spheres, or 'closed islands' (a). The spheres coalesce and open to the endocardium (b), forming a progressive electrical wavefront spreading outwards and transversely (c) through the ventricular free wall.*

When the wave of depolarisation moves towards a positive pole, the deflection is positive; when it moves away from the positive pole, or towards a negative pole, the deflection is negative. In an isolated muscle strip, depolarisation (an advancing wave of positive charge) and repolarisation (a wave of negative charge) both take place from the endocardium to epicardium. The result is that the polarity of repolarisation in the muscle strip is the opposite to that of depolarisation.

In the intact human heart, however, depolarisation also takes place from endocardium to epicardium but repolarisation takes place from epicardium to endocardium, the reverse. Here, polarity of repolarisation is the same as for depolarisation. A small number of individuals, however, especially athletes, may have their repolarisation process as in the isolated muscle strip, so in these individuals T wave inversion may be seen in many leads, particularly the precordial leads.

Thus, depolarisation begins on the left side of the interventricular septum and spreads outwards through the free walls of the ventricles. From an electrocardiographic point of view, the ventricles consist of three muscle masses, the interventricular septum and the free walls (muscle masses) of the right and left ventricles (Fig. 15.3).

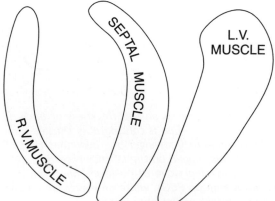

Figure 15.3. *The ventricle may be considered electrographically as three separate muscle masses, as shown.*

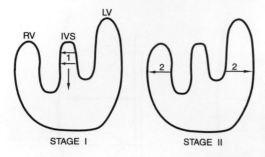

Figure 15.4. Activation of ventricular muscle proceeds first from the interventricular septum (IVS) (1), then spreads across the rest of the muscle mass (2).

The standard surface-recorded ECG is the sum of the potential electrical forces recorded in various planes. Activation of the interventricular septum occurs first (stage 1) and is followed by activation of the rest of the muscle mass (stage 2) (Fig. 15.4).

Because the mass of the left ventricle (LV) is much greater than that of the right vebtricle (RV), the electrical potential from the LV overrides that of the RV on surface ECG electrodes (Fig. 15.5).

Standard ECG leads and electrocardiographic interpretation

Einthoven's triangle (Fig. 15.6) is derived from leads placed on the right and left wrists and the left ankle. The standard ECG is made up of 12 leads: Three standard bipolar leads I, II and III derived from Einthoven's equilateral triangle, plus three augmented extremity leads, which are uni-polar leads and are prefixed with the letter 'a', plus six chest 'V' leads.

The augmented uni-polar leads on the arms and legs are seen as an extension of the torso and record activity from each peripheral electrode (Fig. 15.7). A brief description of the 12 basic ECG leads follows.

I   Lead I connects the left and right wrists
II   Lead II connects the right arm and left ankle
III   Lead III connects the left arm and left ankle

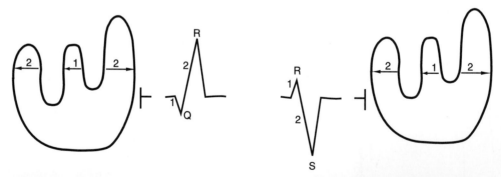

Figure 15.5. The size of the electrical potential depends on the thickness of each of the three muscle masses. As the left ventricular wall mass is considerably thicker than that of the right ventricle, its signal is correspondingly stronger and overrides that of the right ventricle on the ECG trace. An electrode placed on the LV thus records a nett positive deflection with depolarisation (an advancing wave of positive charge moving towards the electrode causes a positive deflection on ECG), while an electrode on the RV records a nett negative deflection (the dominant effect here is a nett positive wave moving away from this electrode).

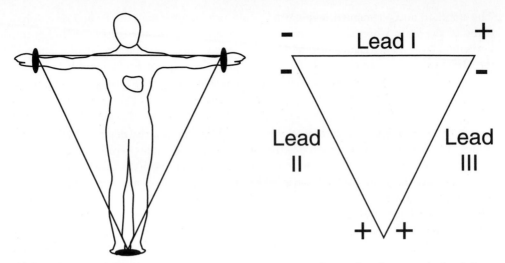

Figure 15.6. Einthoven's triangle, showing the three lines of reference derived from the limb leads.

aVR	The right arm augmented unipolar lead effectively records conduction from the right shoulder
aVL	The left arm augmented unipolar lead records conduction from the left shoulder
aVF	The left leg augmented unipolar lead records conduction from the left thigh
V1	This lead is placed on the 4th right intercostal space, 2.5 cm from the midline of the sternum
V2	This lead is placed on the 4th left intercostal space, 2.5 cm from the middle of the sternum
V3	This lead is placed halfway between V2 and V4
V4	This lead is placed on the 5th left intercostal space in the mid-clavicular line
V5	This lead is placed on the anterior axillary line at the same level as V4
V6	This lead is placed on the mid-axillary line at the same level as V5.

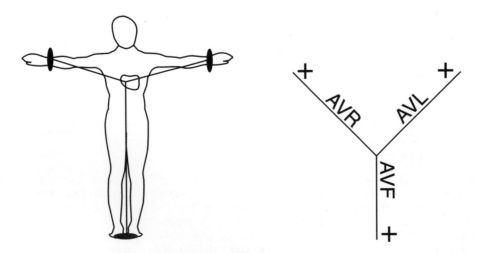

Figure 15.7. Three additional lines of reference formed from the augmented limb leads.

The standard and augmented unipolar leads are oriented through the frontal or coronal plane of the body, whereas the precordial unipolar or V leads are oriented through the horizontal body plane (Fig. 15.8). The Hexagonal reference system is an amalgamation of the orientation of the standard bipolar and augmented unipolar leads, placed through a central point of the heart, and is used to calculate the electrical axis of the heart (Fig. 15.9).

PQRST complex

The PQRST complex is a recording of the electrical cardiac activity detected by skin electrodes. The P wave represents atrial activation, the QRS complex represents ventricular depolarisation, and the T wave represents ventricular repolarisation. Atrial repolarisation can occasionally be seen as a 'ta' wave interposed in the QRS complex, but is generally lost in the stronger T wave.

The P–R interval (or P–Q interval) represents the time from onset of atrial depolarisation to that of ventricular depolarisation, where the impulse has travelled through the atria and down the specialised internodal pathway to the A–V node. It then traverses the His Bundle, the three bundle branches, the left posterior, left anterior and right tracts, and the Purkinje system, finally activating the electrical endocardial surface of the Sodi-Pallares system.

QRS complex

The QRS complex (Fig. 15.10) is the nett resultant electrical potential generated from ventricular depolarisation as seen by the appropriate surface electrode. Activation in the ventricle commences in the left side of the interventricular septum and spreads to the right and left surface, then activates the ventricle. Activation proceeds in the anterior and posterior regions adjacent to the septum (the resultant waveform is electrically neutral) and then traverses the apical and lateral walls of both ventricles. The last areas activated are the lower portion of the interventricular septum and the low posterior wall adjoining it.

QRS interval

This is usually 0.06–0.10 msecs in adults, tends to last longer in men and should be measured from the widest QRS complex, usually found in the mid-precordial leads.

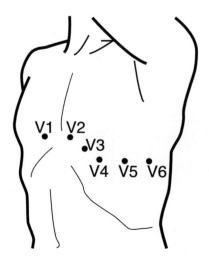

Figure 15.8. *Position of the six chest electrodes, the 'V' leads, in the horizontal plane.*

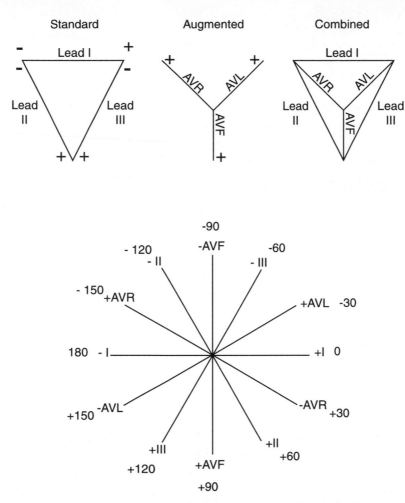

Figure 15.9. *Amalgamation of the standard and augmented limb leads to form the hexagonal reference system in the frontal plane.*

QRS axis

Axis is the direction of the dominant line of electrical excitation through the heart. It lies between −30° to +90° in adults and −30° to +110° in children and adolescents. A slight variation can occur in the same individual from time to time. Axis determines whether conduction is affected by factors such as infarction and hypertrophy and can be judged roughly by inspecting the direction of the R waves in leads I to III (Fig. 15.11). To obtain a more accurate assessment the hexagonal system may be used (Fig. 15.12).

First, the lead with the greatest deflection (tallest R wave), represents the major direction of electrical axis. To determine the angle more precisely, this lead is compared with the most equiphasic leads where the R and S deflections are equal. The electrical axis lies at 90° to the direction of the latter lead.

Fig. 15.13 illustrates an example. In this case the lead with the tallest positive R wave is lead II, so the major direction of electrical axis is in this direction, which is +60°. The most equiphasic lead is aVL (the axis of aVL is −30°). The electrical axis of the heart therefore lies at 90° to the aVL lead, and is +60°.

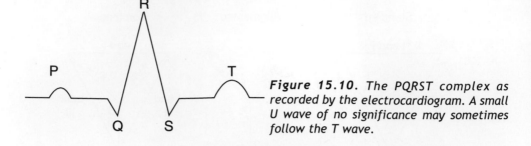

Figure 15.10. The PQRST complex as recorded by the electrocardiogram. A small U wave of no significance may sometimes follow the T wave.

Myocardial infarction and ischaemia

The hallmark of myocardial infarction is the development of pathological Q waves. These are waves greater than 0.04 seconds in width and more than one-third the height of the R wave, or complete loss of the R wave with replacement by a Q wave. Q waves are present when 40% or more of the transmural thickness of the myocardial wall is infarcted or necrotic (Fig. 15.14).

Necrotic or scar tissue is electrically inactive so that an electrical 'window' appears when an electrode is placed over the infarct. In Fig. 15.14, the interventricular septum and right ventricular free wall are recorded from an electrode facing the left ventricular free wall. When cardiac tissue is ischaemic or injured, it becomes electrically negative, whereas the adjacent normal tissue remains positively charged. As a consequence, a negative current of injury is recorded from the injured surface by an electrode facing it, and a continuous positive current is recorded by an electrode facing the normal tissue adjacent to the injured tissue (Fig. 15.15a).

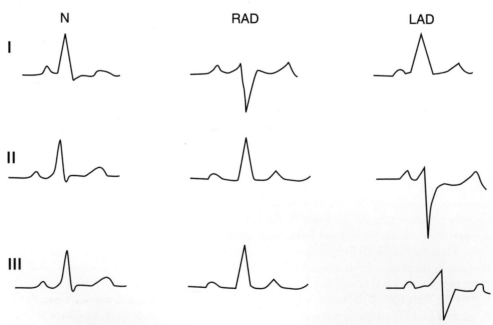

Figure 15.11. Direction of the QRS complex is determined by the axis of the heart. At left is its appearance with a normal axis (N), in the middle is its appearance with right axis deviation (RAD), and at right is its appearance with left axis deviation (LAD).

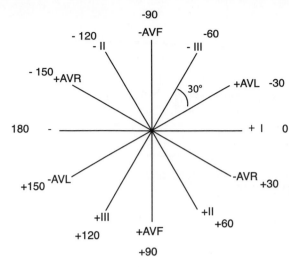

Figure 15.12. Summary of hexagonal system in the frontal plane, showing the relative position and charge of the six limb leads. Each line is separated by 30°, allowing angles to be estimated.

In widespread sub-endocardial ischaemia or unstable angina the whole endocardium is negatively charged. The ECG shows widespread varying ST depression due to an elevated baseline resulting from the continuous positive current (Fig. 15.15b) transmitted from the normal tissue adjacent to the injured tissue. The changes occur because the continuous current related to injury affects the resting electrical baseline, but with depolarisation the true electrical baseline is re-assumed.

Myocardial infarction, however, is not usually an all-or-nothing situation. The region involved in necrosis usually contains patches of injured, ischaemic or even normal tissue. Adjacent to the most damaged portion is a surrounding area of injured tissue, and adjacent to that is ischaemic tissue (Fig. 15.16).

The site of infarction relates to the coronary artery involved. Extended infarction relates to the position of the coronary lesion, such that the more proximal the lesion, generally the more extensive the infarction (taking into consideration other mitigating

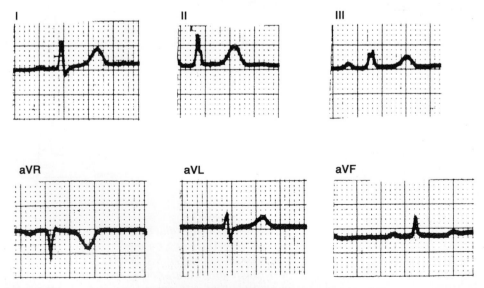

Figure 15.13. Example of QRS direction with an axis rotated to +60°.

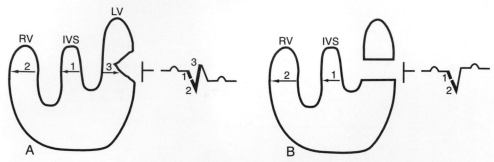

Figure 15.14. *(A) An electrode placed over an infarcted segment of myocardium (3) records the nett current in regions (1) and (2) as moving away from the electrode, i.e. segment (3) is transparent electrically, hence forming pathological Q waves. (A positive charge moving away from a positive electrode records a negative deflection on ECG.) The illustration in (B) depicts a transmural infarct with only a QS complex. There is no R wave.*

tors such as use of thrombolytic therapy, the extent of the luminal thrombotic occlusion, the presence or absence of diabetes mellitus, degree of collateralisation and other factors). Anterior infarction usually involves the left anterior descending artery, inferior infarction usually involves the right coronary artery, and posterior infarction involves the area usually supplied by the left circumflex artery. However, there are variations to this. If a diagonal branch of the left anterior descending artery occludes, T wave inversion is usually seen only in left anterior descending territory. A distal left anterior descending artery occlusion causing apical infarction usually involves T wave inversion in the apico-lateral leads. The proximal circumflex branches, when occluded, are often electrocardiographically silent on a standard ECG. To diagnose these, chest leads V7 to V12 are used. These are at the same level as lead V6 and 5 cm (2 inches) apart, coursing posteriorly around the chest.

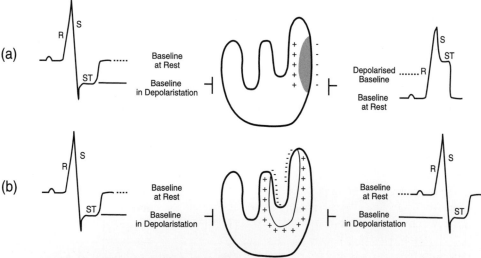

Figure 15.15. *(a) Depiction of an ECG tracing of a myocardial infarct, where an electrode facing a region of infarction registers S-T elevation, and an electrode away from the infarction registers S-T depression ('reciprocal' change in S-T level). (b) This shows an ECG tracing in myocardial ischaemia without infarction, and is more widespread. An electrode over the ischaemic region and another one away from it both record S-T segment depression.*

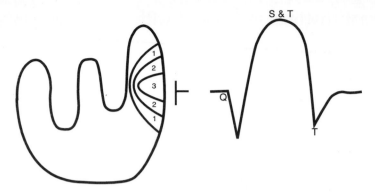

Figure 15.16. Appearance of QRS complex with a Q wave caused by an infarct. At left is the infarcted region in wall of ventricle (1 = ischaemia, 2 = injury, 3 = necrosis).

Patients suffering their first infarct in the left coronary system have a 60% chance of multi-vessel disease, whereas patients with a right coronary artery presentation have a 60% chance of single vessel coronary artery disease. The following is a summary of the major infarction patterns, and their association with the coronary blood supply and corresponding ECG changes.

Anterior infarction involves the left anterior descending artery and/or its major branches, with changes in leads V2–V4.

Septal infarction involves the proximal left anterior descending artery and its septal branches, with changes in leads V2–V3.

High lateral infarction involves the obtuse marginal branch of circumflex, e.g. intermediate artery or a very proximal diagonal branch of the left anterior descending artery, with changes in leads I and aVL.

Lateral infarction involves the distal diagonal branches of the left anterior descending artery, distal circumflex or distal right coronary artery branches, with changes in leads V5–V6.

Inferior infarction usually involves the right coronary artery, but occasionally the circumflex (when dominant, in about 10% of cases) supplies the inferior surface (usually supplied by the posterior descending artery); changes in leads II, III and aVF.

Inferior infarction can show some variation in ECG pattern such that:

a) Sometime after the event Q waves may only be seen in III/aVF, whereas acutely they were present in all inferior leads; this indicates that the infarct is infero-basal, affecting the proximal portion of the inferior left ventricular wall and the interventricular septum.

b) S–T depression may be noted at the same time in leads V1–V4, which is usually a mirror image of S–T elevation in the posterior leads. This implies extension of the infarct upwards along the posterior wall due to:

    i)   a right coronary artery with numerous postero-lateral branches extending up the posterior wall of the heart, or

    ii) the circumflex artery is dominant, supplying the posterior descending branch (PDA).

c) There may be coexisting S–T changes in V5–V6 due to involvement of the lateral wall, from a posterolateral branch or a large PDA running to the apex.

Atrial infarction is unusual and occurs in the context of a large ventricular infarction. It is diagnosed by elevation of the P–R segment, at times with a change in P wave morphology. In acute pericarditis there may be depression of the P–R segment.

Abnormal rhythms associated with myocardial infarction

Sinus node abnormalities

Sinus bradycardia

This may be due to:

a) Ischaemia of the SA node, causing local acidosis depressing nodal automaticity, or elevation of adenosine causing a negative intropic effect, or

b) Intense vagal stimulation, which can be reversed by administration of atropine. Brady-cardia is up to three times more common in infero-posterior infarction, compared to anterior infarction. It is most likely to occur early in acute infarction (<3 hours), and is associated with a higher incidence of ventricular fibrillation, possibly as ventricular threshold is reduced with a bradycardia or because ventricular ectopics may be pre-cipitated by long R–R intervals.

Sinus tachycardia

This is usually due to left ventricular failure but includes fever, coexistent pericarditis, anxi-ety, pulmonary embolus and other ailments. When sinus tachycardia is present there is usually a higher incidence of AV block (1° [first degree], 2° [second degree] and 3° [third degree] AV block).

Sinus arrest

This is a rare occurrence (and to be differentiated from SA block) and only occurs in infe-rior infarction with occlusion of the right coronary artery very proximally.

Atrial dysrrhythmias

Atrial ectopics

These are very common in acute myocardial infarction; they are due to either atrial is-chaemia or atrial distension arising from heart failure with elevated LV diastolic pressure.

Atrial fibrillation

This occurs in up to 10% of patients with acute myocardial infarction or with cardiac failure. It may be coexistent in patients with atrial disease or with damage from ischaemia, hypertension, chronic airways disease or other ailments. Atrial flutter and atrial tachycar-dia are very rare in acute myocardial infarction, when it causes haemodynamic impair-ment due to rapid ventricular response. It may be treated with amiodarone (with intrave-nous loading), or judicious use of beta-blockers or electrical cardioversion.

Ventricular and nodal (junctional) rhythms

Nodal escape rhythm and idionodal tachycardia

These are inherently escape rhythms that occur when there are periods of sinus arrest, sinus bradycardia or abnormalities of impulse conduction with SA block or AV block. These rhythms are reasonably frequent in acute myocardial infarction, particularly infe-rior infarction, as this is often associated with disorders of the SA node causing sinus arrest, sinus bradycardia or SA block. Nodal escape rhythm usually occurs at a rate of 50–60 beats per minute. Idionodal tachycardia occurs at faster rates, usually 70–100 beats a minute. The causes of the relative tachycardia from the AV nodal region (which has automa-ticity) are the same as the causes of sinus tachycardia.

Ventricular ectopic beats

These occur in virtually all patients with acute myocardial infarction and they are of little prognostic significance, although it is considered that those arriving from the left ventricle are more likely to precipitate ventricular fibrillation. In the past there have been recommendations for pharmacological suppression of ventricular ectopy, but controlled trials have shown that doing so has not prevented ventricular fibrillation. Most coronary units now do not prophylactically suppress these ectopics.

Ventricular tachycardia

Ventricular tachycardia consists of a series of three or more consecutive ventricular ectopic beats, which occur at a rate faster than the underlying sinus rhythm. Three to ten escape beats are common in the first 36 hours after an acute myocardial infarction and are of little prognostic significance. However, rapid polymorphic ventricular tachycardia in the first 36 hours following infarction is of prognostic significance. Patients with a *torsade de pointes* (TDP) pattern should have attention paid to the pro-arrhythmic effects of existing anti-arrhythmic therapy. TDP is also associated with the use of phenothiazines, tricyclic antidepressants, erythromycin-based antihistamines, hypokalaemia and hypomagnesaemia. When polymorphic ventricular tachycardia is due solely to the myocardial infarction it usually responds well to anti-arrhythmic therapy.

Idioventricular tachycardia

This is frequently seen in acute myocardial infarction and often occurs following thrombolytic therapy, when reperfusion of the coronary artery involved takes place. This rhythm rarely results in ventricular fibrillation and does not usually require treatment. However, because of loss of the atrial contraction, cardiac output can be significantly impaired by up to 20%, causing symptomatic hypotension and cardiac failure. Under these circumstances it should be treated with either anti-arrhythmic drugs or atropine.

Ventricular fibrillation

Prevention of death from dysrhythmia is one of the major aims in acute coronary care. Ventricular fibrillation is often induced by electrolyte abnormalities and is more common the more extensive the myocardial infarction. The incidence in patients with acute myocardial infarction decreased from 5–7% in the early 1970s to <2% in the late 1980s. This is partly due to use of beta-blockers in acute myocardial infarction, more vigorous and effective treatment of cardiac failure, and correction of electrolyte imbalances. Clinical trials have shown that ventricular premature beats are unreliable predictors of the development of ventricular fibrillation.

Conduction disturbances in acute myocardial infarction

1° atrioventricular block

This is a delay in conduction of the P wave from the SA node to the AV node and is evident as a prolonged P–Q interval. It is seen in inferior infarction involving the AV node, where it is a benign finding, and less frequently in anterior infarction with septal involvement causing His Bundle delay. In this situation it indicates a far more extensive infarction.

2° atrioventricular block

This is also called Mobitz Type I, or Wenckebach block. The mechanism is similar to that of 1° AV block and is evident as one or more 'dropped' QRS beats following failure of a P wave to conduct to the AV node. It is common to see a patient's rhythm progress from 1° AV block to Wenckebach block and then back, although Wenckebach block may be present for some time (>24 hours) before reverting to 1° block. The QRS complex usually remains narrow except in the presence of anterior infarction, when left anterior hemi-block or right bundle branch block may develop. In this situation the course may be more complicated.

Mobitz Type II block is a progressive lengthening of the P–Q interval with a subsequent 'dropped' QRS beat. It is due to ischaemia of the septal infra-nodal conduction pathway in anterior infarction and may be associated with a narrow or wide QRS complex. In the latter, due to bundle branch block, the prognosis is poor. Mobitz Type II may progress to 3° AV block and require temporary pacemaker insertion.

3° atrioventricular block

This is complete conduction failure and results in ventricular standstill, evident as a prolonged flat ECG signal. It may occur in inferior or anterior myocardial infarction. The mechanisms differ and have different prognostic implications. In inferior infarction it is the result of necrosis or ischaemia of the AV node (with or without vagal stimulation) and may progress from 1° AV block to 2° AV block (Mobitz Type I) to 3° AV block. Usually it is benign and haemodynamics are maintained, although a temporary pacemaker may at times be required. In anterior myocardial infarction the prognosis is much poorer due to the extensive nature of the infarct. Rather than having a gradual onset, as in inferior infarction, it may be of abrupt onset with major haemodynamic impairment. A temporary pacemaker is usually required to maintain haemodynamics and often a permanent pacemaker is required if the patient survives.

Hemi blocks

Left anterior hemi-block may occur in antero-septal infarction and is of little significance unless right bundle branch block also develops. In this situation (bi-fascicular block) high grade AV block (Mobitz Type II or 3° AV block) may develop, requiring a temporary pacemaker implantation.

Bundle branch block

This is failure of either the right or left bundle branch to conduct, and is seen as a widened QRS complex. When occurring in the context of acute myocardial infarction it usually indicates extensive infarction with significant haemodynamic impairment. A full prognosis is often associated with Mobitz Type II or 3° AV block and requires temporary pacemaker/permanent pacemaker.

Pseudo-infarct patterns on standard ECG

These are cardiac conditions where the standard resting ECG may be confused with an ischaemic pattern. Following is a brief description of the various types encountered.

Wolff-Parkinson-White syndrome

The delta wave can form Q/Q waves in the inferior, anterior and posterior leads, mimicking infarction patterns.

Hypertrophic cardiomyopathy

This can occur with or without obstruction of the left ventricular outflow tract and is associated not only with cardiac failure but also with ventricular dysrhythmias and, at times, atrial dysrhythmias. The resting ECG can show Q waves due to hypertrophy and also S–T elevation or S–T/T wave changes with depression, thus mimicking hyperacute infarction (S–T elevation), old infarction (Q waves) or ischaemia (S–T/T changes).

Chronic obstructive airways disease and right ventricular hypertrophy

These conditions may be associated with weak R wave development in the inferior and early precordial leads, mimicking old infarction.

Pulmonary emboli

This may be associated with T wave changes due to right ventricular strain suggesting ischaemia. At times, Q waves may develop in lead III, suggesting old infarction. If chronic recurrent pulmonary emboli occur, then right ventricular hypertrophy with clockwise precordial rotation and slow R wave development in V1–V4 may result, suggesting old antero-septal myocardial infarction.

Thoracic cage deformity

This condition, especially *pectus excavatum*, which causes flattening or compression of the heart with movement to the left, causes slow R wave development in leads V1–V4, suggesting anterior infarction.

Miscellaneous

a) Pericarditis (S–T and T wave changes)
b) Acute intracranial catastrophe (S–T/T wave changes, bradyarrhythmia, and $1°$, $2°$ and $3°$ AV block)
c) Cholecystic disease (S–T/T wave changes)
d) Mitral valve prolapse (S–T/T wave changes)
e) Hypokalaemia (S–T/T wave changes, $1°$ AV block, atrial and ventricular dysrhythmias).
f) Cardiac infiltration (e.g sarcoid, amyloid, haemochromatosis) may cause S–T/T wave changes and, in the septal leads, loss of R wave resulting in Q wave formation suggestive of old antero-septal infarction.

Figure 15.17 contains a selection of sample ECG tracings showing some of the characteristics described above.

Figure 15.17a shows Q waves in leads III and aVF and T wave changes in leads I, aVL, V_1–V_4. Changes suggest an old inferior infarction and antero-septal ischaemia. However, the patient has normal coronary arteries and hypertrophic cardiomyopathy.

Figure 15.17b shows an ECG of a patient with an apical form of hypertrophic cardiomyopathy; T wave changes in leads I, V_1 to aVL, V_2–V_6, suggest antero-apicolateral ischaemia. This patient also has normal coronary arteries and proven apical hypertrophy.

The trace in Fig. 15.17c shows T wave changes in leads I, aVL, V_4–V_6, V_1–V_3. All changes are suggestive of lateral ischaemia with or without hyper-acute changes anteriorly. This patient has normal coronary arteries and apical hypertrophy.

The ECG in Fig 15.17d shows that this patient has had a previous antero-apicoseptal infarction and has a RSR pattern in V_4, which is said to indicate apical aneurysm.

The ECG in Fig. 15.17e is from a patient with Q waves in leads III, aVF consistent with and old inferior infarction, Q waves in leads I, V_3 and a small RSR in V_4. Again she has had a previous antero-apicoseptal infarction and the RSR in V_4 indicates apical aneurysm. There are S–T/T wave changes in leads I, aVL, V_5 and V_6 consistent with lateral ischaemia.

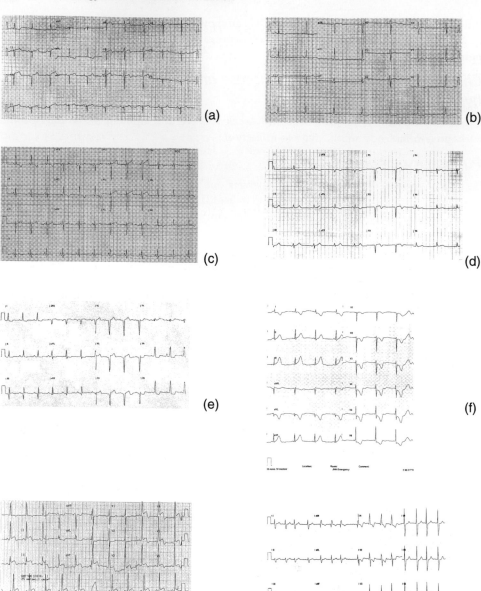

Figure 15.17. Compilation of sample ECG tracings showing various pseudo-infarct patterns. See text for description.

The ECG in Fig. 15.17f was taken from a patient who presented to hospital with severe central pre-cordial chest pain, and was found to have normal coronary arteries. A subsequent VQ scan showed massive pulmonary embolus. Her T wave changes in leads I, aVL, V_1–V_6 could easily be mistaken for myocardial ischaemia.

The ECG in Fig. 15.17g is from a patient who presented to hospital on numerous occasions with severe chest pain and it was treated as myocardial infarction. Her ECG showed dominant R waves in V_1 and V_2 suggestive of an old posterior infarction, and S–T elevation inferiorly and apicolaterally, which can be mistaken for hyper acute infarction. In fact she has normal coronary arteries and hypertrophic cardiomyopathy.

The ECG in Fig. 15.17h shows that this patient has atrial fibrillation and right bundle branch block but there is a small q wave in leads V_1–V_3, as well as a Q wave in III and aVF. This patient has had previous inferior infarction and, in the presence of right bundle branch block, also shows a previous septal infarction.

References

1.   Sodi-Pallares D, Barbato E, Delmar A. Relationship between the intrinsic deflection and the subepicardial activation. Experimental study. *Am Heart J* 1950; **39**:387–99.
2.   Sodi-Pallares D, Bisteni A, Medrano GA, Cisneros AF. Activation of the free left ventricular wall in the dog's heart; in normal condition and in left bundle branch block. *Am Heart J* 1955; **49**:587–602.
3.   Sodi-Pallares D, Medrano GA, De Micheli A *et al.* Unipolar QS morphology and Purkinje potential of the free left ventricular wall. The concepts of electrical endocardium. *Circulation* 1961; **23**:836–46.
4.   Sodi-Pallares D, Rodriguez MI. Morphology of the unipolar leads recorded at the septal surfaces. Its application to the diagnosis of left bundle branch block complicated by myocardial infarction. *Am Heart J* 1952; **43**:27–41.
5.   Durrer D, Dam RT van, Freud GE *et al.* Total excitation of the isolated human heart. *Circulation* 1970:**41**:899.

Further reading

Lipman BS, Massie E, Kleiger E, Robert E. *Clinical scalar electrocardiography,* 6th ed. Chicago: Year Book Medical Publishers Inc 1972.
Chung EK. *Electrocardiography—Practical applications and vectoral principles,* 3rd ed. New York: Harper and Row 1980.
Te-Chuan C, Nylans TK. *Electrocardiography in clinical practice–Adult and paediatric,* 4th ed. Philadelphia: WB Saunders 1996.
Schamroth L. *The electrocardiology of coronary artery disease,* 2nd ed. Oxford: Blackwell Scientific Publications 1984.
Schamroth, L. *An introduction to electrocardiography,* 7th ed. Oxford: Blackwell Scientific Publications 1990.

Chapter 16

Coronary Angiography

Techniques and tools of the trade

Thomas Gavaghan

C ardiac catheterisation has evolved over the last three decades into a sophisticated, highly specialised and low-risk diagnostic procedure that requires considerable skills, intensive training and dedicated support staff. The diversity of catheters from various companies, and improvements in imaging equipment through digital cardiac technology, have made this a predictably safe, reliable and accurate test in the investigation of the cardiac patient. This chapter discusses the indications, equipment and various technical aspects in the performance of cardiac catheterisation and coronary angiography.

Indications for cardiac catheterisation

The most common reason for elective coronary angiography is the diagnosis of coronary artery disease in the patient with chest pain and significant abnormality on non-invasive testing of myocardial perfusion. The more urgent indications for coronary angiography involve patients with unstable angina or acute myocardial infarction and, increasingly, those with recurrent angina after previous coronary artery bypass surgery. Cardiac catheterisation is valuable in the investigation of valvular and congenital cardiac abnormalities and to assess the patient with cardiomyopathy. A summary of recently revised guidelines for cardiac catheterisation presented by the American Heart Association (AHA) and the American College of Cardiologists (ACC) subcommittee on coronary angiography is shown in Table 16.1.

Vascular access

The importance of a thorough and meticulous approach to the insertion of angiography catheters into the vascular system cannot be overemphasised. This one step, completed successfully, enables the operator to perform the insertion and manipulation of diagnostic catheters with remarkable efficiency and accuracy and minimise the potential complications of a prolonged procedure.

Traditionally, the arterial and venous circulation has been entered by direct surgical approach or by the percutaneous approach. Today, most investigators use the percutaneous method due to greater speed in entering the vessel and the relative lack of training in surgical cutdown procedures among modern training diagnosticians.

Table 16.1. Specific indications for cardiac catheterisation*

1.   Patients with known or suspected coronary artery disease
a.   Asymptomatic patients
b.   Symptomatic patients
Stable angina
Unstable coronary syndromes
Post-revascularisation ischaemia
Suspected acute myocardial infarct and S-T segment elevation or left bundle-branch block, and to undergo PTCA
Acute myocardial infarct in patient who has not undergone primary PTCA
Suspected acute myocardial infarct without S-T segment elevation or left bundle-branch block
In-hospital management of Q wave or non-Q wave myocardial infarct
Atypical chest pain in cardiac ischaemia
Evaluation before or after non-cardiac surgery
2.   Valvular heart disease
3.   Congestive cardiac failure
4.   Other conditions (e.g. selected aortic disease such as aortic dissection or aneurysm with known coronary artery disease, or hypertrophic cardiomyopathy)

* As recommended by the American Heart Association and the American College of Cardiologists
Diagnostic coronary angiography is now frequently followed by additional procedures including:
i)   adjunctive pharmacological treatments (nitroglycerine, verapamil and thrombolytic drugs);
ii)   intracoronary ultrasound (IVUS) to accurately quantify coronary atherosclerosis and the effects of coronary interventions;
iii) insertion of a coronary doppler flow wire to study the haemodynamic significance of a coronary stenosis and for evaluation of interventional techniques (angioplasty, stenting, rotational atherectomy and Excimer laser ablation).

Surgical cutdown is primarily used to access the brachial artery directly. There are a variety of catheters which can be used to perform coronary angiography by the Sones technique.

Percutaneous technique. Sites for arterial puncture include femoral, radial, brachial and axillary arteries, as shown in Fig. 16.1.

Prior to formal draping of the patient, laboratory personnel should accurately assess the patient's peripheral vascular status for later comparison after removal of the arterial sheath. Depending on the arm or leg approach, proper positioning of the patient toward the head of the catheter table and a stable, comfortable position of the patient's arms allow smooth progress through the procedure.

Femoral artery

After appropriate skin sterilisation and draping of the right or left groin with sterile, disposable angiographic setup packages, the artery is palpated immediately beneath the inguinal skin crease, using the middle and index fingers of the left hand. Local anaesthetic (1% or 2% xylocaine) is infiltrated into the skin 1 or 2 cm distal to the point of anticipated arterial puncture. Further infiltration is performed down to the arterial surface, using frequent aspiration to avoid injecting directly into the artery. Up to 15 ml is used to adequately anaesthetise this area and assist in the possible deployment of a percutaneous vascular closure device at the end of the procedure. A 3 mm incision is made using a scalpel blade, and a subcutaneous tunnel is opened with blunt dissection from curved arterial forceps.

A sharp 18-gauge needle is held between thumb and index finger of the right hand and firm palpation is made with the left hand to stabilise the femoral artery above and below the skin incision. With the needle tip bevel directed upwards the needle is slowly advanced at an angle of 40° to 45° with the horizontal plane, and usually a firm pulsatile resistance is felt as the needle abuts the wall of the vessel. Further gentle advancement is required and then a strong pulsatile jet of blood indicates that the needle has entered the

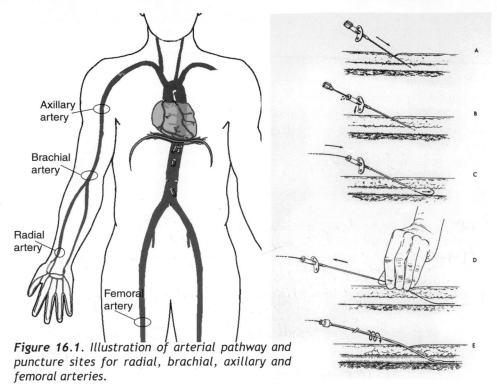

Figure 16.1. *Illustration of arterial pathway and puncture sites for radial, brachial, axillary and femoral arteries.*

Figure 16.2. *The Seldinger technique. A, the vessel is punctured with the needle at a 30°-40° angle. B, the stylet is removed and free blood flow is observed; the angle of the needle is then reduced. C, the flexible tip of the guidewire is passed through the needle into the vessel. D, the needle is removed over the wire while firm pressure is applied at the site. E, the tip of the catheter is passed over the wire and advanced into the vessel with a rotating motion. (Reproduced with permission from Tilkian AG, Daly EK: Cardiovascular procedures: diagnostic techniques and therapeutic procedures. St. Louis: Mosby 1986, courtesy of Mosby-Year Book Inc).*

true lumen of the artery. As indicated in Fig. 16.2, while stabilising the needle with the left hand, a soft J-tipped guidewire is passed through the needle under fluoroscopic guidance 15–20 cm into the proximal vessel without resistance. The introducing needle is then withdrawn, while pressure is maintained over the puncture site with the left hand. An appropriately sized sheath and dilator are passed along the clean guidewire with a forward, twisting motion into the femoral artery. In the patient with significant tortuosity of the iliac artery it may be advantageous to use a 23–30 cm long sheath in order to facilitate subsequent catheter exchanges and to improve torque control of the distal end of the diagnostic catheter.

Radial artery

This approach is possible if the patient has an easily palpable radial pulse and a negative Allen test (intact ipsilateral ulnar circulation). The radial artery is a small-calibre vessel and has a tendency to spasm upon instrumentation. Using the Seldinger technique, the 18-gauge needle is very carefully advanced at 45° into the radial artery and, upon bleed-back, a very soft 0.018" guidewire is advanced into the vessel, then a 5F or 6F sheath is passed smoothly into the artery up to the full length of the sheath.

This may be associated with considerable patient discomfort. Use of intra-arterial xylocaine and nitroglycerine at the time of cannulation of the vessel may alleviate this spasm.

Brachial and axillary arteries

These approaches are less commonly utilised because of the difficulty in securing adequate haemostasis after removal of the sheath. Both sites are nonetheless valuable in the patient with inaccessible femoral vessels and with inadequate collateral perfusion of the hand.

Venous access for right heart catheterisation is possible via the major central veins (subclavian and internal jugular) as well as femoral and antecubital veins. The percutaneous approach is similar to that for arterial access, but aspiration on the venous needle for brisk drawback of blood is necessary to confirm that the tip of the needle is intravascular before proceeding to insert the guidewire and sheath.

During coronary angiography some operators use a small dose of heparin (2000 U–5000 U) given IV or directly into the arterial sheath immediately after it is inserted. This provides protection against the possibility of thrombus forming in the catheter or sheath during a prolonged procedure.

Selection of diagnostic catheters

Once there is stable arterial and/or venous access, it is necessary to choose the appropriate size, length and shape of diagnostic catheters. Ideally one would choose a catheter with good torque control to allow accurate transmission of manipulative movement from the hub of the catheter to the distal tip, and a catheter which has moderate stiffness, sufficient radio-opacity, good memory and an adequate internal lumen to facilitate injection of contrast. Diagnostic catheters vary in size from 4F to 9F; most diagnostic studies are performed with 5F or 6F catheters. There is a lower risk of femoral haematoma with 5F catheters, which has implications for out-patient angiography in the current cost-conscious health-care environment.

There is great variety in subtle characteristics (stiffness, radio-opacity, torque control and memory) among catheters of various companies and it is only possible to find the best individual feel by trialling the products of several companies for comparative purposes.

The guidewire provides the safest means by which an open-ended catheter can be passed from a distal insertion point along the circulatory tree to the vessel to be examined. There is a large selection available; the most commonly used wires include the 0.035 or 0.038 inch J-tipped standard wire, the 0.035" movable core wire (with variable length distal flexible tip) and the 0.038" teflon-coated Glidewire in patients with marked tortuosity or atherosclerotic disease of the iliac system. These wires are usually curved and soft in the tip and stiffer in the shaft to avoid any trauma to the vessel wall and yet allow smooth passage of the catheter to the region of interest. The straight-tipped Glidewire is often used inside a pigtail or Judkins right catheter as a means of crossing the aortic valve in significant aortic stenosis.

Coronary angiographic catheters

A sample range of specialist diagnostic catheters available is demonstrated in Fig. 16.3.

Femoral approach

The Judkins left and right coronary catheters have preformed curves that allow relatively easy positioning of the catheters in the ostium of the relevant coronary artery. Judkins

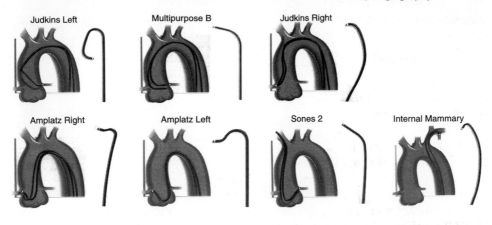

Figure 16.3. *Illustration of various diagnostic catheter types, showing variations in shape and positioning inside the aortic arch. (Reproduced courtesy of Cordis/Johnson and Johnson Medical).*

catheters are available in differently sized curves according to the size of the aortic root and, to a lesser degree, the take-off of the coronary artery.

The Amplatz left and right coronary catheters are again preshaped catheters that are used for angiography of both native coronary vessels and difficult graft studies. These catheters can be used for angiography via the radial and brachial approach. In all cases, however, there is a higher incidence of coronary dissection due to the rather aggressive hook shape of the distal end of the catheter.

The Multipurpose catheter is designed such that it is capable of selectively catheterising both left and right coronary arteries and can then be used to perform ventriculography without the need to exchange to other diagnostic catheters. This inherently requires greater manipulative skills and involves longer fluoroscopy times, making the Multipurpose catheter a second choice for most operators. Coronary vein graft catheters (left and right) are specifically designed to cater for the high, anterior origin of the left grafts and the vertically oriented take-off of right grafts. In difficult cases it is often possible to selectively cannulate the grafts using Amplatz and/or Multipurpose catheters.

The internal mammary artery graft catheter is designed to fit the acute inferior take-off of either mammary artery and may be useful in the catheterisation of left coronary grafts.

Brachial approach

The Sones catheter is a straight catheter with a tapered tip, which is advanced carefully over a guidewire around the tortuous brachiocephalic vessels to the proximal aorta and then manipulated into both left and right coronary arteries. This requires considerable training before adequate competency is achieved.

Amplatz and Multipurpose catheters are acceptable alternatives for coronary angiography from the right brachial approach and, due to their preformed shape, these catheters usually sit securely in the ostium of the coronary artery once intubated. Amplatz catheters are well suited to cannulate a superiorly directed high take-off left main coronary artery and to engage the origin of both left and right bypass grafts (venous or free pedicle arterial grafts).

Radial approach

The preshaped Judkins and Amplatz coronary catheters and the Multipurpose catheter are used to perform coronary angiography from the radial artery. The larger left Amplatz coronary catheter (AL3, AL4) is the most effective for reliable cannulation of the left coronary artery. It requires initial placement over the guidewire formed into a large loop in the proximal aortic root and then, with gentle advancement, into the left coronary artery. At all times the catheters must by withdrawn over a guidewire to prevent any trauma to the small calibre radial artery. Multipurpose, right Amplatz or Kiemeneij catheters can be used for angiography of the right coronary artery.

Ventriculography catheters

Femoral approach

Typically the multiple side-hole Pigtail catheter is passed retrogradely through the aortic valve into the body of the left ventricle.

Brachial and radial approach

The multipurpose, NIH, pigtail or Sones catheters can be used for left ventriculography from these approaches. Catheters with a single endhole should not be used for ventriculography because of the risk of myocardial perforation.

Techniques of angiography

General principles

Manifold management

A two- or three-port plastic disposable manifold is commonly used for diagnostic and/or interventional coronary procedures. The manifold acts as an airtight closed junction between the catheter, pressure manometer, radio-opaque dye line, infusion port and injecting port. Rigid attention throughout the procedure to ensure that the line and manifold are free of air minimises the chance of significant air embolism to the coronary bed or aorta. The injection syringe should be held constantly in a downward-sloping direction to prevent inadvertent injection of air bubbles during image acquisition. Accurate arterial waveform recognition is necessary during angiography in order to detect damping of the pressure trace. This may indicate air in the system or possible catheter tip impaction against the arterial intima or an ostial obstruction. Further injection of dye under force may precipitate intimal dissection. Usually, gentle withdrawal of the catheter resolves this problem without injury to the vessel wall.

Contrast injection

All angiographic contrast media currently in use are derivatives of tri-iodinated benzene. In recent years, improved patient tolerance and a lower incidence of adverse effects has favoured an increased preference for non-ionic hydrophylic agents with low viscosity and low osmolarity and osmolality, particularly for patients with renal impairment. In most angiography suites ionic agents are no longer used. The incidence of renal failure requiring dialysis after contrast administration is greatly increased in diabetics and patients with a history of renal failure. Contrast-induced acute renal failure following angiography can occur in up to 5% of in-patients with healthy kidneys, and contrast administration still accounts for 12% of hospital-acquired cases of renal failure. Concern over potential toxicity and osmotic load stress restricts dosages given to a conservative level. True ana-phylactoid responses are not dose-dependent.

Contrast media (often called dye) can be injected either manually through a refillable syringe or via a power-automated injector. Contrast is usually injected at 2–4 ml/sec with volumes of 3–6 ml for the right coronary and 6–10 ml for the left coronary artery. During faster heart rates, a higher rate of injection may be required.

Catheter manipulation

After the syringe and manifold have been correctly set up and the pressure trace is clear and pulsatile, the operator must concentrate on placement of the diagnostic catheter into the relevant artery under fluoroscopic control in a specified x-ray viewing plane. Manipulation of the catheter is usually done by one of two methods.

Method 1: The operator may elect to have the scrub nurse stabilise the manifold/syringe with manual support while the doctor uses the right hand to rotate the hub of the catheter and the left hand to provide forward or backward motion to the catheter after it enters the femoral, brachial or radial sheath.

Method 2: The doctor may prefer to support the manifold and catheter hub assembly in the right hand and use the left hand for forward/backward motion on the catheter shaft as it enters the sheath. With this approach the manifold is stabilised between the third, fourth and fifth fingers of the right hand and right palm, leaving the thumb and index finger to provide rotation of the hub as desired. Although greater dexterity is required with this approach, it allows for smoother, more subtle movement of the diagnostic catheter during a difficult cannulation. It is essential to recognise that one-to-one torque transmission from the hub to the distal catheter tip is greatly facilitated by gentle back and forth movement on the catheter with the left hand while rotating the hub with the right

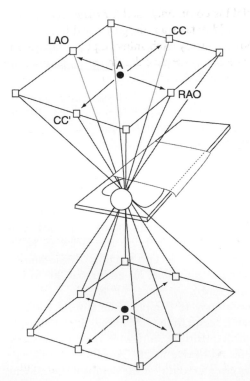

Figure 16.4. Positioning of x-ray camera around the patient, illustrating the various viewing planes and angiographic projections (RAO = right anterior oblique, LAO = left anterior oblique, A = anterior, P = posterior, CC = caudo-cranial, and CC' = cranio-caudal). The cardiologist's preference for determining U-arm orientation in relation to position of the image intensifier rather than the generator is followed.

hand. This tends to avoid the sudden whip-like rotation of the catheter tip resulting from excess build-up of non-transmitted torque.

Panning

Most operators acquire coronary images using the 5–6 inch (17 cm) field size to enable sufficient magnification of the coronary arteriogram and reduce the image distortion from overlying lung and diaphragm. In order to account for the reduced field of view, it is necessary for the operator to move (or pan) the table during the latter third of each imaging sequence to follow the flow of dye from the proximal to the more distal segments of each coronary artery. This requires practice in the various viewing planes and is essential for accurate assessment of late filling collateral vessels and unsuspected anatomical variants. Generally, in the right anterior oblique (RAO) view, the table is moved slowly towards the operator and slightly cranially. In the left anterior oblique (LAO) view the table is panned in a cranial direction. Fig. 16.4 illustrates the viewing planes formed by positioning the x-ray source and image intensifier at various angles around the patient.

Cardiologists refer to the orientation of the U-arm according to the position of the image intensifier (above the table) in relation to the patient's left side as the LAO projection, with the generator (below the table) on the patient's right side. Radiologists refer to the position of the generator in relation to the patient's left (with the image intensifier on the patient's right) as the LAO projection. Hence, the terms RAO and LAO to a cardiologist mean the opposite to a radiologist. The same applies to the terms caudo-cranial and cranio-caudal. The terminology used in this text refers to the cardiologist's viewpoint, as in Fig.16.4.

Angiographic views

In most modern cardiac catheterisation laboratories the x-ray source (the generator) is beneath the table and the camera (image intensifier) is above the patient. In the LAO projection the image intensifier is rotated in the transverse plane to the left of the patient. On the resulting angiogram the spine is usually seen on the right side of the image. The RAO projection is the opposite and entails rotation of the image intensifier to the patient's right, the spine being seen on the left side of the subsequent images. In specific cases the image intensifier is then rotated toward the patient's head (cranial) or feet (caudal) in order to accurately outline otherwise overlapping vessels.

As a general rule, cranial views are helpful for assessment of the left anterior descending coronary artery (LAD) and the caudal views for the left circumflex artery (LCX). For graft angiography the standard views are important, with emphasis on the left lateral view for distal LAD anastomoses, LAO cranial for distal right coronary artery anastomoses and RAO/LAO caudal for left circumflex anastomoses.

Left ventriculography provides essential information on ventricular contractility, particularly in cases of myocardial infarction and cardiomyopathy, along with aortic and mitral valve function. When left ventriculography is performed, the standard view is 30° RAO for single plane assessment and calculation of the ejection fraction. For additional information on regional left ventricular function or shunting, an additional 30° to 60° LAO view provides complete biplane ventriculography.

At times it is necessary to perform aortography to complete the cardiac catheter investigation. The proximal and arch aortogram is set up in the LAO using digital subtraction angiography as the preferred mode of acquisition, and with the lowest x-ray magnification (largest field size). Usually 40–50 ml of dye at 20–25 ml/sec is sufficient with a power injector. The aortogram provides essential data for the complete assessment of aortic valve disease, aortic dissection, aortic aneurysm, coarctation of the aorta and patent ductus arteriosus.

Coronary anatomy

The key to identifying coronary artery anatomy lies in mentally forming a 3-D image of the heart from the 2-D pictures presented on screen. The heart may be considered in 3-D as an oval football shape, with two imaginary planes of reference transsecting the football transversely and longitudinally (Fig. 16.5). The LAD courses along the longitudinal plane, running along the seam of the football before curving anteriorly, while the LCX courses clockwise around the circumference of the football in the transverse plane, tracking along the atrio-ventricular groove. The right coronary artery (RCA) runs counter-clockwise along the same transverse plane as the LCX, branching distally to form the posterior descending and posterolateral branches (Fig. 16.5).

The LAD can be identified in the RAO view by the septal perforators tracking downwards at right angles from its main trunk, with the diagonal branches extending to the right. In the LAO views, septal vessels project towards the left of the LAD, the diagonals to the right. The LCX gives rise to the obtuse marginal and lateral ventricular branches.

The RCA is anatomically less complex and can be readily identified in any view. The conus and right atrial branches arise proximally from the RCA. Distally, the point at which the RCA bifurcates into the posterior descending and posterolateral branches is called the crux. The main trunk of the posterior descending branch of the RCA lies in the same longitudinal plane as the LAD. The main trunks of the LCX and RCA lie along the same transverse plane.

Standard viewing planes for left and right coronary arteries are shown in Table 16.2.

Table 16.2. Standard viewing planes for angiographic examination of left and right coronary arteries

Coronary segment	Standard views	Other views
Left Main	RAO caudal	AP
	LAO cranial	
	LAO caudal	
Proximal LAD	LAO cranial	AP caudal
	RAO cranial	
Mid LAD	LAO cranial	AP cranial
Distal LAD	RAO cranial	lateral
Diagonal	LAO cranial	LAO caudal
	RAO cranial	
Proximal LCX,	RAO caudal	AP caudal
Intermediate,	LAO caudal	
Obtuse marginal		
Left posterolateral,	LAO cranial	LAO caudal
PDA	RAO cranial	
Proximal RCA	LAO	lateral
Mid RCA	LAO	lateral
Distal RCA	LAO cranial	lateral
	AP cranial	
PDA, Posterolateral	LAO cranial	RAO cranial
	AP cranial	

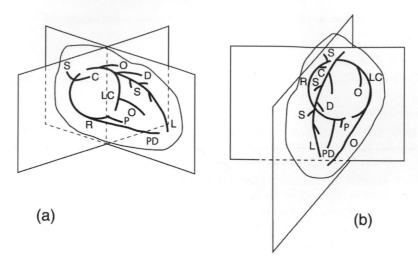

Figure 16.5. Basic coronary anatomy and its orientation in relation to transverse and longitudinal planes of cross-section. (a): right anterior oblique view, (b): left anterior oblique view (R = right coronary artery, LC = left circumflex coronary artery, L = left anterior descending coronary artery, D = diagonal branch, l = lateral branch, S = septal branch).

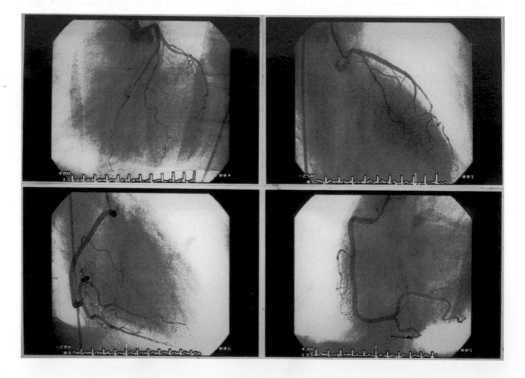

Figure 16.6. Typical angiographic presentation of left and right coronary arteries. Clockwise from top left: Left coronary artery in LAO projection; left coronary artery in RAO projection; right coronary artery in LAO projection; right coronary artery in RAO projection with cranial tilt. Exact angulation is shown by number at bottom left corner of each frame.

The angiographic anatomy of normal left and right coronary arteries is shown in Fig. 16.6.

Selective coronary angiography

Femoral technique

After successful insertion of the femoral artery sheath, a preshaped left and right catheter (usually Judkins or Amplatz design) or a multipurpose catheter can be used for selective angiography of the coronary vessels. The appropriate catheter with preloaded 0.035 inch guidewire is inserted through the femoral sheath and, under fluoroscopic guidance, the wire is gently advanced ahead of the catheter along the abdominal aorta, around the aortic arch and to the mid ascending aorta. The diagnostic catheter is positioned just above the sinuses of Valsalva and the wire is withdrawn carefully. After meticulous aspiration and flushing technique to ensure that no air bubbles or thrombus lie within the system, the catheter assembly is now ready for manipulation into the relevant coronary artery.

The Judkins catheters

Selection of the appropriate left Judkins catheter (JL3.5, JL4.0, JL5.0, JL6.0) depends primarily on the operator's assessment of the size of the aortic root. A small female often requires a JL3.5 catheter whereas for severe aortic stenosis, Marfan's syndrome or prominent aortic unfolding the JL5 or JL6 is appropriate. The Judkins left catheter requires slow advancement and minimal manipulation to cannulate the left coronary artery (as in Fig. 16.3). Usually inserted in the LAO view, it is important to ensure that the tip of this end-hole catheter is not deeply engaged against the roof of the left main coronary artery with the risk of inducing dissection in this area. Alteration or damping of the pressure wave may indicate such occurrence, hence gentle withdrawal and test injection is required to confirm a safer, more axial orientation with the left main orifice. The Judkins left catheter is then exchanged for the right and is best advanced towards the right coronary in the LAO projection. Initially the catheter is directed toward the left coronary sinus. Gentle clockwise torque on the hub, coupled with a smooth push/pull movement on the catheter shaft, causes the tube to migrate anteriorly and then either into or just below the origin of the right coronary artery. Excessive rotation usually results in the catheter flicking out of the ostium during inspiration, and then the manoeuvre must be repeated. Pre-formed catheters that do not require rotation are now available and are particularly useful in patients with severe peripheral vascular disease or dilated aortas.

The Amplatz catheters

These preshaped catheters have a rounded distal curve leading to a sharply angulated terminal hook for the left coronary and a less sharp hook for the right coronary artery. The most commonly used left coronary Amplatz catheter (AL2) is advanced in the LAO towards the left sinus and then gently moved forward to make the tip climb up towards the left main ostium. This is a more aggressive catheter shape and care is needed when disengaging the left Amplatz by pushing slightly forward to move the catheter tip above the left main coronary for safe removal. The right (modified) Amplatz catheter is inserted in the LAO by the same approach as the right Judkins, starting with clockwise rotation from the left coronary sinus.

The Multipurpose catheter

This catheter makes for a faster and more efficient diagnostic angiogram but does require greater manipulative skills on the part of the operator. The technique is similar to the Sones technique and requires the formation of a terminal loop on the catheter either in the LAO or RAO projection. In the LAO, for cannulation of the left coronary artery the loop is enlarged by forward motion and slight counterclockwise rotation until the catheter tip is near the left main ostium. At this point, slight clockwise rotation moves the tip to the left main and, if desired, the tip may enter the ostium further during inspiration by slight withdrawal and clockwise rotation of the catheter. To approach the right coronary, a less pronounced loop is used in the LAO projection. The catheter tip is directed towards the left sinus and then rotated clockwise from the left cusp until the tip is pointing toward the right sinus and slightly cranially. This usually engages the ostium of the right coronary artery. During inspiration care must be taken taken to avoid deep cannulation of vertical, downward take-off right coronary vessels.

Brachial and radial techniques

The brachial artery is entered by either open cutdown or percutaneous puncture; the radial artery is entered only by percutaneous puncture. Most commonly the Sones catheter (5–6F) is used with the brachial approach and is a multipurpose catheter for coronary angiography and ventriculography. The catheter is usually inserted with a guidewire through the subclavian artery (often acutely angulated and tortuous) into the ascending aorta. The more flexible tip may be preshaped by the operator outside the body, thus allowing easier formation of a loop in the left coronary sinus after withdrawal of the guidewire. In the LAO view, this loop can be enlarged by forward/backward motion and counterclockwise rotation of the catheter until the tip reaches the left main ostium. During inspiration the tip can be 'lifted' into the left ostium by gentle withdrawal and clockwise rotation. After completion of the left coronary runs the Sones catheter tip is withdrawn and a less pronounced loop is formed in the left coronary sinus. A smooth clockwise rotation and gentle push/pull movement of the catheter shaft rotates the tip and loop towards the right coronary sinus and the tip enters the right coronary ostium. The catheter tends to deeply intubate the right coronary artery and may need gentle withdrawal during respiratory movements.

The pre-shaped Amplatz catheters can be used from both brachial and radial approaches but must be inserted over a guidewire. They tend to sit snugly in the ostia of the coronary arteries once engaged.

Selective coronary bypass graft angiography

From the femoral approach graft angiography (either vein grafts or free mammary or radial grafts) can often be performed using the same right Judkins or modified right Amplatz catheters used for the native right coronary injections. These catheters should be placed in the mid-ascending aorta in the LAO view, and clockwise rotation usually causes the catheter to seat in the graft ostium. If the grafts are placed in a more anterior position on the aorta, then a left coronary bypass graft catheter or Amplatz AL2 catheter can be used to find the graft ostium. Right coronary grafts (vertically downward takeoff) can usually be found by the right Judkins, right modified Amplatz or multipurpose catheter rotated clockwise from a slightly more proximal aortic position.

Mammary artery grafts are most often approached from the femoral artery using an acutely angulated preshaped mammary artery catheter. After passage of this catheter to the proximal aortic arch over the preferred guidewire, a reliable method of accessing the left subclavian artery is described. The guidewire is withdrawn approximately 8–10cm into the catheter, then gentle withdrawal of the catheter with mild counterclockwise rotation causes the catheter to access sequentially the right innominate, the left common carotid and then the left subclavian artery. Once at the origin of the left subclavian the guidewire is passed forward into the axillary artery, the mammary catheter is moved forward along the wire just beyond the origin of the left internal mammary artery. After withdrawing the wire and flushing the system, the catheter is carefully withdrawn with slight counterclockwise (anterior) rotation. This frequently causes the catheter tip to subtly drop into the ostium of the mammary artery. Small test injections and occasional minor forward or backward adjustment of the catheter facilitate proper selective injections.

For patients with severe peripheral vascular disease the right and/or left brachial approach is needed to find the mammary arteries, utilizing the same diagnostic catheters. Great care is needed, when intubating the mammary ostium, to avoid dissection or spasm at this delicate area. An overly forceful graft injection may cause intense chest wall burning to the patient.

Further reading

Pepine CJ, Hill JA, Lambert CR. *Diagnostic and therapeutic cardiac catheterization,* 3rd ed. Baltimore: Williams & Wilkins 1998.

Kern MJ. *The cardiac catheterization handbook,* 3rd ed. St.Louis: Mosby 1999.

Baim DS, Grossman W. *Cardiac catheterization, angiography and intervention,* 5th ed. Baltimore: Williams and Wilkins 1996.

Judkins MP. Selective coronary angiography: 1. A percutaneous transfemoral technic. *Radiology* 1967; **89**:815–24.

Judkins MP, Gander M. Prevention of complications of coronary angiography (editorial). *Circulation* 1974; **49**:599–602.

Kiemeneij F, Laarman GJ. Percutaneous transradial artery approach for coronary Palmaz-Schatz stent implantation. *Am Heart J* 1994; **128**:167–74.

Ross J Jr, Brandenburg RO, Dinsmore RE *et al.* ACC/AHA Guidelines for coronary angiography: A report of the American College of Cardiology/American Heart Association Task Force on Assessment of Diagnostic and Therapeutic Cardiovascular Procedures. In press. Previously in: *J Am Coll Cardiol* 1987; **10**:935–50.

Scherberich JE. Do contrast media lead to impaired kidney function? In: Dawson P, Clauss W. *Contrast media in practice. Questions and answers,* 2nd ed. Berlin: Springer 1999, pp. 84–86.

Deray G. Pathophysiology and prevention of contrast media nephrotoxicity. In: Marco J, King SB (eds) *Current concepts on the role of thrombosis in interventional cardiology. Focus on contrast agents.* La Garenne-Colombe: Apex. edt editions medicales 1997.

Chapter 17

Measurement of Cardiac Output and Shunts

Michael P. Feneley

Cardiac output

Cardiac output is the total quantity of blood delivered to the systemic circulation per unit of time, and is generally expressed in litres per minute (L/min). Normal cardiac output at rest for a 70 kg adult is approximately 5 L/min. It is usual to normalise cardiac output measurements for differences in body size by dividing the cardiac output by the body surface area, yielding the cardiac index (L/min/M^2). Trained athletes are capable of increasing cardiac output up to 6-fold at peak exercise. Maximal oxygen delivery to the tissues can be increased further, however, by increasing the amount of oxygen extracted by the tissues from each unit of blood: this is called the extraction reserve, which permits up to a 3-fold increase in oxygen extraction from the blood. When the 6-fold cardiac output reserve is multiplied by the 3-fold extraction reserve, it can be seen that the body has the capacity to increase oxygen delivery to the tissues up to 18-fold above normal resting values. Conversely, it can be seen that the minimum cardiac output compatible with life is one-third the normal resting cardiac output, because below this level the extraction reserve is exhausted.

The Fick Principle

Cardiac output is usually measured in the cardiac catheterisation laboratory either by the Fick oxygen method or the indicator dilution method. Both methods of cardiac output measurement rely on the principle first stated by Adolph Fick in 1870: the amount (A) of any substance taken up or released by an organ is the product of the blood flow to the organ (Q) and the difference between the concentration of the substance in blood on the arterial (C_A) and venous (C_V) sides of the organ:

$$A = Q \times (C_A - C_V) \qquad (1)$$

By rearranging Equation 1, it can be seen that blood flow through an organ can be determined by measuring the amount of any substance taken up or released by the organ and the arterio-venous concentration difference of the substance:

$$Q = \frac{A}{C_A - C_V} \qquad (2)$$

Fick oxygen method

This method of measuring cardiac output applies the Fick principle to uptake of oxygen from the lungs. It relies on the fact that under steady-state conditions, uptake of oxygen from the lungs into the blood (A) is equal to the uptake of oxygen from room air by the lungs. The arterio-venous oxygen content difference across the lungs (C_A - C_V) is taken to be the difference between blood samples drawn from the pulmonary artery and the left ventricle (or any systemic artery). Use of left ventricular or systemic arterial blood in place of pulmonary venous blood is a matter of sampling convenience. Doing so ignores the small contribution of bronchial and thebesian venous drainage, but this involves minimal error. In the presence of a right-to-left shunt, however (see below), systemic arterial oxygen content cannot be substituted for the true pulmonary venous oxygen content.

Two methods are in common use in cardiac catheterisation laboratories to measure oxygen uptake from room air by the lungs:

1. The Douglas bag method: In this method, a collection bag (the Douglas bag) attached to a mouthpiece via a 3-way valve is used to collect all of the patient's expired air over a precisely measured time period, usually 3 minutes. Prior to inserting the mouthpiece, the technician must ensure that a nose clip is correctly placed so that all expired air passes through the mouthpiece. For the same reason, the technician should ensure that the patient's lips are firmly clasped over the mouthpiece. The 3-way valve should first be adjusted to permit the patient to breathe room air quietly for no less than 30 seconds before the valve is adjusted to direct the expired air into the bag and the collection period begins. Because the lungs have a large reservoir capacity, the assumption of the method that oxygen uptake from room air is equal to oxygen uptake from the lungs to the blood is valid only under **steady-state** conditions. For this reason, it is important that the room be quiet and the patient's breathing pattern undisturbed throughout the collection period.

The amount (A in Equation 1) of oxygen taken in by the lungs is then calculated as the product of the volume (Q) of the expired air collected and the difference in oxygen concentration between room air and expired air. The volume of expired air is measured with a spirometer. The oxygen content of the samples of room air and expired air can be measured directly with a fuel-cell technique, or derived from measurements of the partial pressure of oxygen (pO_2) in the samples. The total amount of oxygen consumed during the 3-minute collection period is then divided by 3 to express the oxygen consumption in ml/min.

Oxygen content of the pulmonary arterial and systemic blood samples can be measured directly with a fuel-cell technique. This is more accurate than the older technique of reflectance oximetry, which is still widely used (see Chapter 5). Reflectance oximetry measures the fraction of total haemoglobin that is oxygenated. The oxygen content is then calculated as the product of this fraction and the oxygen-carrying capacity of the patient's blood (assumed to be the total haemoglobin concentration x 1.36 ml O_2/gm haemoglobin). Leaving aside the approximation of the assumed oxygen-carrying capacity, the reflectance oximetry method is inaccurate in the presence of abnormal haemoglobins or if some haemoglobin is bound to carbon monoxide (e.g. smokers).

Pulmonary blood flow is then calculated, according to Equation 2, by dividing the measured oxygen consumption by the arterio-venous oxygen difference. In the absence of a shunt, pulmonary blood flow is equal to the total cardiac output.

Sample calculations: Cardiac output by the Fick method

To calculate cardiac output by the Fick method, the following data were collected from a patient, and blood samples taken from the left ventricle (LV) and pulmonary artery (PA).

Height, weight, age and sex can be used to determine surface area and to estimate oxygen consumption from morphometric charts as an alternative to a Douglas bag collection.

Height: 152 cm   Weight: 50 kg   Age: 68 y   Sex: F

Surface area (SA): 1.45 M^2

Oxygen consumption: 200 ml/min

Haemoglobin (Hb): 12.5 g%

Oxygen-carrying capacity of blood: $= 12.5 \times 1.36 = 17.0$ ml/100ml, or Vol%

LV saturation: 97.3 %   LV O_2 content: $= 17.0 \times 0.973 = 16.5$ Vol%

PA saturation: 68.7%   PA O_2 content: $= 17.0 \times 0.687 = 11.7$ Vol%

Arterio-venous (A-V) O_2 difference: $= 16.5 - 11.7 = 4.8$ Vol%

Cardiac output (CO, or Q) can then be calculated according to Equation (2):

CO = O_2 consumption / AV O_2 difference $= 200/4.8 = 42$ dL/min $= 4.2$ L/min

Cardiac index (CI) = CO/SA $= 4.2/1.45 = 2.9$ L/min/M^2

2. Polarographic oxygen method: This is an alternative to the older Douglas bag method of measuring oxygen consumption. The patient is connected by a hood or face mask to a servo-controlled unit that maintains a unidirectional flow of air from the laboratory through the hood or mask and into the polarographic oxygen sensor. The flow rate is automatically adjusted to maintain the oxygen content of air detected by the sensor at a constant level. As a consequence of this design, the only variable determining the patient's oxygen consumption under steady-state conditions is the speed of the blower in the servo-control unit, because the remaining determinants are constants.

Indicator dilution methods

Thermodilution is now more commonly used than the older indocyanine green method, but the principle behind all indicator dilution methods is the same. These methods also rely on the Fick principle. In these methods, a specified amount of a substance (A) is injected as rapidly as possible at one point in the circulation and the concentration (C) of the substance is then measured continuously as a function of time (t) at some point downstream from the injection site. Figure 17.1 shows an example of the type of curve resulting from plotting continuous measurements of concentration over time at the downstream site. Because all of the substance injected (A) must pass the measurement site, blood flow rate can be calculated as a variation of Equation 2:

$$Q = \frac{A}{\int C(t)dt} \tag{3}$$

where the denominator of Equation 3 is the integral of concentration with respect to time for the period of time that it takes for all of the substance injected to pass the measurement point **for the first time**. This integral is equivalent to the area under the curve indicated in Fig. 17.1. Note that there is a second hump in Fig. 17.1 that occurs because after all the injected substance passes the measurement point for the first time ('first pass'), it then recirculates and passes the measurement point again. It is important, therefore, to determine the area under the concentration-time curve only for that period of time corresponding to the first pass of the substance. This is done by converting the concentration-time curve to a logarithmic concentration scale, which permits linear extrapolation to be used to accurately define the time at which the first pass is completed, but these measurement operations are now automated. One advantage of the thermodilution technique is that there is essentially no recirculation of the injectate, which simplifies calculation of the area under the concentration-time curve.

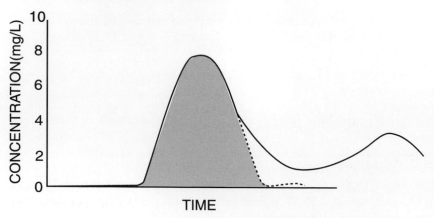

Figure 17.1. *Graph of concentration-time curve, as measured by the indicator dilution technique for determination of cardiac output. Detection of the indicator reaches a peak on its first pass, then declines. There is a smaller second hump, indicating detection of a second pass as the indicator recirculates. With thermodilution techniques, temperature is the indicator and there is no second pass. Shaded area indicates extrapolated estimate of the area under the curve for the first pass.*

In the indocyanine green method, a 1 ml sample (usual concentration 5 mg/ml) is injected into the pulmonary artery and blood is withdrawn at a constant rate from the femoral artery (or any other systemic artery) and passed through a densitometer cuvette to generate the concentration-time curve.

In the thermodilution method, the 'indicator' is a known volume of a cold solution, such as 5% dextrose, which is injected at a proximal site, such as the superior vena cava. The temperature of the injectate is measured before injection. The temperature at the distal site, usually the pulmonary artery, is measured continuously with a thermistor on the catheter. The amount of 'cold' injected (A in Equation 3) is the product of (a) volume of the injectate, (b) temperature difference between blood and injectate, and (c) the ratio of the products of specific gravity and specific heat of blood and injectate, respectively (this ratio is 1.08 for 5% dextrose). This calculated amount of 'cold' is then divided by the area under the temperature-time curve in the pulmonary artery (equivalent to the concentration-time area in the denominator of Equation 3) to yield the cardiac output. The final value is usually multiplied by a correction factor (0.825) to account for warming of the injectate in the catheter prior to injection.

Advantages of the thermodilution method over the indocyanine green method include not only the virtual absence of recirculation but also the simplicity of the 'cold' indicator, absence of a need for systemic arterial blood sampling and, consequently, the ease with which multiple measurements can be made. This last is an important advantage, as thermodilution cardiac output determination should be based on at least three consecutive measurements.

Bioimpedance cardiography

Non-invasive determination of cardiac output is possible by means of echocardiography (*vide infra*) or by thoracic electrical bioimpedance (TEB), a form of electrical impedance plethysmography. TEB can determine cardiac output, stroke volume, systemic vascular resistance, thoracic fluid level, certain indices of myocardial contractility, and other haemodynamic parameters. A small alternating current is sent through the thorax. Sensors on the sides of the neck and chest detect changes in impedance (resistance) along the aorta, recording changes in blood volume and flow with each heartbeat, while a pressure cuff on the upper arm automatically measures arterial blood pressure. Transfer function analysis is then used to convert these signals into standard haematological values to provide continuous analysis of haemodynamic status. TEB is a relatively new technology and is not widely used in the cardiac catheterisation laboratory. Nevertheless, it provides a viable alternative to right heart catheterisation for monitoring high-risk or critically ill candidates who require haemodynamic monitoring.

Cardiac shunts

Shunt measurements are based on a variation of the Fick oxygen method discussed above. In the presence of an intracardiac shunt, the outputs of the left and right heart are no longer equal. In order to measure the size of the shunt, therefore, it is necessary to measure pulmonary blood flow (Q_p) and systemic blood flow (Q_s) separately. Pulmonary blood flow measurement is identical to the measurement described above for the cardiac output determination by the standard Fick oxygen method: that is, oxygen consumption divided by the pulmonary arterio-venous oxygen content difference. As noted above, the pulmonary venous oxygen content can be approximated from a left ventricular or systemic arterial blood sample provided there is no evidence of a right-to-left shunt, which would be suggested by a systemic oxygen saturation less than 95%. If a right-to-left shunt is suspected, a direct sample from one of the pulmonary veins (often possible in the presence of an atrial septal defect) should be used; otherwise, an assumed value for the pulmonary venous oxygen content can be calculated as the product of an assumed saturation of 98% x oxygen-carrying capacity (see above).

Systemic blood flow in the presence of an intracardiac shunt is calculated by dividing the oxygen consumption by the systemic arterio-venous oxygen content difference, which is the difference between the systemic arterial oxygen content and the mixed venous oxygen content **in the chamber immediately proximal to the shunt.**

In order to localise the site of the shunt, it is necessary to perform an oximetry run. This is done by placing an end-hole catheter in the right or left pulmonary artery. The catheter is then withdrawn through the right heart, taking sequential 2 ml heparinised blood samples for oxygen saturation and oxygen content measurements at each of the following sites: right or left pulmonary artery, main pulmonary artery, right ventricular outflow tract, mid-right ventricle, right ventricular inflow tract, low-,mid- and high-right atrium, low superior vena cava (junction with right atrium), high superior vena cava, high inferior vena cava, and low inferior vena cava. Oximetry samples should also be taken from the left ventricle and any arterial site distal to the insertion of the ductus arteriosus into the aorta (usually the femoral artery). From these samples, it is possible to identify the site of a 'step-up' in oxygen saturation, indicating the presence of a left-to-right shunt.

In the presence of a patent ductus arteriosus, the 'step-up' would occur in the pulmonary artery. In this case, the average of the right ventricular blood samples should be used as the mixed venous oxygen content in the calculation of systemic blood flow because the right ventricle is the chamber immediately proximal to the shunt. In the case of a left-to-right shunt through a ventricular septal defect, the 'step-up' would occur in the right ventricle. In this case, the appropriate value for mixed venous oxygen content to be used in the calculation of systemic blood flow would be the average of the right atrial measurements because the right atrium is the chamber immediately proximal to the shunt. In the case of a left-to-right shunt through an atrial septal defect, the 'step-up' would occur in the right atrium. In this case, both the superior and inferior venae cavae are the sites proximal to the level of the shunt, so that the mixed venous oxygen content value to be used for the calculation of systemic blood flow should be the average of the measurements made in both venae cavae. There is empirical evidence that the most accurate method of performing this averaging process is to add three-quarters of the superior vena caval value to one-quarter of the inferior vena caval measurement.

Once pulmonary blood flow (Q_p) and systemic blood flow (Q_s) have been calculated, the absolute value of the left-to-right shunt is given by Q_p - Q_s in litres/min. The shunt size is more commonly reported, however, as the ratio Q_p/Q_s. Because the value for oxygen consumption is common to both Q_p and Q_s measurements, this common value cancels out in the Q_p/Q_s ratio: that is, in order to determine the shunt size as the Q_p/Q_s ratio, it is not actually necessary to measure oxygen consumption. Size of a shunt can be calculated directly from the oximetry data. A Q_p/Q_s ratio less than 1.5 indicates a small left-to-right shunt that may not warrant surgical intervention, but the threshold for intervention to close intracardiac shunts is becoming lower, particularly in the case of atrial septal defects, because of the availability of percutaneous closure methods.

Sample shunt calculations

Left-to-right shunt

Cardiac output calculations are not necessary to determine whether a shunt is present or not. A blood oximetry run is sufficient, as in the following example.

Site	O$_2$ saturation (%)	O$_2$ content (Vol%)
SVC1	69.5	9.9
SVC2	67.5	9.7
IVC	75.8	10.8
RA	87.1	12.5
RV	87.1	12.5
PA1	86.8	12.4
PA2	87.2	12.5
PV	98.4	14.1
Arterial	97.9	14.0

(where SVC = superior vena cava, IVC = inferior vena cava, RA = right atrium, RV = right ventricle, PA = pulmonary artery, PV = pulmonary vein. HB is 10.5 g%, O$_2$ capacity is 14.3 Vol% and O$_2$ consumption is 220 ml/min).

The key issue is to determine whether there is a sudden rise in saturation in a right heart chamber. In the above example, there is a sudden step-up in saturation in the RA sample, indicating a shunt (caused by flow of oxygenated left atrial blood into the right atrium across an atrial septal defect). In a normal heart, right heart saturations should remain relatively constant, apart from variations caused by streamlining effects of blood flow. The critical values in calculating the size of a shunt are taken as the arterial sample, and venous samples before (venae cavae) and after the shunt (PA). An accurate measure of true mixed venous blood (MV) saturation before the shunt is given by the average of 3 SVC and 1 IVC samples [(68.5+68.5+68.5+75.8 / 4) = 281.3/4 = 70.3%]. In this example, the average PA saturation is 87.0% and the arterial saturation is 97.9%.

IVC saturation is frequently higher than SVC, indicating the sample has come from the renal stream. If IVC saturation is lower than SVC, the IVC sample has come from the hepatic stream and should be discarded. Taking the average of 3 SVC samples and 1 IVC overcomes this sampling variability and provides a true mixed venous sample when right atrial saturation cannot be used.

Size of the shunt is reported as the Q_p/Q_s ratio, and can be calculated directly from the pulmonary and systemic A-V differences in the oximetry run. Only the values for arterial, PA and MV saturations are necessary for the calculation. Thus:

Pulmonary A–V difference	= (arterial saturation–PA saturation)
	= 97.9–70.3 = 27.6 Vol%
Systemic A–V difference	= (arterial saturation–MV saturation)
	= 97.9 - 87.0 = 10.9 Vol%

Size of shunt is the Q_p/Q_s ratio (27.6/10.9) and is reported as 2.5:1. This means that 2.5 times more blood passes through the right heart than the left.

Bi-directional shunt

A bi-directional shunt is one in which shunting occurs in both directions across any communication between the systemic and pulmonary circulations. The following data from an oximetry run from a patient with Eisenmenger's syndrome demonstrate very low arterial and venous saturations in both systemic and pulmonary systems.

Site	O_2 saturation (%)	O_2 content
SVC1	50.6	12.4
SVC2	51.0	12.5
IVC	54.8	13.4
RA	55.4	13.6
RV	57.8	14.2
PA1	56.3	13.8
PV	91.9	22.5
LA	84.6	20.7
LV	68.1	16.7

(HB is 18.3 g%, O_2 capacity is 24.9 Vol% and O_2 consumption is 255 ml/min). The following formulae for pulmonary blood flow (PBF), systemic blood flow (SBF) and effective pulmonary blood flow (EPBF) are used to calculate cross-cardiac flows, from which to determine the size and direction of a bi-directional shunt (the effective pulmonary blood flow [EPBF] is the flow that would normally occur if no shunt were present).

PBF = O_2 consumption/PV–PA O_2 content = (255/22.5–13.8) = 255/8.7 = 2.9 L/min
SBF = O_2 consumption/LV–MV O_2 content = (255/16.7–12.7) = 255/4 = 6.4 L/min
EPBF = O_2 consumption/PV–MV O_2 content = (255/22.5–12.7) = 255/9.8 = 2.6 L/min
The left-to-right-shunt is the difference PBF–EPBF = (2.9–2.6) = 0.3 L/min
The right-to-left shunt is the difference SBF–EPBF = (6.4–2.6) = 3.8 L/min

In this example, the patient had a predominant right-to-left shunt of 3.8 L/min, with a small left-to-right shunt of 0.3 L/min.

Right-to-left shunt

With a right-to-left shunt, mixing occurs only on the systemic side, so that systemic arterial saturations are reduced without affecting right heart saturations. If systemic arterial saturations are less than 95%, a right-to-left shunt should be suspected. Given that arterial O_2 content is 18.5 Vol%, PV O_2 content is 22.8 Vol%, MV O_2 content is 10.6 Vol%, and PA

O_2 content is 10.6 Vol%, the following calculations can be used determine the shunt (O_2 consumption is 385 ml/min).

PBF = O_2 consumption/PV–PA O_2 content = (385/22.8–10.6) = 385/12.2 = 3.2 L/min
SBF = O_2 consumption/LV–MV O_2 content = (385/18.5–10.6) = 385/7.9 = 4.9 L/min
EPBF = O_2 consumption/PV–MV O_2 content = (385/22.8–10.6) = 385/12.2 = 3.2 L/min
The left-to-right shunt is the difference PBF – EPBF = (3.2–3.2) = 0 L/min
The right-to-left shunt is the difference SBF – EPBF = (4.9–3.2) = 1.7 L/min

As expected, with a pure right-to-left shunt there is no flow from the systemic to the pulmonary side, so the left-to-right flow is zero ml/min, and pulmonary blood flow is identical to the effective pulmonary blood flow (3.2 ml/min). In this example, there is a right-to-left shunt from the pulmonary to the systemic side of 1.7 L/min.

No shunt

When no shunt is present, there is no sudden step-up in any chamber and saturations in the oximetry run do not vary significantly, as in the following example. No additional measurements or calculations are required to confirm this.

Site	O_2 saturation (%)	O_2 content (Vol%)
SVC1	69.5	12.5
IVC	68.2	10.3
HRA	67.9	10.3
MRA	69.8	10.5
LRA	66.7	10.1
RV	67.2	10.2
PA1	67.9	10.3
PA2	66.7	10.1
LV	96.5	14.6

Echocardiographic methods

It should be noted that it is now rare for intracardiac shunts to be detected for the first time at cardiac catheterisation. Diagnosis of intracardiac shunts is now more commonly made by echocardiography. While it has been possible for many years to detect atrial septal defects by peripheral venous injection of agitated saline and observation of some of the resulting bubbles crossing to the left side of the heart, colour Doppler echocardiography has made the detection and localisation of intracardiac shunts a relatively straightforward procedure. Using this technique, the abnormal jet of blood flow across an atrial or ventricular septal defect or across a patent ductus arteriosus can be directly visualised. It is also possible to measure both the cardiac output and the size of an intracardiac shunt using echocardiographic techniques. Total blood flow across any one of the four cardiac valves is equal to the product of the cross-sectional area of the open valve and the velocity-time integral of the blood flow crossing the valve. The cross-sectional area of the annulus of the aortic or pulmonary valve can be determined by two-dimensional echocardiography. It is usual to measure the diameter (D) of the annulus from the cross-sectional image of the valve, then calculate the area as $\pi D^2/4$. The velocity of blood flow across the valve of interest is measured by the Doppler technique, and displayed as a function of time. The echocardiographic machine permits the area under the velocity-time curve for each systolic period (the velocity-time integral) to be determined automatically after the curve is traced. From the product of cross-sectional area and velocity-time integral measurements, the machine automatically calculates stroke volume and multiplies this by heart rate to yield the output of the left or right ventricle in litres/min. In the absence of an intracardiac shunt, the measurement of the output of either ventricle is the same as the total cardiac output. In the presence of an intracardiac shunt, the ratio of pulmonary blood flow to systemic blood flow (Q_p/Q_s) provides an estimate of the shunt size, as described for catheterisation techniques.

Further Reading

Bain DS, Grossman W. *Cardiac catheterization, angiography and intervention*, 5th ed. Baltimore: Williams and Wilkins 1996.

Davidson CJ, Fishman RF, Bonow RO. Cardiac catheterization. In: Braunwald E (ed) *Heart disease: A textbook of cardiovascular medicine*, 5th ed. Philadelphia: WB Saunders 1997.

Feigenbaum H. *Echocardiography*, 5th ed. Philadelphia: Lea and Febiger 1994.

Chapter 18

Measurement of Left Ventricular Function Using Pressure-Volume Loops

Christopher S. Hayward and Raymond P. Kelly

Background

Accurate measurement of myocardial contractility in man is valuable in the investigation of heart failure, in assessment of cardiac performance when significant valvular incompetence is present, and in understanding the mode of action of a wide variety of drugs that act on the cardiovascular system. There are, however, complexities in cardiac function that render measurement of contractility a demanding assessment requiring precision. The complexities of function include the geometric shape of the ventricle (making assessment of individual fibre shortening difficult), the finite time required to initiate contraction in all cells (making contraction only partly synchronous, especially when there is extensive myocardial damage), the sensitivity of myocardial performance to loading conditions, the sensitivity of contractility to alterations in heart rate, and the effect of sympathetic activity.

It is not surprising, therefore, that several methods have been used to develop indices of contractility, each with its own limitations. These indices are conveniently divided into isovolumic and ejection phase indices. The simplest and most frequently used is the maximum rate of pressure development (dP/dt). It is, however, dependent to some extent on loading conditions, especially filling pressure. Ejection phase indices include ejection fraction, mean velocity of circumferential fibre shortening, and aortic flow velocity. These also provide important information about cardiac function but are susceptible to afterload conditions. None of these indices provides information about ventricular compliance or diastolic function.

More comprehensive overall assessment of cardiac pump function may be obtained from on-line simultaneous measurement of left ventricular pressure and volume using pressure micromanometer and multi-electrode volume measurement catheters in the cardiac catheterisation laboratory. Such an approach has a strong physiological foundation. Otto Frank was one of the first physiologists to apply muscle physiology to the heart in a systematic way.[1] Because of geometric differences in fibre orientation compared with isolated muscle strips, Frank recognised that the description of cardiac function in simple terms of time-varying parameters such as pressure or volume was inadequate. Studying the frog ventricle, Frank described cardiac chamber or pump function in terms of simultaneous pressure (P) and volume (V) **independent of time**. Such pressure-volume (P-V) relationships were initially referred to as 'work' diagrams, referring to the work performed by the heart on the blood.[2] Once difficulties in the continuous measurement of ventricular

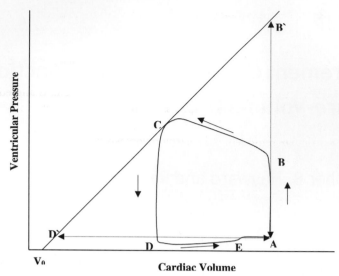

Figure 18.1. *Schematic of generation of P-V loops and an idealised end-systolic P-V relationship (ESPVR). The P-V cycle is performed anticlockwise. Isovolumic contraction begins at A and continues until B when the aortic valve opens and cardiac ejection commences. Following end-systole, C, there is a period of isovolumic relaxation, (CD). At D the left ventricle starts to fill until atrial systole (E) occurs, completing left ventricular filling and the cardiac cycle. AB' and AD' represent hypothetical P-V trajectories generated by isometric and isotonic contractions respectively. The line B'CD' represents the idealised ESPVR.*

volume were overcome[2,3] (pressure recordings having been mastered earlier), a new era of cardiovascular physiology based on analysis of P-V loops began.[4-6]

As seen in Fig. 18.1, the P-V loop is performed anti-clockwise, as described by Sagawa *et al.*[7] Starting at the onset of contraction (or end-diastole, A) pressure can be seen to increase with little change in volume. This phase (AB) corresponds to left ventricular isovolumic contraction. At B the aortic valve opens and cardiac ejection commences. From this point volume decreases with a small variable increase in left ventricular pressure. The shape of the loop during ejection is dependent on the interaction of cardiac contraction with arterial characteristics.[8] At C, the end of systole, the left ventricle starts to relax with a rapid fall in pressure and little change in volume (CD, isovolumic relaxation). At D the left ventricle starts to fill until atrial systole (E) occurs, completing left ventricular filling and the cardiac cycle.

Definition of systolic function using pressure-volume loops

From series of variably preloaded P-V loops, three related indices of chamber function can be derived. They are the end-systolic P-V relationship (ESPVR), the preload recruitable stroke work relationship (PRSWR) and the dP/dt_{max}-end-diastolic volume relationship. Each is derived from simultaneous, continuous measurement of pressure and volume during alteration in cardiac loading conditions by decreasing preload (usually by occlusion of the inferior vena cava, IVC)[9] or increasing afterload (usually pharmacologically by phenylephrine). IVC occlusion has the advantage that a large, rapid change in loading conditions can be achieved before sympathetic reflex responses are evident. It has been shown that methods that increase afterload are associated with a reflex increase in contractility.[9-11]

Continuous left ventricular volumes may be obtained using a conductance catheter,[9,12] from ultrasonic crystals deriving volume from orthogonal pairs of crystals,[13] or from radionucleide ventriculography.[14] For the latter technique, load is altered by pharmacological means (phenylephrine or nitroprusside). By obtaining such on-line recordings, ESPVRs have been extensively used to define inotropic effects of drugs,[15] ischaemia[16] and the effects of ventricular remodelling in cardiomyoplasty.[17]

A.

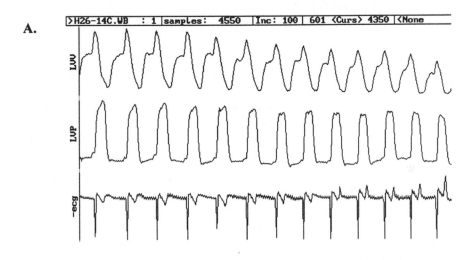

B.

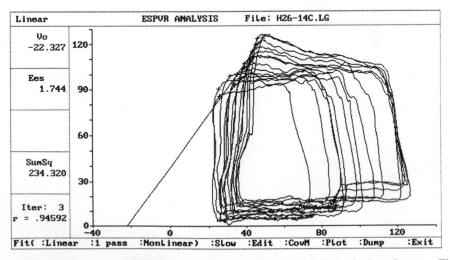

Figure 18.2. Derivation of ESPVR from IVC occlusion using P-V Analysis software. The raw data (A) shows a gradual decrease in both pressure (LVP) and volume (LVV). The ESPVR is calculated by linear regression of the end-systolic points (r=0.95 in this study). The gradual decrease in the size of loops during IVC occlusion is seen in B. Actual recordings are shown.

Derivation of the end-systolic pressure-volume relationship

The ratio of simultaneous pressure and volume defines the elastance (or stiffness) of the ventricle. It can be shown that this increases to a maximum during systole and then decreases to a low value during diastole.[5] If cardiac function is examined in terms of ventricular elastance, end-systole may be defined as the point at which elastance reaches a maximum.[18] This corresponds to point C on the P-V loop diagram (Fig. 18.1). The distinction of end-systole from end-ejection may not be clear under normal conditions, but does become significant in situations of elevated afterload, as may occur with ageing or hypertension.[18,19] The linear ESPVR is then calculated from a series of end-systolic points under varying load (Fig. 18.2).[5,20]

The linearity of the ESPVR has been extensively investigated. A linear relation for end-systolic PV points under variable loading conditions was first suggested in 1957.[21] It has been confirmed in the isolated heart[5] as well as *in vivo*.[22] It is the justification for using only 2–3 loops to characterise the ESPVR.[14,23] Subsequent investigators have found that the relation may be curvilinear at high afterloads, prompting a reappraisal of the significance and usefulness of the derived V_0, the chamber volume at zero pressure.[24] The curvilinearity of the ESPVR has been explained theoretically on the basis of calcium transients,[25] and may explain why extrapolated V_0 values often result in negative volumes.[26] Instead of reporting the volume at zero pressure (V_0), it has been suggested that the calculated volume at operating pressures (such as 100 mmHg) may be used (V_{100}).[27] This has the advantage that extrapolation to V_0 is not required, and minor non-linearities of the ESPVR do not significantly affect the result. Consistent with this, other investigators have found that operating volumes (V_{100}) are more reliable than the extrapolated volume V_0.[28]

The slope of the line is termed the end-systolic elastance (Ees) and the extrapolated intercept, V_0. An increase in Ees has been interpreted as an increase in ventricular chamber performance,[26] an increase in contractility[6,29] and an increase in preload sensitivity.[30] One problem with the ESPVR is that it is sensitive to ventricular size.[26,31] To account for this, various normalising techniques have been suggested including normalising to left ventricular mass,[32] end-diastolic volume (EDV),[33] or body surface area.[6,14,20] However, many commentators are not satisfied that current normalisation techniques have achieved their aim.[31] The ESPVR differs from preload recruitable stroke work (discussed subsequently) in this respect.[34]

One of the greatest difficulties with ESPVR, as with the other 'load-independent measures' of contractility, is that they rely on an accurate assessment of the response of the ventricle to a systematic alteration of loading conditions. Simple extrapolation of the end-systolic P–V ratio through the origin is not valid.[35] As left ventricular pressure and volume can be defined non-invasively throughout systole, research has been directed to non-invasive methods of defining load-independent indices of contractility.[36] The notion for single-beat elastance is derived from the finding that, under different loading as well as inotropic conditions, the normalised elastance time curve is remarkably stable.[37] This adds circumstantial evidence to the suggestion that the P-V loop is a macrostructural representation of cellular and subcellular machinery. Alternative mechanisms for derivation of single beat elastance have been proposed, including mathematical estimation of the isovolumic pressure for a single ejecting beat based on a curve-fitting algorithm.[38]

Preload-recruitable stroke work relationship

The preload recruitable stroke work relationship (PRSWR) is the relationship between stroke work and end-diastolic volume, and an extension of the Frank-Starling concept.[13,39]

The PRSWR is highly linear. Stroke work will increase in a linear fashion with increased preload when preload is defined by end-diastolic volume rather than filling pressure. The non-linear relationship between stroke work and end-diastolic pressure reflects the non-linearity of the relationship between end-diastolic pressure and end-diastolic volume.[13] The degree to which stroke work increases with end-diastolic volume (the slope of the relation, often termed M_{sw}) is dependent on the contractility of the ventricle[13] and is independent of heart rate and size.[34] The independence from size contrasts with ESPVR and allows better comparison of inter-subject responses to the same intervention.

A major advantage of PRSWR is that there is a much greater percentage change in stroke work than end-systolic pressure for any given change in preload (EDV) due to IVC occlusion.[40] This gives the relationship better reproducibility and it tends to be more robust than the ESPVR or the dP/dt_{max}-end-diastolic relationship (described subsequently).[28,34,40] A possible downside of this finding is that some investigators have found M_{sw} to be less sensitive than Ees in responding to inotropic changes,[27,39,41] but this finding is not universal.[42] A limitation of PRSWR is that it does not distinguish diastolic from systolic dysfunction.[26] This is particularly a problem in conditions with steep end-diastolic P-V relationships such as hypertrophy and ischaemia and may complicate assessment of systolic function.[39]

dP/dt$_{max}$-end-diastolic volume relationship

While dP/dt_{max} is preload dependent it is largely independent of afterload. To account for this, a further index incorporating preload was derived. This dP/dt_{max}-end-diastolic volume is derived from the same P-V loops and based on the time-varying elastance model used in the derivation of ESPVR.[43] Because dP/dt_{max} occurs during isovolumic contraction, it provides a conceptual framework to understand left ventricular performance during early systole. Unfortunately, while the relation is sensitive to changes in inotropic state, it suffers from much greater variability than either ESPVR or PRSWR[28,34,40] and is rarely reported independently.

Definition of diastolic function using pressure-volume loops

Just as the definition of the onset and duration of diastole has been debated,[44] accurate quantification of intrinsic diastolic left ventricular function has also been controversial.[45] While diastole was initially considered to be entirely passive, it is now accepted as an energy-dependent process,[46] particularly in its early part. More than systole, it is dependent on factors extrinsic to the left ventricle, including the pericardium, respiration and, via septal interaction, the right ventricle.[47] Because of this, apparent drug effects on diastolic function may be mediated by effects on the venous system, altering preload and thus the degree of pericardial constraint and ventricular interaction, rather than any direct left ventricular relaxation.[48]

End-diastolic pressure-volume relationship

Simple indices of passive ventricular performance have been used to demonstrate chamber stiffness. The simplest of these is diastolic chamber compliance or dV/dP.[46] It has been shown that this relationship is non-linear.[47] As the ventricle fills, therefore, the slope of this relation increases. This relation of end-diastolic pressure and volume across a range of filling pressures defines the end-diastolic P-V relationship (EDPVR).[49] Meaningful comparison of results for compliance, even in the same individual, can therefore only be made

END-SYSTOLIC and END-DIASTOLIC

PRESSURE-VOLUME RELATIONSHIPS

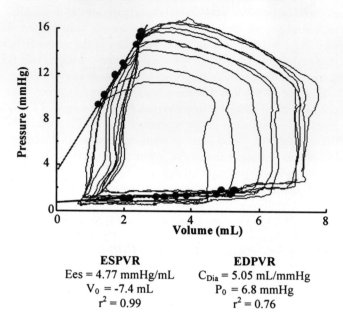

ESPVR	EDPVR
E_{es} = 4.77 mmHg/mL	C_{Dia} = 5.05 mL/mmHg
V_0 = -7.4 mL	P_0 = 6.8 mmHg
r^2 = 0.99	r^2 = 0.76

PRELOAD RECRUITABLE STROKE WORK RELATIONSHIP

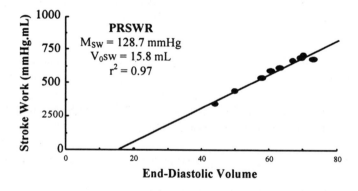

Figure 18.3. Actual recordings of load-independent indices for one subject. The derivation of ESPVR and EDPVR is shown from the end-systolic and end-diastolic points overlying the pressure-volume loops. The preload recruitable stroke work relationship is derived from the stroke work (area within the loop) and EDV for the corresponding loop.

at the same diastolic pressure. As a result of atrial contraction, curve fitting to the entire duration of diastole may be inaccurate.[50] Because of this, clinical studies using EDPVR use the portion of diastolic filling prior to atrial contraction.[51,52]

The entire EDPVR is complex and dependent on cardiac and non-cardiac factors mentioned above. Viscosity or elasticity of the heart is only one of the variables. Marked changes in the slope of the EDPVR in response to haemodynamic interventions may be

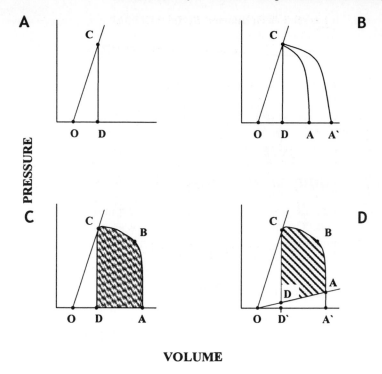

VOLUME

Figure 18.4. Derivation of P-V area and relation to ventricular energetics.
A. Mechanical potential energy at end-systole (DCO), defined by the ESPVR (OC). B.
This area (DCO) is independent of trajectory of contraction (DC, AC or A'C). C. External
mechanical work in an ejecting contraction (ABCD). D. P-V area (ABCD+DCO). Note:
ADO represents the EDPVR.

explained by factors extrinsic to the left ventricle.[48,53] Some authors have suggested that passive characteristics of the left ventricle may only be altered acutely by active ischaemia.[54]

Figure 18.3 shows derivation of the end-systolic and end-diastolic pressure-volume relationships as well as the PRSWR. The linearity of ESPVR, EDPVR and PRSWR is easily appreciated within physiological changes in volume.

Pressure-volume area and ventricular energetics

A further benefit of assessment of left ventricular function using P-V loops is the ability to determine ventricular energetics[13,55] and efficiency.[56] Figure 18.4 shows the derivation of ventricular energy expenditure derived from P-V loops, as described by Suga.[57] From this it can be seen that the end-systolic point (C), the end-systolic volume (D), and the ESPVR define potential energy of contraction. It is independent of the shape of the P-V trajectory. The external mechanical work is defined by the P-V loop (ABCD). The combination of the potential and external mechanical energy defines the pressure-volume area (PVA) which is closely correlated with energy consumption of the left ventricle.[57]

Recognition that the heart performs work in ejecting blood is fundamental to the understanding of ventricular energetics. Since early in the 20th century attempts have been made to quantify this work, in an effort to define the efficiency and energetic cost of cardiac contraction. In 1932 Katz calculated total work from the potential and kinetic energy of the blood leaving the heart, based on the mean ventricular pressure and volume of blood ejected.[58] It has since been shown that the total mechanical energy of contraction of the heart can be described by the area defined within a closed P-V loop.[57] This is made up of both the area inside the loop (defining external work of the heart) as well as the area circumscribed by the ESPVR (defining the potential energy of contraction) (Fig. 18.4).[57]

The significance of this finding is the recognition that the myocardial oxygen consumption/beat is linearly correlated with this P-V area. This empirical relationship between energy consumption and contraction has been verified by other investigators.[8,55,59] The surprising constancy of this relationship suggests a fundamental physical phenomenon of chemo-mechanical energy transduction.[60]

Pressure-volume study protocol

Pressure-volume studies are performed at the completion of routine left heart catheterisation in appropriate patients. The 6F femoral arterial sheath is exchanged for an 8.5F arterial sheath and a 9F femoral venous sheath inserted. An 8F volume catheter (Webster 7212-08, Webster Lab. Inc.) is then inserted into the ventricular cavity under fluoroscopic guidance. Following electrical calibration, a 2F Millar pressure micromanometer (SPC-360, Millar Instruments, Houston TX) is passed through the volume catheter to rest at its tip. Once catheters are in position, simultaneous pressure and volume data are displayed on-line and recorded. Volume calibration is performed off-line using a radio-opaque sphere of known diameter. Alternative methods of volume calibration include determination of cardiac output by thermodilution (obtained by right ventricular catheterisation) for calculation of the measured stroke volume from the ventriculogram. Because the ventricular catheter remains *in situ* for approximately 30–40 minutes, a slow pressurised heparin infusion (2500 Units sodium heparin in 500 mL 5% dextrose) is attached via arterial pressure bag and Tuohy-Borst adapter.

Manipulation of loading conditions

A 35mm vena caval balloon catheter (Cordis 530000A-15565, Cordis Corporation, Miami FL) is used for acute preload reduction. The balloon catheter is passed to the right atrium under fluoroscopic guidance. Inferior vena caval balloon occlusion (IVCBO) is performed in the right atrium by brief inflation of the vena caval balloon with 30–35mL of carbon dioxide for 8–10 seconds or until ventricular ectopy occurs. The catheter is then gently withdrawn to lodge in the mouth of the inferior vena cava. The load-independent indices ESPVR, PRSWR and EDPVR are calculated from IVCBO data. Runs with changes in heart rate of >10% during IVCBO are excluded.

Two main sets of data are recorded using P-V measurements. Continuous pressure and volume data sets in a stable rhythm (10–20 beats) are collected for 'steady-state' analysis. The second set of data involves preload reduction with continuous recording during reducing pressure and volume. An example of the generation of ESPVR by inferior vena caval occlusion in a single subject is shown in Fig. 18.2. The ESPVR is determined by linear regression of the end-systolic points as described above. An iterative procedure is performed from the linear regression of the lines using an initial estimate of V_0 of 0 mL. Subsequent iterations are performed until errors are minimised.[9,22]

End-diastolic relationships are determined from two EDP/EDV points on each P-V loop. The points chosen are those immediately prior to the 'a' wave and a second point at 10% of the filling volume earlier in the same loop.[51] An examination of diastole prior to atrial contraction best reflects passive diastolic properties of the left ventricle. A linear model is assumed for EDPVR as this is simpler and has been shown to be as valid as more complex exponential regression models.[61] Although the slope of the regression describes an

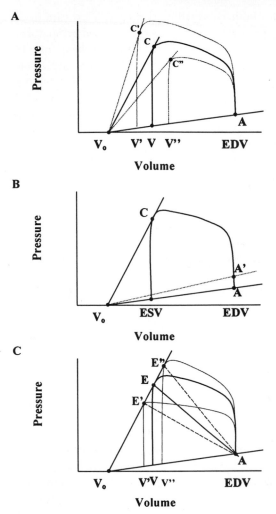

A

B

C

Figure 18.5. A. Effects of changes in inotropic status on stroke volume. In the absence of a change in arterial function or EDV, an increase in contractility results in an increase in stroke volume (EDV-V'). In cardiomyopathy or under the influence of a negative inotrope (EDV-V"), the stroke volume is decreased. End-systolic pressure can also be seen to change in a similar fashion (C', C" respectively) assuming no change in heart rate. B. An impairment of diastolic function, shown as an increase in the slope of the EDPVR (AV$_o$→A'V$_o$), results in a significant rise in EDP in response to a small change in EDV. Stroke volume is not affected. C. If arterial properties change, stroke volume is affected, even in the absence of changes in contractility. Stroke volume falls (EDV-V") in response to an increase in arterial elastance (AE→AE") and increases (EDV-V') if arterial elastance falls (AE→AE').

elastance, the results are usually reported as inverse, chamber compliance, $C_{Dia.}$[48] The equation for diastolic compliance is therefore $V=C_{Dia} \cdot P + V_{oDia}$, where V_{oDia} is the volume axis intercept. Previous studies have shown that a linear description of diastolic compliance is simpler and fits data just as well as exponential curves.[61]

Clinical relevance of information derived from pressure-volume loops

One of the strengths of P-V analysis is that information is available on systolic and diastolic ventricular function as well as its interaction with the arterial tree. The effect of inotropes, exercise, and pericardial disease on ventricular filling and stroke volume may also be easily understood. Figure 18.5 shows the effect of a change in inotropy on the PV loop. A positive inotrope (in isolation) increases stroke volume with a small associated increase in stroke work, whereas a negative inotrope can be seen to decrease stroke volume. These effects are independent of end-diastolic volume, which in this simplified model remains constant. In cardiomyopathic states (with intrinsically lower contractility and therefore lower Ees), the response is to increase end-diastolic volume to maintain stroke volume. The reflex sympathetic response in cardiac failure increases both contractility (Ees) and heart rate in an attempt to maintain cardiac output. In response to exercise, with increased sympathetic tone, increased stroke volume is maintained in the face of an increase in heart rate by increasing contractility. In patients without contractile reserve (who are already under sympathetic stimulation due to cardiomyopathy) the heart is unable to respond in this manner, limiting stroke volume and thereby exercise tolerance.

The effect of a decrease in diastolic compliance (increase in passive diastolic stiffness), as may be found in states of left ventricular hypertrophy or ischaemia, is to increase the ventricular filling pressure required to achieve the same volume. This can occur in the absence of systolic function, as shown in Fig. 18.5b. Pericardial constriction imposes a similar limitation on ventricular filling.

Perhaps the most significant haemodynamic breakthrough that P-V loop analysis allows is integration of information concerning arterial function with that concerning the left ventricle. This integration is termed ventriculo-vascular coupling. Other methods used to characterise ventricular function are implicitly dependent on arterial function, as ventricular ejection has long been recognised to depend on the afterload imposed on it by the arterial tree.[62] As arterial impedance, commonly accepted as the most appropriate method of determining afterload,[63] requires invasively obtained aortic pressure and flow, it is not commonly measured. Effective arterial elastance (Ea), derived from P-V loops, incorporates much of the information available from the aortic impedance spectrum,[64] and is considered a reasonable alternative to the definition of afterload.[64,65] A major benefit of this arterial elastance is that it is expressed in the same units and defined by the same method as ventricular elastance, allowing an obvious and direct introduction into the concept of ventriculo-vascular coupling.[66] The effect of an isolated change in arterial stiffness as expressed by arterial elastance is shown in Fig. 18.5c. It can be seen that stroke volume is therefore sensitive to both contractile state (Ees) and arterial compliance (Ea). Numerous drug studies have used this fact to compare and contrast ventricular with vascular effects.[67] The dependence of ventricular function on arterial properties is involved in the use of nitroglycerine to unload the failing heart.[68] From Fig. 18.5c, it can be seen that the decrease in arterial elastance may increase stroke volume without any change in ventricular function being required.

References

1. Frank O, (translated by Chapman CB, Wasserman E). Zur Dynamik des Herzmuskels. (On the dynamics of cardiac muscle, Reproduced in *Am Heart J* 1959; **58**:282-317,467-78). *Z Biol* 1895; **32**:370-447.
2. Katz AM, Katz LN, Williams FL. Registration of left ventricular volume curves in the dog with the systemic circulation intact. *Circ Res* 1955; **3**:588-93.
3. Baan J, Van Der Velde ET, De Bruib Hg *et al.* Continuous measurement of left ventricular volume in animals and humans by conductance catheter. *Circulation* 1984; **70**:812-23.
4. Katz LN. The performance of the heart. (Lewis A. Connor Memorial Lecture). *Circulation* 1960; **21**:483-98.
5. Suga H, Sagawa K. Instantaneous pressure-volume relationships and their ratio in the excised, supported canine left ventricle. *Circ Res* 1974; **35**:117-26.
6. Grossman W, Braunwald E, Mann T, McLaurin LP, Green LH. Contractile state of the left ventricle in man as evaluated from end-systolic pressure-volume relations. *Circulation* 1977; **56**(5):845-52.
7. Sagawa K, Maughan WL, Suga H, Sunagawa K. *Cardiac contraction and the pressure volume relationship*. New York: Oxford University Press 1988.

8.   Kelly RP, Tunin R, Kass DA. Effect of reduced aortic compliance on cardiac efficiency and contractile function of in situ canine left ventricle. *Circ Res* 1992; **71**:490-502.

9.   Kass DA, Yamazaki T, Burkhoff D, Maughan WL, Sagawa K. Determination of left ventricular end-systolic pressure-volume relationships by the conductance (volume) catheter technique. *Circulation* 1986; **73**:586-95.

10. Burkhoff D, de Tombe PP, Hunter WC, Kass DA. Contractile strength and mechanical efficiency of left ventricle are enhanced by physiological afterload. *Am J Physiol* 1991; **260**:H569-H578.

11. Baan J, van der Velde ET, Steendijk P. Ventricular pressure-volume relations in vivo. *Eur Heart J* 1992; **13**(supE):2-6.

12. Burkhoff D, van der Velde E, Kass D, Baan J, Maughan WL, Sagawa K. Accuracy of volume measurement by conductance catheter in isolated, ejecting canine hearts. *Circulation* 1985; **72**(2):440-7.

13. Glower DD, Spratt JA, Snow ND, Kabas JS, Sabiston DC, Rankin JS. Linearity of the Frank-Starling relationship in the intact heart: the concept of preload recruitable stroke work. *Circulation* 1985; **71**:994-1009.

14. McKay RG, Aroesty JM, Heller GV, et al. Left ventricular pressure-volume diagrams and end-systolic pressure-volume relations in human beings. *J Am Coll Cardiol* 1984; **3**(2 Pt 1):301-12.

15. Cheng C-P, Noda T, Nordlander M, Ohno M, Little W. Comparison of effects of dihydropyridine calcium antagonists on left ventricular systolic and diastolic performance. *J Pharmacol Exp Ther* 1994; **268**:1232-41.

16. Kass DA, Marino P, Maughan WL, Sagawa K. Determinants of end-systolic pressure-volume relations during acute regional ischemia in situ. *Circulation* 1989; **80**:1783-94.

17. Kass DA, Baughman KL, Pak PH *et al.* Reverse remodeling from cardiomyoplasty in human heart failure. External constraint versus active assist. *Circulation* 1995; **91**:2314-318.

18. Suga H. End-systolic pressure volume relations. *Circulation* 1979; **59**:419-20.

19. Nishioka O, Maruyama Y, Ashikawa K, et al. Effects of changes in afterload impedance on left ventricular ejection in isolated canine hearts: dissociation of end ejection from end systole. *Cardiovasc Res* 1987; **21**:107-18.

20. Sagawa K. The end-systolic pressure-volume relation of the ventricle: definition, modifications, and clinical use. *Circulation* 1981; **63**:1223-27.

21. Holt JP. Regulation of the degree of emptying of the left ventricle by the force of ventricular contraction. *Circ Res* 1957; **5**:281-87.

22. Kass DA, Midei M, Graves W, Brinker JA, Maughan WL. Use of a conductance (volume) catheter and transient inferior vena caval occlusion for rapid determination of pressure-volume relationships in man. *Cathet Cardiovasc Diagn* 1988; **15**:192-202.

23. Mehmel HC, Stockins B, Ruffman K, Olshausen Kv, Schuler G, Kubler W. The linearity of the end-systolic pressure-volume relationship in man and its sensitivity for assessment of left ventricular function. *Circulation* 1981; **63**:1216-22.

24. van der Velde ET, Burkhoff D, Steendijk P, Karsdon J, Sagawa K, Baan J. Nonlinearity and load sensitivity of end-systolic pressure-volume relation of canine left ventricle in vivo. *Circulation* 1991; **83**(1):315-27.

25. Burkhoff D. Explaining load dependence of ventricular contractile properties with a model of excitation-contraction coupling. *J Mol Cell Cardiol* 1994; **26**(8):959-78.

26. Kass DA, Maughan WL. From Emax to pressure-volume relations: a broader view. *Circulation* 1988; **77**:1203-12.

27. Little WC, Cheng CP, Mumma M, Igarashi Y, Vinten-Johansen J, Johnston WE. Comparison of measures of left ventricular contractile performance derived from pressure-volume loops in conscious dogs. *Circulation* 1989; **80**(5):1378-87.

28. Rahko P. Comparative efficacy of three indexes of left ventricular performance derived from pressure-volume loops in heart failure induced by tachypacing. *J Am Coll Cardiol* 1994; **23**:209-18.

29. Cohen-Solal A, Dahan M, Guiomard A, Baleynaud S, Laperche T, Himbert D, Gourgon R. Effects of aging on left ventricle-arterial coupling in man. *Arch Mal Coeur Vaiss* 1993; **86**(8):1095-7.

30. Chen C-H, Nakayama M, Nevo E, Fetics BJ, Kass DA. Age-related ventricular-vascular stiffening: effects of preload sensitivity. *Circulation* 1997; **96**(8):I-199 (Abstract).

31. Mirsky I. An appraisal of ventricular myocardial function variables based on the elastance concept. *J Am Coll Cardiol* 1989; **14**:354.

32. Suga H, Hisano R, Goto Y, Yamada O. Normalization of end-systolic pressure-volume relation and Emax of different sized hearts. Jpn *Circulation* J 1984; **48**(2):136-43.

33. Sagawa K. The ventricular pressure volume diagram revisited. *Circ Res* 1978; 43:677.

34. Takeuchi M, Odake M, Takaoka H, Hayashi Y, Yokoyama M. Comparison between preload recruitable stroke work and the end-systolic pressure-volume relationship in man. *Eur Heart J* 1992; **13**(supE):80-84.

35. Starling MR, Montgomery DG, Walsh RA. Load dependence of the single beat maximal pressure (stress)/volume ratios in humans. *J Am Coll Cardiol* 1989; **14**:345-353.

36. Fetics BJ, Nevo E, Nakayama M, Wong EY, Pak PH, Maughan WL, Chen C-H. Total non-invasive estimation of left ventricular end-systolic elastance from steady state data. *Circulation* 1997; **96**(8):I-640 (Abstract).

37. Senzaki H, Chen C-H, Kass DA. Single beat estimation of end-systolic pressure-volume relation in humans. A new method with the potential for noninvasive application. *Circulation* 1996; **94**:2497-06.

38. Takeuchi M, Igarashi Y, Tomimoto S *et al*. Single-beat estimation of the slope of the end-systolic pressure-volume relation in the human left ventricle. *Circulation* 1991; **83**(1):202-12.

39. Foex P, Leone BJ. Pressure-volume loops: a dynamic approach to the assessment of ventricular function. *J Cardiothor Vasc Anesth* 1994; **8**:84-96.

40. Feneley MP, Skelton TN, Kisslo KB, Davis JW, Bashore TM, Rankin JS. Comparison of preload recruitable stroke work, end-systolic pressure-volume and dP/dtmax-end diastolic volume relations as indexes of left ventricular contractile performance in patients undergoing routine cardiac catheterisation. *J Am Coll Cardiol* 1992; **19**:1522-30.

41. Starling MR. Responsiveness of the time varying elastance to alterations in left ventricular contractile state in man. *Am Heart J* 1989; **118**:1266-76.

42. Kass DA, Maughan WL, Guo ZM, Kong A, Sunagawa K, Sagawa K. Comparative influence of load versus inotropic states on indexes of ventricular contractility: experimental and theoretical analysis based on pressure-volume relationships. *Circulation* 1987; **76**:1422-36.

43. Little WC. The left ventricular dP/dtmax-end-diastolic volume relation in closed-chest dogs. *Circ Res* 1985; **56**(6):808-15.

44. Brutsaert DL, Rademaker FE, Sys SU. Triple control of relaxation: implications in cardiac disease. *Circulation* 1984; **69**:190-96.

45. Glantz SA. Computing indices of diastolic stiffness has been counterproductive. *Fed Proc* 1980; **39**(2):162-8.

46. Grossman W, McLaurin LP. Diastolic properties of the left ventricle. Ann Int Med 1976; **84**:645-53.

47. Janicki JS, Weber KT. Factors influencing the diastolic pressure-volume relation of the cardiac ventricles. *Fed Proc* 1980; **39**:133-40.

48. Kass DA, Wolff MR, Ting C-T, Lui C-P, Chang M-S, Lawrence W, Maughan WL. Diastolic compliance of hypertrophied ventricle is not acutely altered by pharmacological agents influencing active processes. Ann Int Med 1993; **119**:466-73.

49. Templeton GH, Ecker RR, Mitchell JH. Left ventricular stiffness during diastole and systole: the influence of changes in volume and inotropic state. *Cardiovasc Res* 1972; **6**(1):95-100.

50. Gaasch WH, Cole JS, Quinones MA, Alexander JK. Dynamic determinants of left ventricular diastolic pressure-volume relations in man. *Circulation* 1975; **51**:317-23.

51. Lui C-P, Ting C-T, Yang T-M *et al*. Reduced left ventricular compliance in human mitral stenosis. Role of reversible internal constraint. *Circulation* 1992; **85**:1447-56.

52. Hayward CS, Kalnins WV, Rogers P, Feneley MP, Macdonald PS, Kelly RP. Effect of inhaled nitric oxide on normal left ventricular hemodynamics. *J Am Coll Cardiol* 1997; **30**(1):49-56.

53. Pak PH, Maughan WL, Baughman KL, Kass DA. Marked discordance between dynamic and passive diastolic pressure-volume relations in idiopathic hypertrophic cardiomyopathy. *Circulation* 1996; **94**:52-60.

54. Rankin JS, Arentzen CE, Ring WS, Edwards CH, McHale PA, Anderson RW. The diastolic mechanical properties of the intact left ventricle. *Fed Proc* 1980; **39**:141-47.

55. Takaoka H, Takeuchi M, Odake M, Yokoyama M. Assessment of myocardial oxygen consumption (VO2) and systolic pressure-volume area (PVA) in human hearts. *Eur Heart J* 1992; **13**(supE):85-90.

56. de Tombe PP, Jones S, Burkhoff D, Hunter WC, Kass DA. Ventricular stroke work and efficiency both remain nearly optimal despite altered loading conditions. *Am J Physiol* 1993; **264**:H1817-H1824.

57. Suga H. Total mechanical energy of a ventricle model and cardiac oxygen consumption. *Am J Physiol* 1979; **236**(3):H498-505.

58. Katz LN. Observations on the external work of the isolated turtle heart. *Am J Physiol* 1932; 99:579-597.

59. Nozawa T, Cheng CP, Noda T, Little WC. Relation between left ventricular oxygen consumption and pressure- volume area in conscious dogs. *Circulation* 1994; **89**(2):810-7.

60. Gibbs CL, Chapman JB. Cardiac mechanics and energetics: chemomechanical transduction in cardiac muscle. *Am J Physiol* 1985; **249**(2 Pt 2):H199-206.

61. Kass DA, Midei M, Brinker J, Maughan WL. Influence of coronary occlusion during PTCA on end-systolic and end-diastolic pressure-volume relations in humans. *Circulation* 1990; **81**:447-60.

62. Elzinga G, Westerhof N. Pressure and flow generated by the left ventricle against different impedance. *Circ Res* 1973; **32**:178-86.

63. Nichols WW, Pepine CJ, Geiser EA, Conti CR. Vascular load defined by the aortic input impedance spectrum. *Fed Proc* 1980; **39**:196-201.

64. Kelly RP, Ting C-T, Yang T-M, Liu C-P, Maughan WL, Chang M-S, Kass DA. Effective arterial elastance as index of arterial vascular load in humans. *Circulation* 1992; **86**:513-21.

65. Sunagawa K, Maughan WL, Burkhoff D, Sagawa K. Left ventricular interaction with arterial load studied in isolated canine ventricle. *Am J Physiol* 1983; **245**:H773-H780.

66. Sunagawa K, Maughan WL, Sagawa K. Optimal arterial resistance for the maximal stroke work studied in isolated canine left ventricle. *Circ Res* 1985; **56**(4):586-95.

67. Kameyama T, Asanoi H, Ishizaka S, Sasayama S. Ventricular load optimization by unloading therapy in patients with heart failure. *J Am Coll Cardiol* 1991; **17**(1):199-207.

68. Haber HL, Simek CL, Bergin JD, Sadun A, Gimple LW, Powers ER, Feldman MD. Bolus intravenous nitroglycerin predominantly reduces afterload in patients with excessive arterial elastance. *J Am Coll Cardiol* 1993; **22**(1):251-7.

Chapter 19

Non-invasive Assessment of Ischaemic Heart Disease

Neville Sammel

Cardiac catheterisation remains the 'gold standard' by which coronary artery disease (CAD) is diagnosed and evaluated. Diagnostic angiography can unequivocally pinpoint the nature, location and severity of CAD. Patients who present with typical symptoms of ischaemic heart disease (IHD) are therefore often referred directly for coronary angiography. Although reliable, it is nonetheless an invasive, labour-intensive and expensive procedure which, by virtue of its popularity, is placing an increasing burden on the health care system. For many patients, the presenting diagnosis of IHD is uncertain on clinical grounds and many of these will be referred for non-invasive testing.

Non-invasive assessment of IHD provides an alternative to cardiac catheterisation for suitable cases and often confirms or refutes the diagnosis of CAD. In some cases it can also provide information about the functional capacity of the heart. By comparison with coronary angiography, all non-invasive tests have a certain proportion of false positive and false negative results and this information needs to be considered in the patient's overall management. The clinician thus requires a thorough understanding of specific advantages and disadvantages of individual tests and their limitatons, with selection of each test depending on a number of factors including clinical presentation, the resting electrocardiogram (ECG) and the patient's ability to exercise.

There are three major forms of non-invasive testing:
1. Exercise stress testing
2. Radioisotope scanning
3. Stress echocardiography.

Exercise stress testing (EST)

Exercise stress testing is widely available and is usually used as a screening test for coronary artery disease.[1-3] It may also be of value in assessment of exercise capacity and in diagnosis and evaluation of exercise-induced arrhythmias. If exercise stress testing were undertaken for diagnostic reasons the resting ECG should be normal as exercise-induced changes cannot be interpreted in the presence of an abnormal resting ECG. The patient should also be capable of adequate exercise.

Protocols

The patient may be exercised on either a treadmill or exercise bicycle. A treadmill is more popular as a form of exercise, as some patients have poor coordination and have difficulty using the bicycle. Most patients are exercised according to the Bruce protocol, which is well established and researched. The advantage of the Bruce protocol is the ability to achieve high levels of exercise relatively quickly. One disadvantage of the standard Bruce protocol is its inability to cater for patients with reduced exercise capacity (e.g. after myocardial infarction). This disadvantage is to some extent overcome by the addition of two earlier stages (stages 0 and ½) known as the Modified Bruce Protocol. In patients with poor exercise capacitiy (e.g. heart failure), protocols such as the Congestive Heart Failure (Modified Naughton) protocol may be more appropriate. Other protocols include the Balke-Ware, Stanford and Asymptomatic Cardiac Ischaemia Pilot (ACIP).

Different levels of exercise can be correlated with metabolic equivalents or METS . One MET is the oxygen uptake at rest, which is equivalent to 3.5 ml/kg/min. Different stages of the various protocols can be correlated with various activities based on the METS achieved. This can assist in assessing a patient's functional capacity for everyday activities. Examples of METS are:

1 MET	Resting	8 METS	Jogging slowly
2 METS	Level walking at 3KPH	9 METS	Sawing wood
3 METS	Sailing	10 METS	Heavy labour
4 METS	Raking leaves	11 METS	Cross-country skiing
5 METS	Walking briskly	12 METS	Squash
6 METS	Light backpacking	13 METS	Rowing
7 METS	Climbing hills	16 METS	Endurance athletes

Tables 19.1–19.3 provide examples of protocols.

Table 19.1. Modified Bruce Protocol – 3 minute stages

Stage	Speed (kph)	Slope (%)	METS
0	2.7	0	2
½	2.7	5	3
1	2.7	10	4
2	4.0	12	7
3	5.4	14	10
4	6.7	16	13
5	8.0	18	16
6	8.8	20	19
7	9.6	22	22

Table 19.2. Modified Naughton Protocol – 1 minute stages

Stage	Speed (kph)	Slope (%)	METS
1	1.6	0.0	1
2	2.4	0.0	2
3	3.2	3.5	3
4	3.2	7.0	4
5	3.2	10.5	5
6	4.8	7.5	6
7	4.8	10.0	7
8	4.8	12.5	8
9	4.8	15.0	9
10	5.5	14.0	10

Table 19.3. Bicycle Ergometer Protocol

Watts (for 70kg body weight)	METS
25	2
50	4
75	5
100	6
125	8
150	9
175	10
200	11
225	12
250	14

Diagnosis of coronary artery disease

EST may provide considerable information about the patient, such as the following:

1. S–T segment changes
2. Exercise capabilities
3. Reproduction of symptoms
4. Blood pressure response to exercise
5. Exercise-induced arrhythmias.

An EST is said to be positive if the patient develops 1mm or more of horizontal or downsloping S–T depression, as illustrated in Fig. 19.1 (the significance of S–T changes and their correlation with ischaemia is explained in Chapter 9).

ST segment changes on exercise cannot be interpreted unless the resting ECG is normal, since an exaggeration of resting S–T segment changes is commonly seen, even in patients with no obstructive coronary disease. It is also necessary to achieve an adequate level of exercise. The decision that the patient has exercised satisfactorily is largely based on the objective opinion of the person conducting the stress test that the patient has achieved close to his or her maximal effort. A maximal heart rate can be calculated from the formula 200–0.6 x age and also provides a rough guide of the patient's level of exercise.

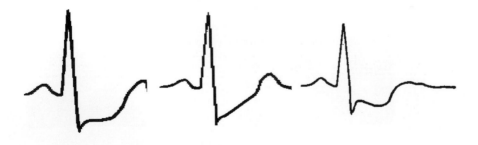

Horizontal S–T   **Upsloping S–T**   **Downsloping**
depression   **depression**   **S–T depression**

Figure 19.1. Examples of S-T depression. Horizontal and downsloping S-T segments are suggestive of ischaemia, whereas upsloping S-T segments may be a normal variant.

Apart from S–T segment changes, other factors on EST that would support the diagnosis of CAD are (a) reproduction of symptoms with exercise, (b) inability to exercise adequately and (c) fall in blood pressure. It is normal for blood pressure to increase with exercise; if blood pressure falls or fails to rise with exercise, this would support diagnosis of IHD. This observation, however, is a non-specific finding as blood pressure is often difficult to record with exercise and other factors (e.g. antianginal and antihypertensive drugs) will affect blood pressure response to exercise.

Comparison with coronary angiography

Numerous studies have compared results of exercise stress testing based on S–T segment changes with coronary angiography. In most cases CAD has been defined as a stenosis of 70% or more in at least one coronary artery. It has been shown that the accuracy of exercise stress testing depends largely on patient selection (Baye's Theorem). Baye's theorem (given a positive test result) calculates the post-test probability of a disease from the known prevalence of the disease, and the sensitivity and specificity of the diagnostic test. Before referring a patient for exercise stress testing, the referring physician should have some idea of the pre-test probability of CAD, based on clinical assessment and the resting ECG.

In patients with an intermediate pre-test probability of CAD, exercise stress testing has shown to have a sensitivity of approximately 70% (30% false negatives) and a specificity of approximately 80% (20% false positive). In patients with a low pre-test probability of IHD, the specificity will fall; in patients with a high pre-test probability of IHD, an EST is often unhelpful as a negative result does not rule out CAD with any degree of certainty (sensitivity and specificity are explained in Chapter 33).

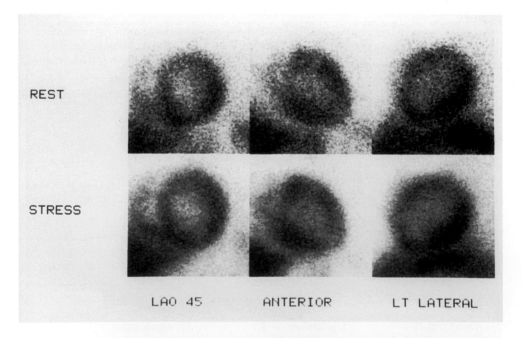

Figure 19.2. *Reversible defect of left ventricular apex caused by lesion in left anterior descending coronary artery, as shown in anterior view (middle) by reduced tracer uptake during exercise.*

Radioisotope scanning

Coronary artery disease can also be diagnosed and assessed with radioisotope myocardial perfusion imaging,[4-6] which depends on detection of a variation in perfusion in different parts of the left ventricular myocardium. Radioisotope perfusion agents are injected, following which the myocardium is scanned for distribution of the agent. A comparison is made of myocardial perfusion for patients at rest and under stress. Figure 19.2 is an example of a sestamibi scan from a patient with a reversible anterior lesion.

Role of myocardial perfusion imaging

Myocardial perfusion imaging can be used in situations where standard exercise stress testing is contraindicated. Unlike standard EST, it is not necessary to have a normal resting ECG for interpretation of the test. It can also be used in patients who are unable to exercise, as pharmacologically induced stress can be used in conjunction with radioisotope imaging. There are many patients in this category, which includes the elderly and those with peripheral vascular disease or orthopaedic conditions.

If information is required about left ventricular function, this can be obtained by using technetiun-99m based compounds. Radioisotope imaging also assists in localising and assessing the severity of myocardial ischaemia in patients with known CAD.

Comparison with coronary angiography

As with standard EST, diagnostic accuracy depends on selection of patients according to Baye's Theorem. Sensitivity and specificity are generally better than with the standard EST. In patients with an intermediate pre-test probability of CAD, most series have reported sensitivities of approximately 90% (10% false negatives) and specificities of approximately 90% (10 % false positives). In patients with a low pre-test probability of CAD, the specificity will be lower. There is little diagnostic value in patients with a high pre-test probability of CAD, as a negative test cannot exclude CAD with confidence.

In a small number of patients with severe widespread disease (e.g. disease of the left main coronary artery), a radioisotope test may be negative. Accordingly, patients should be referred directly for coronary angiography if there is a high pre-test probability of CAD or if severe disease (e.g. left main coronary disease) is suspected.

Myocardial perfusion agents

Thallium-201 (^{201}Tl)

Thallium-201 has been available for many years and has been well evaluated. It has a biological half-life of approximately 58 hours. ^{201}Tl usually redistributes in the myocardium within 2 hours, which allows assessment of myocardial perfusion both with stress and at rest with a single injection. ^{201}Tl is injected into a peripheral vein at peak stress (exercise or pharmacological), following which immediate myocardial imaging is undertaken. This is compared with myocardial imaging at rest, which is usually performed about 4 hours later. In some cases optimal redistribution has not occurred at 4 hours and better information can be obtained by either reinjecting ^{201}Tl before rest imaging or by repeating rest imaging at 24 hours.

Technetium -99m Labelled Compound (^{99m}Tc)

Technetium -99m - sestamibi (^{99m}Tc-sestamibi) is the most widely used agent in this group. Other agents include ^{99m}Tc-tetrofosmin and ^{99m}Tc-furofosmin. The biological half-life of

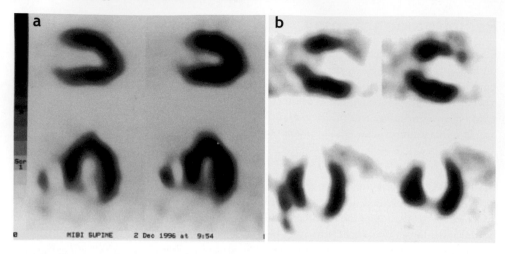

Figure 19.3. Sestamibi stress scan of gated slice of left ventricle in diastole (left) and systole (right), demonstrating *a.* normal left ventricular contraction and *b.* impaired left ventricular contraction, as shown by reduced contrast at apex. Top view is the vertical long axis, bottom view is the horizontal long axis.

technetium-labelled compounds is approximately 6 hours. Unlike Thallium-201, technetium-labelled compounds redistribute poorly in the myocardium and separate injections are required to compare the radioisotope uptake at rest and with stress. This makes it possible to delay imaging for several hours after the isotope has been injected. This can be of practical value in assessing chest pain in the emergency department, as the isotope can be injected during chest pain and imaging can take place some hours later at a time that may be more convenient. If the chest pain is due to myocardial ischaemia then there will be reduced radioisotope uptake in the distribution of the affected vessel, e.g. reduced uptake in the interventricular septum in patients with disease of the left anterior descending artery.

A major advantage of technetium-labelled compounds over thallium imaging is the ability to assess left ventricular contractility by ECG gating (Fig 19.3a,b). This is achieved by imaging the left ventricular wall at several phases of the cardiac cycle and displaying the average image over many cycles. The ability to provide information from both perfusion and function in a single test has made technetium imaging the preferred option in most centres.

Stress imaging

Occasionally, rest images only are required (e.g. during chest pain in the emergency department). In most cases, however, an assessment is made by comparing perfusion images taken at rest and with stress. There are currently four methods of stressing the patient:

1. Exercise
2. Dipyridamole
3. Adenosine
4. Dobutamine

If the patient is able to exercise then this is the preferred option, as the patient's exercise performance may provide important additional information. Exercise is undertaken in the same way as for standard exercise testing.

In patients unable to exercise, the pharmacological agents of choice are dipyridamole and adenosine. Both agents are given intravenously and cause widespread arteriolar dilatation, including dilatation of the coronary arteries. In patients with coronary atherosclerosis, the stenosed vessel is unable to dilate to the extent of the normal coronary vessel and this will result in a relative reduction in perfusion of the stenosed vessel. The two agents act in a similar way, but may aggravate asthma and heart block and are contraindicated in both conditions. Adenosine has a shorter half-life than dipyridamole and may be safer in some situations (e.g. after myocardial infarction).

A small proportion of patients may be unsuitable for both exercise and dipyridamole or adenosine and will need to be stressed with intravenous dobutamine. Results of perfusion imaging with dobutamine are not quite as good as other forms of stress, but this agent is still a valuable alternative. Dobutamine stresses the heart by causing a sinus tachycardia that increases myocardial oxygen demands.

Interpretation of myocardial perfusion imaging

The interpretation of myocardial perfusion imaging requires a comparison of images taken at rest and with stress. There are four major categories, as outlined in Table 19.4.

Table 19.4. Major categories of myocardial perfusion imaging

Radioisotope Imaging	Implications
1. Normal stress and rest scan	No significant CAD
2. Abnormal stress scan and normal rest scan	Myocardial ischaemia
3. Abnormal stress scan with no improvement at rest	Myocardial infarction without residual ischaemia
4. Abnormal stress scan with partial improvement at rest	Myocardial infarction with residual ischaemia

Myocardial viability scanning

Myocardial revascularisation (coronary bypass surgery or angioplasty) is usually undertaken to relieve angina or to abolish myocardial ischaemia. In some patients with impaired left ventricular contractility, revascularisation may be indicated to improve left ventricular function even in the absence of angina or myocardial ischaemia. In these patients it is necessary to identify 'hibernating myocardium', i.e. myocardium that is not contracting but is still viable and can be expected to contract when perfusion is restored. Hibernating myocardium can be identified when there is uptake of a radioisotope-labelled metabolic agent, e.g. fluorine-18 fluorodeoxyglucose (FDG) with no uptake or reduced uptake of a perfusion agent, e.g. technetium sestamibi.[7]

Stress echocardiography

The diagnosis of myocardial infarction can usually be made on standard echocardiography. These patients demonstrate a regional wall abnormality, sometimes associated with left ventricular wall thinning. For detection of myocardial ischaemia, stress echocardiography is required.[8-11] In patients with normal hearts, there will be an increase in left ventricular contractility with exercise or pharmacological stress (e.g. dobutamine). In patients with myocardial ischaemia, left ventricular contractility will not improve with exercise and in most cases a regional wall abnormality will develop.

The indications for stress echocardiography are similar to those for radioisotope perfusion imaging. Patients unsuitable for standard EST because of abnormal resting

ECG or inability to exercise may be suitable for stress echocardiography. Stress echocardiography may also be of value when 'balanced ischaemia' due to multivessel coronary disease is suspected.

Sensitivity and specificity are similar to radioisotope perfusion imaging. Radioisotope imaging may be more sensitive for single vessel disease, while stress echo may be less likely to miss severe diffuse disease (e.g. left main coronary disease).

Exercise is the preferred mode of stress, as the patient's exercise performance provides additional clinical data. With exercise echocardiography, a comparison is made of images taken at rest and immediately after exercise. In patients unable to exercise, intravenous dobutamine is the most commonly used pharmacological stress. Imaging is performed at rest and compared with images taken during the dobutamine infusion. Atrial pacing and intravenous dipyridamole are less commonly used to induce stress.

The echocardiogram is also useful in identifying viable myocardium. Myocardium is likely to be viable if wall thickness is retained and/or myocardial contractility improves with dobutamine or exercise.

Coronary artery calcification scanning

Computed tomography with rapid scanning times has been used to assess calcification in the region of the coronary arteries. Electron beam computed tomography has been the most widely evaluated technique, although helical tomography is also commonly used. Assessment of this technique to detect significant CAD in patients undergoing coronary angiography has demonstrated sensitivities of >95% but low specificities of <50%. The precise indication for this test is still under evaluation but should not be considered as anything more than a screening test for CAD. It may also be useful in coronary risk factor management, e.g. deciding whether to prescribe a lipid-lowering agent.[12]

Selection of non-invasive testing for CAD

Based on Baye's Theorem, non-invasive testing for CAD may be misleading and has little place in diagnosing patients with very low or very high pre-test probabilities of CAD. In other groups, standard exercise stress testing should be considered for patients with normal resting ECGs who are able to exercise satisfactorily. In patients who are able to exercise and have abnormal resting ECGs, exercise radioisotope imaging or exercise echocardiography should be performed, the choice depending on local expertise and preference. In patients unable to exercise, the non- invasive tests of choice are either radioisotope imaging or echocardiography with pharmacological stress.

Non-invasive tests are very valuable in the investigation and management of CAD but, despite optimal techniques and careful patient selection, there will always be a small percentage of false positives and false negatives. Accordingly, patients with convincing or persistent symptoms usually require coronary angiography.

References

1.   Fletcher GF, Balady G, Froelicher VF *et al*. Exercise Standards. A statement for healthcare professionals from the American Heart Association. *Circulation* 1995; **91**:580-615.
2.   Pina IL, Balady GJ, Hanson P *et al*. Guidelines for clinical exercise stress testing laboratories. A statement for healthcare professionals from the Committee on Exercise and Cardiac Rehabilitation, American Heart association. *Circulation* 1995; **91**:912-21.

3. Froelicher VF, Myers J, Follansbee WP, Labovitz AJ. *Exercise and the Heart*, 3rd ed. St Louis: Mosby-Year Book 1993.
4. Berman DS, Kiat HS, Van Train KF *et al.* Myocardial perfusion imaging with technetium-99m sestamibi: Comparative analysis of analysis of available imaging protocols. *J Nucl Med* 1994; **35**:681-8.
5. The Cardiovascular Imaging Committee, American College of Cardiology; The Committee on Advanced Cardiac Imaging and Technology, Council of Clinical Cardiology, American Heart Association and the Board of Directors, Cardiovascular Council, Society of Nuclear Medicine ACC/AHA/SNM Policy Statement: Standardisation of cardiac tomographic imaging. *J Nucl Cardiol* 1994; **1**:117.
6. Sinusas AJ, Bergin JD, Edwards NC *et al.* Redistribution of ^{99m}Tc-Sestamibi and Tl in presence of severe coronary artery stenosis. *Circulation* 1994; **89**:2332-41.
7. Bax JJ, Cornel JH, Visser FC *et al.* Prediction of recovery of myocardial dysfunction after revascularization. Comparison of fluorine-18 fluorodeoxyglucose/thallium-201 SPECT, thallium-201 stress-reinjection SPECT and dobutamine echocardiography. *J Am Coll Cardiol* 1996; **28**:558-64.
8. Quinones MA, Verani MS, Haichin RM *et al.* Exercise echocardiograpy verses 201 Tl single photon emission computed tomography in evaluation of coronary artery disease. *Circulation* 1992; **85**:1026-31.
9. Rober VL, Pellikka PA, Oh JK *et al.* Identification of multivessel coronary artery disease by exercise echocardiography. *J Am Coll Cardiol* 1994; **24**:109-14.
10. Previtali M, Lanzarini L, Fetiveau R *et al.* A. Comparison of dobutamine stress echocardiography dipyridamole stress echocardiography and exercise stress testing for diagnosis of coronary artery disease. *Am J Cardiol* 1993; **72**:865-70.
11. Iliceto S, Sorino M, D'Ambrosio G *et al.* Detection of coronary artery disease by two dimensional echocardiography and transesophageal atrial pacing. *J Am Coll Cardiol* 1985; **5**:1188-97.
12. WexlerL, Brundage B, Crouse J *et al.* American Heart Association Scientific Statement. Coronary artery calcification: pathophysiology, epidemiology, imaging methods, and clinical implications. *Circulation* 1996; **94**:1175-2292.

Chapter 20

Catheter-based Reperfusion in Acute Myocardial Infarction

Derek Chew and Mark Horrigan

Introduction

Following the thrombolytic trials of the last two decades, reperfusion therapy is now established as an integral part of the management of acute myocardial infarction (AMI) in patients presenting with S–T segment elevation. During the last decade, the results of multicentre studies comparing fibrinolytic therapy with angioplasty have prompted increasing use of catheter-based reperfusion techniques. Percutaneous transluminal coronary angioplasty (PTCA) for patients with AMI is commonly performed and regarded by many centres as the treatment of choice. Coronary stents, antiplatelet agents and novel devices have provided new ways to address the pathophysiology underlying acute coronary occlusion, aiming for rapid and complete reperfusion. This chapter provides an overview of the current status of percutaneous revascularisation techniques, with emphasis on important practical and technical issues for health professionals treating patients with acute myocardial infarction.

Studies comparing primary angioplasty with thrombolytic therapy

Although PTCA as primary therapy for acute infarction was first described by Hartzler et al in 1983,[1] it was initially investigated as an adjunct to **intracoronary** thrombolysis. The results of large trials assessing its usefulness following **intravenous** thrombolysis were disappointing[2-4] with increased mortality and major complications following combined therapy (Table 20.1). These results have been attributed to thrombin generation and platelet activation by thrombolytic agents, producing a locally prothrombotic environment[5,6] predisposed to ischaemic complications.

The published results describing primary angioplasty without antecedent thrombolysis were more promising.[7,8] Eckman et al. reviewed the outcomes of 2073 patients undergoing angioplasty for acute myocardial infarction, including those ineligible for thrombolysis and those with cardiogenic shock. Infarct-related artery (IRA) patency was attained in 91%, with a hospital mortality of 8.3% and one- and five-year survival rates of 95% and 84%, respectively.[8] In the Primary Angioplasty Registry,[9,10] patients similar to those randomised in thrombolytic trials underwent PTCA within 1–3 hours of symptom onset. Patency was restored in 99%, with low hospital mortality and rates of emergency bypass

Table 20.1. Overview of initial studies of PTCA with antecedent thrombolysis.

	t-PA + PTCA (%)	t-PA only (%)	Odds Ratio
TAMI, n=197			
Death	4.0	1.0	4.0
Emergency CABG	7.1	2.0	3.6
ECSG, n=367			
Death	7.0	3.0	2.3
TIMI IIA, n=389			
Death	7.2	5.7	1.7
Emergency CABG	4.3	1.9	2.3

KEY: t-PA, tissue plasminogen activator; PTCA, percutaneous transluminal coronary angioplasty; TAMI, Thrombolysis and Angioplasty in Myocardial Infraction; ECSG, the European Cooperative Study Group; TIMI IIA, Thrombolysis in Myocardial Infarction IIA; CABG, coronary artery bypass grafting.

surgery, reinfarction and stroke. These results formed the basis for randomised trials comparing PTCA with thrombolytic therapy.

The Primary Angioplasty in Myocardial Infarction trial (PAMI) randomised 395 patients to thrombolysis or to coronary angiography with a view to immediate angioplasty.[11] In the invasive group, 90% underwent PTCA with a procedural success rate of 97%; emergency bypass surgery for failed angioplasty was not required. Following angioplasty, in-hospital mortality and reinfarction rates were lower than in the group assigned to thrombolysis. No cerebral haemorrhages were observed, compared with a 2% rate among patients receiving thrombolytic agents. A meta-analysis[12] of PAMI and similar studies[13,14] showed reduced in-hospital death and reinfarction.

The largest randomised trial of primary angioplasty was the GUSTO IIb angioplasty substudy[15] which compared invasive management (n=565) with intravenous t-PA (n=573). The time to first balloon inflation (1.3 hrs) was 40 min longer than the 'door to needle' time. The composite endpoint of death, recurrent infarction and disabling stroke was significantly reduced in the angioplasty group at 30 days (9.6% vs 13.6%, p=0.033). However, at 6 months there was little difference between the two groups. This attrition may in part have been due to restenosis, which occurred in 40–45% of cases.

Weaver and colleagues performed a meta-analysis of 2606 patients enrolled in 10 randomised trials comparing thrombolysis with primary angioplasty.[16] Angioplasty was associated with lower rates of death (4.4% vs. 6.5%), re-infarction (2.9% vs. 5.3%) and stroke. The mortality benefit was independent of thrombolytic regimens. With the proviso that the procedural success rates reported in these trials are reproducible, the data suggest that an extra 46 deaths and non-fatal re-infarctions per 1000 patients can be prevented by use of primary angioplasty (Table 20.2).

In a retrospective community-based study from the Myocardial Infarction Triage and Intervention (MITI) Registry,[17] Every and co-workers[18] compared the outcomes of 1050 patients undergoing primary angioplasty with a similar group of 2095 patients receiving thrombolytic therapy. As in the GUSTO IIb sub-study, the time to initiation of reperfusion therapy in the PTCA group was 42 minutes longer than in patients receiving thrombolytic therapy. Prior bypass surgery and contraindications to thrombolysis were more frequent in the primary angioplasty group. In-hospital mortality was 5.5% in both groups and no survival advantage was observed in either group at 4 years. However, 74%

Table 20.2. Meta-analysis of outcomes in a population of 2606 patients randomised to receive primary angioplasty or fibrinolytic therapy*

Study Group	Drug	Rates (%)		Odds Ratio (95% CI)	P-Value
		PTCA	Fibrinolytic Therapy		
Mortality					
	SK	4.0	5.9	0.66 (0.29-1.50)	0.38
	t-PA	3.5	5.7	0.60 (0.24-1.41)	0.28
	Acc. t-PA	5.0	7.2	0.68 (0.42-1.08)	0.10
	pooled	4.4	6.5	0.66 (0.46- 0.94)	0.02
Death + Non-fatal Reinfarction					
	SK	5.6	13.0	0.40 (0.21-0.75)	0.003
	t-PA	5.6	10.3	0.51 (0.26-0.99)	0.05
	Acc. t-PA	8.7	12.0	0.70 (0.48-1.08)	0.05
	pooled	7.2	11.9	0.58 (0.44-0.76)	<0.001
Stroke *pooled*		0.7	2.0	0.35 (0.14-0.77)	0.007
I.C.H. *pooled*		0.1	1.1	0.07 (0.00-0.43)	<0.001

*Adapted from: Weaver WD, Simes RJ, Betriu A *et al.* Comparison of primary coronary angioplasty and intravenous thrombolytic therapy for acute myocardial infarction. A quantitative review. *JAMA* 1997; 278:2093-2098, with permission.
KEY: SK = Streptokinase, t-PA = recombinant tissue plasminogen activator, Acc. = accelerated, C.I. = confidence intervals, PTCA = percutaneous transluminal coronary angioplasty.

of the thrombolytic group underwent subsequent angiography, with revascularisation procedures in 77%. A report from the Second Registry of Myocardial Infarction[19] described similar outcomes.

The overview of the randomised trials suggests that primary angioplasty provides additional benefit over thrombolysis, with reductions in 30-day mortality, re-infarction and haemorrhagic stroke. The fact that these benefits were not observed in community studies may be due to small real differences between strategies, less operator experience, lower institutional volumes, and a high incidence of subsequent revascularisation procedures in patients initially treated with thrombolytic drugs. In the thrombolytic literature, time to reperfusion is a critical determinant of outcome; a similar relationship for primary PTCA was observed in the GUSTO IIb trial.[15] The MITI and NRMI-2 registry data reflect 'real world' clinical experience. Primary infarct angioplasty is a therapy in evolution; most of the current literature was published prior to the widespread use of stents and abciximab, both of which are now ubiquitous in infarct angioplasty.

Stenting

Although randomised trials demonstrate significant benefits of angioplasty over thrombolysis therapy, recurrent ischaemia (10–15% of patients) and re-infarction (3–5% of patients) in hospital are common and target vessel revascularisation (TVR) is required in up to 35% by 6 months[20] after PTCA. Angiographic studies suggest 6-month restenosis rates of 40–45%; late re-occlusion occurs in up to 14% of cases.[21–25] Several groups have reported experience of coronary stenting in acute myocardial infarction.[26-31] Suryapranata and co-workers[27] studied 227 patients, comparing angioplasty and bail-out stenting with elective stenting. Of the population screened for the study, 50% were excluded because of diffuse target vessel disease, side branch involvement, or a target vessel less than 3.0 mm in diameter. Abciximab was not used. In the stent group, recurrent infarction and TVR rates were significantly reduced, and event-free survival at 6 months was increased from 80% to 95%. Similar results were reported in GRAMI and other trials.[28-30]

In the Florence Randomised Elective Stenting in Acute Coronary Occlusion (FRESCO) Trial[31] 227 patients underwent primary angioplasty; 150 patients with optimal angioplasty results (residual stenosis <30% and TIMI grade 3 flow in the target vessel) were randomised to no further treatment or additional stent deployment. In the stent group, recurrent ischaemia at 30 days was reduced from 15% to 3% and the 6-month TVR rate was reduced from 25% to 7% when compared with those patients treated by balloon dilatation alone. Angiographic follow-up in 143 patients demonstrated restenosis or reocclusion in 3% of the stent group and 17% of the angioplasty group. At 6 months, restenosis was less frequent among patients receiving stents (17% versus 43%; p=0.001). Although these results are promising, reference vessel diameters were large and patients with smaller vessels and more complex anatomy were excluded.

The PAMI-Stent trial confirmed the lower need for repeat revascularisation in patients treated by balloon dilatation and stenting. Although there was a marginally lower TIMI 3 rate, and somewhat higher mortality in the stent group (3.5% vs 1.8%, p=NS), event-free survival was significantly better at 6 months in these patients.[32]

Glycoprotein IIbIIIa inhibition

There is now a large body of clinical trial experience with glycoprotein IIbIIa inhibition in angioplasty and acute coronary syndromes, including myocardial infarction. Abciximab alone may cause 'platelet lysis' in acute myocardial infarction,[33,34] and may attenuate or prevent 'no-reflow' and abnormal flow conditions commonly observed during primary angioplasty.[35] Lefkovits and co-workers studied 66 patients undergoing primary or rescue angioplasty in the EPIC trial.[36,37] Among patients receiving abciximab, death, recurrent infarction and TVR were reduced from 26% to 5% at 30 days. At 6 months there was a 46% event rate in the placebo arm, and no further events in the abciximab bolus and infusion arm. Azar *et al* reported results in 182 patients undergoing primary angioplasty.[38] In 103 patients receiving abciximab, there was a risk reduction of 51% for death, re-infarction, unstable angina and TVR at 7 months.

In the RAPPORT Trial, Brenner and co-workers randomly assigned 483 patients undergoing primary PTCA for myocardial infarction to abciximab or placebo.[39] Benefits were of relatively short duration in those randomised to receive abciximab. However, among patients who **actually received** abciximab as intended, there was a 74% reduction in death and other ischaemic complications, with persisting benefit at 6 months. Preliminary data from the CADILLAC trial[40] also support the use of IIb/IIIa antagonist therapy in patients treated by balloon angioplasty alone or coronary stenting. In this trial, 2625 patients were randomly asigned to PTCA, PTCA and abciximab, stent alone or stent and abciximab. In-hospital outcomes were remarkably good in each of the four groups. Recurrent ischaemia occurred less frequently in patients who received abciximab. Timi III flow was marginally lower in patients stented without abciximab but this was not statistically significant.

Specific patient subgroups

Cardiogenic shock

Cardiogenic shock complicating myocardial infarction has a high mortality, particularly in the elderly, and its incidence has remained stable for decades[41,42] The number of patients with cardiogenic shock studied in trials comparing thrombolysis and primary PTCA has been small. In the GISSI trial,[43] mortality was 70% in both the placebo and intravenous streptokinase groups, and a reperfusion rate of only 44% has been reported using **intracoronary** streptokinase.[44] In the GUSTO-III trial,[45] efficacy of t-PA and r-PA in treatment and prevention of shock were similar, with 30-day mortality rates of 58–64% for patients presenting with shock. Data from the GISSI-2 trial[46] also suggest that t-PA may be less effective for those presenting in cardiogenic shock. Pooled data from 18 series with 626 patients showed a PTCA success rate of 73%, with a 54% survival to hospital discharge. Hospital mortality was 30% for those with successful PTCA and 70% for those in whom intervention was unsuccessful, with very poor results in patients over 75 years of age.

The SHOCK Trial[47,48] compared interventional and conservative strategies in 302 patients with cardiogenic shock. Shock occurred 5–6 hours after the onset of infarction. Intra-aortic balloon pump (IABP) counterpulsation was performed in 86% of patients in both groups and almost all patients were treated according to their randomisation strategy. There was a trend to lower 30-day mortality in the invasive group, and mortality was 50% in the invasive group compared with 63% (p=0.027) in the conservatively treated group at 6 months. For patients less than 75 years of age, 30-day mortality reduction was greater (56.8% vs 41.4%, p=0.01), while in patients 75 years and older, mortality in the intervention group was worse at 75% compared with 53% in the medical group. Early revascularisation has not proved to be the definitive solution to the problem of cardiogenic shock, however in patients under 75 years of age it seems to offer an advantage over conservative therapy and should be offered where possible.[49]

Complicated inferior infarction

Although the reduced mortality of inferior infarction is well established,[50] data on patients with right ventricular infarction or praecordial lead ST segment depression has only been available recently. Ribichini and co-workers[51] examined outcomes in 110 patients with inferior myocardial infarction and praecordial ST-segment depression. Rates of death, re-infarction and target vessel revascularisation at one year were also significantly reduced in the primary angioplasty arm (11% vs 52.7%, p<0.0001). Patients receiving stents showed a trend toward reduced in-hospital mortality and re-infarction, and recurrent angina and TVR were significantly reduced. In an observational series of 53 patients, Bowers and colleagues assessed the impact of primary angioplasty in right ventricular infarction.[52] Failure to restore normal flow in the right coronary artery and branches was associated with persistently elevated filling pressures, prolonged hypotension and increased hospital death. Mortality for patients with right ventricular infarction and haemodynamic compromise may be as high as 38%. However, the impact of thrombolytic therapy on right ventricular infraction has not been assessed in prospective trials,[53,54] and primary angioplasty and thrombolysis have not been compared in randomised trials. However, rapid reperfusion often results in resolution of haemodynamic and conduction abnormalities, and angioplasty facilitates pacing and invasive haemodynamic monitoring.

Patients ineligible for fibrinolytic therapy

Many studies have demonstrated increased mortality in patients who are ineligible for thrombolysis.[55] In patients presenting with ST segment elevation and contra-indications to thrombolysis (particularly those with recent strokes or surgery), angioplasty provides another option for reperfusion therapy, with a lower risk of serious bleeding. With the exception of cardiogenic shock, benefits for patients presenting 12 or more hours after the onset of infarction or without ST segment elevation are less clear. The Medicine versus Angiography in Thrombolytic Exclusion (MATE) Trial[56] randomised 201 patients with less than 24 hours of symptoms to early triage angiography or conventional medical therapy. In the invasive arm, 58% were revascularised, while 37% of the conservative arm went on to revascularisation. Earlier revascularisation in the invasive group was associated with a 45% reduction in hospital death and recurrent myocardial infarction. At 21 months there was no difference in rates of revascularisation, recurrent myocardial infarction and all-cause mortality. In patients without S–T segment elevation or those who present outside the usual window for fibrinolytic therapy, the need for catheter-based reperfusion should be assessed on an individual basis, with consideration of early angiography for those with haemodynamic compromise or ongoing symptoms resistant to medical management.

Saphenous vein grafts, previous bypass grafts

Several large studies suggest that patients with previous bypass surgery presenting with acute myocardial infarction have more advanced coronary disease and increased morbidity and mortality.[57,58] In the GUSTO trial, 35% of patients with previous CABG surgery had saphenous vein culprit lesions, the majority of occlusions occurring in native vessels (Table 20.3). In the largest published series of acute vein graft cases, the procedural success rate was 86% compared with 95% in native vessels.[59] Patients with saphenous graft occlusions responded poorly to thrombolytic therapy.[53] A strong case can thus be made for urgent catheterisation with a view to mechanical intervention in such cases. Performance of PTCA in saphenous grafts is associated with a risk of embolisation of thrombus and grummous debris, frequently associated with no-reflow or slow flow conditions. Abciximab is of limited benefit in preventing these complications. Utility of extraction atherectomy, rheolytic catheters, covered stents and filter devices is being evaluated at present, but acute vein graft intervention remains hampered by a high incidence of procedural complications.

The elderly

With increasing age, mortality and morbidity rates increase regardless of treatment.[60] Despite the favourable risk-benefit ratio of thrombolytic therapy in this group, many clinicians remain reluctant to offer reperfusion therapy because of the increased incidence of intracranial haemorrhage.[61] Data from the PAMI trial suggest that there is a strong trend toward lower mortality in patients over 65 years of age,[11] yet sub-analysis of the GUSTO-IIb study data did not demonstrate different outcomes for the elderly.[62] It is still considered that treatment of elderly patients is associated with an increased risk of adverse outcomes. However, the potential benefits should lead to careful consideration of angioplasty on an individual basis, particularly in patients at increased risk.

Delayed, incomplete and failed reperfusion

It is now clear that reduced delay in institution of reperfusion therapy translates to reduced mortality.[17,50] Improved left ventricular contraction has been demonstrated where catheter-based reperfusion was instituted within 2 hours of the onset of symptoms.[63,64] In-

Table 20.3. Clinical characteristics of patients with and without previous bypass surgery in GUSTO-I*

Characteristic (%)	Prior CABG (n = 1784)	No CABG (n = 39110)	P-value
Prior myocardial infarct	65.0	14.2	< 0.0001
Prior Angina	77.8	35.0	< 0.0001
24-hour mortality	3.5	2.6	< 0.03
30-day mortality	10.7	6.4	< 0.0001
1-year mortality	15.8	8.0	< 0.0001
Cardiogenic shock	9.0	5.8	< 0.0001
Pulmonary oedema	22.3	16.0	< 0.0001
Recurrent ischaemia	25.8	19.7	< 0.0001
Reinfarction	5.9	3.9	< 0.0001

*Adapted from: De Franco AC *et al.* Substantial (three-fold) benefit of accelerated t-PA over standard thrombolytic therapy (sterptokinase) in patients with prior bypass surgery and acute MI: Results of the GUSTO Trial. *J Am Coll Cardiol* 1994; 23:1A-484A, with permission from the American College of Cardiology.

hospital and 30-day mortality advantages were also observed, concordant with data from fibrinolytic trials.[50] Beyond 2 hours, no significant improvement in outcomes was observed. The time to treatment in the PAMI trial was 60 minutes, while in larger, multicentre studies it ranged from 102–114 min, possibly accounting for the smaller net benefits observed.[15,19,65] Strong evidence from the fibrinolytic literature indicates that complete reperfusion is important to maximise mortality reduction.[66] Using myocardial contrast echocardiography, Ito and colleagues[67] demonstrated that tissue no-reflow is common and may occur even with **angiographically normal flow** in more than 25% of cases. Agati and co-workers[68] compared microvascular perfusion at one month in patients who had undergone mechanical and fibrinolytic reperfusion therapy. Even in patients with TIMI grade 3 flow, a greater proportion of those who had been treated with t-PA exhibited microvascular dysfunction, suggesting that angioplasty may promote more complete reperfusion.

Rescue angioplasty and the impact of IIb/IIIa plus fibrinolytic regimens

When fibrinolytic therapy is unsuccessful, invasive therapy remains a viable option for reperfusion. The clinical diagnosis of reperfusion is unreliable and only accurate when relief of pain and complete resolution of S–T segment elevation are observed.[69] Because of the inherent delays to rescue angioplasty, such therapy is usually considered only when persistent chest pain and S–T segment elevation are accompanied by haemodynamic deterioration. Numerous studies exist and have been summarised in detail.[70,71]

Technical success is achieved in more than 80% of cases, and more commonly after treatment with streptokinase and urokinase, which generate FDPs with anti IIb IIIa effects.[70] Ellis and co-workers reported results of a trial in which 150 patients with persisting occlusion during first anterior infarcts were randomised to invasive or conservative therapy.[71] Mortality was reduced from 9.9% to 5.2% and the combined incidence of death or heart failure was reduced from 16.4% to 6.5% with invasive therapy. The exercise ejection fraction at follow-up was significantly better in the invasive group. In practice, the greatest problems with rescue angioplasty are the lack of an accurate non-invasive test for reperfusion and the often lengthy delays to eventual reperfusion. Although the risk of bleeding is greater due to the combination of fibrinolytics, heparin, aspirin and often abciximab in the presence of femoral vascular instrumentation, it should be considered in those for whom thrombolysis has failed, especially where the infarct is large or where haemodynamic compromise is present.

Practical considerations

Assessment and indications

Although somewhat controversial, it is generally considered that primary angioplasty has most to offer patients with large infarcts and circulatory compromise or frank cardiogenic shock. In patients at lower risk, management is expedited and safe early discharge[71] may save health dollars. A list of indications is presented in Table 20.4. Once the decision is made to proceed, all delays in obtaining reperfusion must be avoided. While transfer for infarct angioplasty is usually reserved for compromised patients with failed reperfusion after thrombolysis, Zijlstra and co-workers have demonstrated that small delays exist only for patients transferred from smaller community hospitals to centres experienced with primary angioplasty.[73] Time lost in transfer may be offset in bypassing emergency departments and with earlier notification of the catheterisation laboratory.

Transfer and preparation

Once the decision to perform angiography has been made, the catheterisation suite should be notified and prepared as soon as possible. If not already given, aspirin 300 mg should be taken by the patient and 5000–10 000 U heparin should be administered intravenously. To avoid delay, placement of additional lines, urinary catheterisation and investigations such as chest x-rays should be deferred. When the patient is placed on the catheterisation table, balloon pump leads should be attatched if there is a significant chance of haemodynamic instability. Cardiogenic shock and pulmonary oedema are strong indications for IABP counterpulsation, which is generally instituted unless arterial access is impossible or hazardous. Significant left heart failure, hypotension or poor tissue perfusion should lead to prophylactic IABP counterpulsation prior to coronary angiography. Temporary RV pacing should be established prior to intervention where infarction is associated with AV block and bradycardia. Coronary angiography may be best performed with ionic contrast media that are known to cause less platelet activation.[74] To minimise contrast dosage, ventricular angiography can be deferred or avoided but initial measurement

Table 20.4. Indications for invasive management in acute myocardial infarction

Absolute	Cardiogenic shock < 75 years of age
Strong	Killip class III or IV status
	Prior contralateral Q-wave infarction
	Patients ineligible for fibrinolytic therapy
	'Right place, right time' indication
Relative	Suggestive clinical presentation with non-diagnostic ECG
	Patients with previous coronary bypass surgery
Uncertain	Presentation > 6 hours after onset of symptoms
	Cardiogenic shock > 75 years of age

of the left ventricular end-diastolic pressure is invaluable in determining fluid administration during angioplasty. Establishment of venous access is convenient if temporary pacing is required, as it allows rapid fluid administration and provides convenient access for a pulmonary artery catheter for invasive haemodynamic monitoring during and after angioplasty.

Angioplasty

If a culprit lesion cannot be identifed, it may be imprudent to proceed for fear of treating the wrong lesion and risking simultaneous ischaemia in two vascular territories. Multivessel angioplasty is usually reserved for cases of refractory cardiogenic shock. If spontaneous recanalisation has occurred with normal flow, and a residual stenosis is less than 50%, it is reasonable not to intervene, but the operator may wish to administer a soluble IIb/IIIa inhibitor. Cyclic flow variation is often observed during myocardial infarction. Frequently, a contrast injection or passage of the angioplasty guide wire will produce reflow in the target vessel, facilitating treatment. Use of abciximab is highly desirable during primary angioplasty, but expensive on a routine basis. It is of particular importance to use the drug prior to balloon inflation rather than on an ad hoc basis. The authors usually wire the lesion after administration of aspirin and heparin. If normal flow is not re-established or if there is visible thrombus, abciximab is administered prior to the first balloon inflation. Balloon dilatation should initially be performed at low pressure to re-establish flow. High pressure dilatation, particularly during stent deployment, is frequently associated with distal embolism and a 'no-reflow' situation in which abnormal flow conditions are associated with recurrent or worsening ischaemic pain and S–T segment elevation. In the right coronary artery this may be associated with profound hypotension and bradycardia, which usually respond to atropine and bolus injections of pressor agents. Slow flow and no-flow conditions are usually treated with intracoronary nitroglycerine. Verapamil should be used with extreme caution because of the potential for myocardial depression and bradycardia. Following percutaneous intervention, routine post-procedural and post-infarct mangement are instituted.

New concepts and technical developments

Use of coronary stents and IIb/IIIa inhibitors is now ubiquitous in infarct angioplasty. The most recent conceptual development in the medical management of acute infarction is combined IIb/IIIa inhibition with thrombolysis. Preliminary dose-finding studies[75] have demonstrated superior reperfusion rates using this approach, and major clinical trials are underway. The concept of 'angioplasty friendly' lysis, the combination of a relatively fibrin-specific fibrinolytic agent with abciximab or other intravenous IIb/IIIa inhibitors, has also been developed.[76] It is anticipated that IIb/IIIa inhibition will attenuate or abolish the undesirable consequences of thrombolytic platelet activation seen in early studies and create a haematological milieu conducive to rescue angioplasty. Other new developments include extraction and rheolytic catheters that remove large thrombi from vessels where conventional angioplasty is difficult or impossible. This may significantly enhance outcomes of procedures in saphenous grafts and the right coronary trunk, where gross thrombus formation with potential for embolism and slow flow is frequently encountered.

Conclusion

Primary angioplasty is an attractive reperfusion option for patients presenting with acute coronary occlusion. Clinical results are constantly improving, and with continual biological and technological advances there is great potential for further development. While its widespread application will remain limited globally by logistical constraints, catheter-based reperfusion offers superior outcomes in experienced centres. The challenge facing cardiologists will be to define its most effective role in treatment of myocardial infarction.

References

1.   Hartzler GO, Rutherford BD, McConahay DR *et al.* Percutaneous transluminal coronary angioplasty with and without thrombolytic therapy for the treatment of acute myocardial infarction. *Am Heart J* 1983; **106**:965–73.

2.   Topol EJ, Califf Rm, George BS *et al.* A randomised trial of immediate versus delayed elective angioplasty after intravenous tissue plasminogen activator in acute myocardial infarction. *N Engl J Med* 1987; **317**:581–88.

3.   Simoons ML, Arnold AER, Betriu A *et al.* Thrombolysis with t-PA in acute myocardial infarction: No beneficial effects of immediate PTCA. *Lancet* 1988; **1**:197–203.

4.   The TIMI Study Group. Comparison of invasive and conservative strategies following intravenous tissue plasminogen activator in acute myocardial infarction: Results of the Thrombolysis in Myocardial Infarction (TIMI) II Trial. *N Engl J Med* 1989; **320**:618–28.

5.   Topol, EJ. Toward a new frontier in myocardial reperfusion therapy: Emerging platelet preeminence. *Circulation* 1998; **97**:211–18.

6.   Topol EJ. Catheter-based reperfusion for acute myocardial infarction. In: *Textbook of interventional cardiology*, 3rd ed. Philadelphia: Saunders 1998.

7.   O'Keefe J Jr, Rutherford BD *et al.* Early and late results of coronary angioplasty without antecedent thrombolytic therapy for acute myocardial infarction. *Am J Cardiol* 1989; 64:1221–30.

8.   Eckman MH, Wong JB, Salem DN *et al.* Direct Angioplasty for Myocardial Infarction: A review of outcomes in clinical subsets. *Ann Intern Med* 1992; **117**:667–76.

9.   O'Neil WW, Brodie BR, Ivanhoe R *et al.* Primary coronary angioplasty for acute myocardial infarction (the Primary Angioplasty Registry). *Am J Cardiol* 1994; **73**:627–34.

10.   Brodie BR, Grines CL, Ivanhoe R *et al.* Six month clinical and angiographic follow-up after direct angioplasty for acute myocardial infarction: Final results from the Primary Angioplasty Registry.

11.   Grines CL, Browne KF, Marco J *et al.* A comparison of immediate angioplasty with thrombolytic therapy for acute myocardial infarction. *N Engl J Med* 1993; **328**:673–79.

12.   Simari R, Berger PB, Bell MR *et al.* Coronary angioplasty in acute myocardial infarction: primary, immediate adjunctive, rescue or deferred adjunctive approach? *Mayo Clin Proc* 1994; **69**:346–58.

13.   Gibbons RJ, Holmes DR, Reeder GS *et al.* Immediate angioplasty compared with the administration of a thrombolytic agent followed by conservative treatment for myocardial infarction. *N Engl J Med* 1993; **328**:685–91.

14.   Zijlstra F, Jan de Boer M, Hoorntje JC *et al.* A comparison of immediate coronary angioplasty with intravenous streptokinase in acute myocardial infarction. *N Engl J Med.* 1993; **328**:680–84.

15.   GUSTO IIb Angioplasty Substudy Investigators. A clinical trial comparing primary coronary angioplasty with tissue plasminogen activator for acute myocardial infarction. *N Engl J Med* 1997; **336**:1621–28.

16.   Weaver WD, Simes RJ, Betriu A *et al.* Comparison of primary coronary angioplasty and intravenous thrombolytic therapy for acute myocardial infarction. A quantitative review. *JAMA* 1997; **278**:2093–98.

17.   Weaver WD, Eisenberg MS, Martin JS *et al.* Myocardial Infarction Triage and Intervention Project-Phase I: patient characteristics and feasibility of prehospital initiation of thrombolytic therapy. *N Engl J Med* 1990; **15**:625–31.

18.   Every NR, Parsons LS, Hlatky M *et al.* A comparison of thrombolytic therapy with primary coronary angioplasty for acute myocardial infarction. *N Engl J Med* 1996; **335**:1253–60.

19.   Tiefenbrunn AJ, Chandra N, French WJ *et al*. Clinical experience with primary percutaneous transluminal coronary angioplasty compared with Alteplase (recombinant tissue-type plasminogen activator) in patients with acute myocardial infarction. A report from the Second National Registry of Myocardial Infarction (NRMI-2). *J Am Coll Cardiol* 1998; **31**:1240–45.

20.   Stone GW, Grines CL, Topol EJ. Update on percutaneous transluminal coronary angioplasty for acute myocardial infarction. In: Topol E, Serruys P (eds). *Current review of interventional cardiology*, 2nd ed. Philadelphia: Current Medicine 1995, 1–56.

21.   Simonton CA, Mark DB, Hinohara T *et al*. Late restenosis after emergent coronary angioplasty for acute myocardial infarction: comparison with elective coronary angioplasty. *J Am Coll Cardiol* 1988; **11**:698–705.

22.   Nakaqawa Y, Iwasaki Y, Kimura T *et al*. Serial Angiographic follow up after successful angioplasty for acute myocardial infarction. *Am J Cardiol* 1996; **78**; 980–84.

23.   Kake I, Fujita M, Fudo T *et al*. Relation between preexistent coronary collateral circulation and the incidence of restenosis after successful primary coronary angioplasty for acute myocardial infarction. *J Am Coll Cardiol* 1996; **27**:1688–92.

24.   Waldecker B, Waas W, Haberbosch W *et al*. Long-term follow-up after direct percutaneous transluminal coronary angioplasty for acute myocardial infarction. *J Am Coll Cardiol* 1998; **32**; 1320.25.

25.   Zijlstra F, de Boer M, Beukema W *et al*. Mortality, reinfarction, left ventricular ejection fraction and cost following reperfusion therapies for acute myocardial infarction. Eur Heart J 1996; **17**:382–87.

26.   Stone GW, Brodie BR, Griffin JJ *et al*. Prospective, multicentre study for the safety and feasibility of primary stenting in acute myocardial infarction: In-hospital and 30 day results from the PAMI Stent Pilot Trial. *J Am Coll Cardiol* 1998; **31**:23–70.

27.   Suryapranata H, van't Hof AW, Hoorntje JC *et al*. Randomised comparision of coronary stenting with balloon angioplasty in selected patients with acute myocardial infarction. *Circulation* 1998; **97**; 2502–25.

28.   Rodriguez A, Bernardi V, Fernandes M *et al*. In-hospital and late results of coronary stents versus conventional balloon angioplasty in acute myocardial infarction (GRAMI trial). *Am J Cardiol* 1998; **81**:1286–91.

29.   Benzuly KH, O'Neil WW, Gangadharan V *et al*. Stenting in acute myocardial infarction (STAMI): Bailout, conditional and planned stents. *J Am Coll Cardiol* 1997; **29**:Suppl A:456A.

30.   Siato S, Hosokawa G, Suzuki S, for the Japanese PASTA Trial study group. Primary stent implantation is superior to balloon angioplasty in acute myocardial infarction.: results from the Japanese PASTA (Primary Angioplasty versus Stent Implantation in Acute Myocardial Infarction) trial. *J Am Coll Cardiol* 1997; **29**:Suppl A:390A.

31.   Antoniucci D, Santoro GM, Bolognese L *et al*. A clinical trial comparing primary stenting of the infarct related artery with optimal primary angioplasty for acute myocardial infarction. Results from the Florence Elective Stenting in Acute Coronary Occlusions (FRESCO) Trial. *J Am Coll Cardiol* 1998; **31**:1234–39.

32.   Grines CL, Cox DA, Stone GW *et al*. Coronary angioplasty with or without stent implantation for acutemyocardial infarction. Stent primary angioplasty in myocardial infarction study group. *N Engl J Med* 1999; **341;** (26)1949–56.

33.   Gold HK, Garabedian HD, Dinsmore RE *et al*. Restoration of coronary flow in myocardial infarction by intravenous chimeric 7E3 antibody without exogenous plasminogen activators: observations in animals and humans. *Circulation* 1997; **95**:1755–59.

34.   Cigarroa JE, Ferrell MA, Collen DJ *et al*. Enhanced endogenous coronary thrombolysis during acute myocardial infarction following selective platelet receptor blockade with ReoPro. *Circulation* 1997; **94** (supp I):1-552.

35.   Rawistscher D, Levin TN, Cohen I *et al*. Rapid reversal of no-reflow using abciximab after coronary device intervention. *Cathet Cardiovasc Diagn* 1997; **42**:187–90.

36.   The EPIC Investigators. Use of a monoclonal antibody directed against the platelet glycoprotein IIb/IIIa receptor for high risk coronary angioplasty. *N Engl J Med* 1994; **330**:956–61.

37. Lefkovits J, Ivanhoe RJ, Califf RM *et al*. Effects of a platelet glycoprotein IIb/IIIa receptor blockade by a chimeric monoclonal antibody (Abciximab) on acute and six-month outcomes after percutaneous transluminal coronary angioplasty for acute myocardial infarction. *Am J Cardiol* 1996; **77**:1045–51.

38. Azar RR, McKay RG, Thompson PD *et al*. Abciximab in primary coronary angioplasty for acute myocardial infarction improves short-and medium term outcomes. *J Am Coll Cardiol* 1998; **32**:1996–2002.

39. Brener SJ, Barr LA, Burchenal JE *et al*. Randomised placebo-controlled trial of platelet glyco-protein IIb/IIIa blockade with primary angioplasty for acute myocardial infarction. *Circulation* 1998; **98**:734–41.

40. Stone G. Interim CADILLAC. Results underscore success rates of PTCA and stenting. American Heart Association Meeeting, November 1999.

41. Goldberg RJ, Gore JM, Alpert JS *et al*. Cardiogenic shock after acute myocardial infarction: Incidence and mortality from a community-wide perspective, 1975 to 1988. *N Engl J Med* 1991; **325**:1117–22.

42. Califf RM, and Bengtson, JR. Cardiogenic shock. *N Engl J Med* 1994; **330**:1724.

43. Gruppo Italiano per lo Studio della Streptochinasi nell'Infarcto Miocardico (GISSI): Effective-ness of intravenous thrombolytic treatment in acute myocardial infarction. *Lancet* 1986; **1**:397–402.

44. Kennedy JW, Gensini GG, Timmis GC *et al*. Acute myocardial infarction treated with intracoronary streptokinase: a report of the Society for Cardiac Angiography. *Am J Cardiol* 1985; **55**:871–77.

45. The GUSTO-III investigators: An international, multicenter, randomized comparison of reteplase with alteplase for acute myocardial infarction. *N Engl J Med* 1997; **337**:1118–23.

46. Gruppo Italiano per lo Studio della Sopravvienza nell'Infarcto Miocardico: GISSI-2: A facto-rial randomised trial of alteplase versus streptokinase and heparin versus no heparin among 12,490 patients with acute myocardial infarction. *Lancet* 1990; **336**:65–71.

47. Hochman JS, Boland J, Sleeper LA *et al*. Current spectrum of cardiogenic shock and effect of early revascularisation on mortality: Results of an International Registry: SHOCK Registry Investigators. *Circulation* 1995; **91**:873–81.

48. Hochman JS, Sleeper LA, Webb JG *et al*. Early revascularization in acute myocardial infarction comlicatied by cardiogenic shock. *N Engl J Med* 1999; **341**:625–34.

49. Ryan TJ. Early revascularization in cardiogenic shock—a positive view of a negative trial. *N Engl J Med* 1999; **341**:687–8.

50. Fibrinolytic Therapy Trialists' (FTT) Collaborative Group: Indications for fibrinolytic therapy in suspected acute myocardial infarction: collaborative overview of mortality and major mor-bidity results from randomised trials of more than 1000 patients. *Lancet* 1994; **343**:311–22.

51. Ribichini F, Steffenino G, Dellavalle A *et al*. Comparison of thrombolytic therapy and primary coronary angioplasty with liberal stenting for inferior myocardial infarction with precordial ST-segment depression. *J Am Coll Cardiol*. 1998; **32**:1687–94.

52. Bowers T, O'Neill W, Grines C *et al*. Effect of reperfusion on biventricular function and sur-vival after right ventricular infarction. *N Engl J Med* 1998; **338**; 933–40.

53. White H, and Van de Werf FJ. Thrombolysis for acute myocardial infarction. *Circulation* 1998; **97**:1632–46.

54. Bates ER. Revisiting reperfusion therapy for inferior myocardial infarction. *J Am Coll Cardiol*. 1997; **30**:334–42.

55. Cragg, DR, Feidman HZ, Bonema JD *et al*. Outcome of patients with acute myocardial infarc-tion who are ineligible for thrombolytic therapy. *Ann Intern Med* 1991; **115**:173–77.

56. McCullough PA, O; Neill WW, Graham M *et al*. A prospective randomised trial of triage angiography in acute coronary syndromes ineligible for thrombolysis. *J Am Col Cardiol* 1998; **32**:596–605.

57. Davis KB, Alderman EL, Kosinski AS *et al*. Early mortality of acute myocardial infarction in patients with and without prior coronary revascularisation surgery: a Coronary Artery Surgery Study Registry study. *Circulation* 1992; **85**:2100–09.

58. De Franco AC, Abramowitz B, Krichbaum D *et al.* Substantial (three-fold) benefit of accelerated t-PA over standard thrombolytic therapy in patients with prior bypass surgery and acute MI: Results of the GUSTO Trial. *J Am Coll Cardiol* 1994; **23**:1A–484A.

59. O'Keefe JO, Bailey WL, Rutherford BD, Hartzler GO. Primary angioplasty for acute myocardial infarction in 1000 consecutive patients. *Am J Cardiol* 1993; **72**:107G–115G.

60. The GUSTO Investigators. An international randomized trial comparing four thrombolytic strategies for acute myocardial infarction. *N Engl J Med* 1993; **329**:673–82.

61. Weaver WD, Litwin PE, Martin JS *et al.* Effect of age on use of thrombolytic therapy and mortality in acute myocardial infarction: the MITI project group. *J Am Coll Cardiol.* 1991; **18**:657–62.

62. Holmes DR, White HD, Peiper KS *et al.* Effect of age on outcome with primary angioplasty versus thrombolysis. *J Am Coll Cardiol* 1999; **33**:412–19.

63. De Boer MJ, Hoorntje JCA, Ottervanger JP *et al.* Immediate coronary angioplasty versus intravenous streptokinase in acute myocardial infarction: left ventricular ejection fraction, hospital mortality and reinfarction. *JACC* 1994; **23**(5):1004–08.

64. Brodie BR, Stuckey TD, Wall TC *et al.* Importance of time to reperfusion for 30-day and late survival and recovery of left ventricular function after primary angioplasty for acute myocardial infarction. *J Am Coll Cardiol* 1998; **32**:1312–19.

65. Weaver WD, Cerquiera M, Hallstrom AP *et al.* Pre-hospital initiated vs hospital initiated thrombolytic therapy: The Myocardial Infarction Triage and Intervention trial. *JAMA* 1993; **270**:1211–16.

66. The GUSTO Angiographic Investigators. The effects of tissue plasminogen activator, steptokinase or both on coronary artery patency, left ventricular function and survival after acute myocardial infarction. *N Engl J Med* 1993; **329**:1615–22.

67. Ito H, Okamura A, Iwakura K *et al.* Myocardial perfusion patterns related to thrombolysis in myocardial infarction perfusion grades after coronary angioplasty in patients with anterior wall myocardial infarction. *Circulation* 1996; **93**:1993–99.

68. Agati L, Voci P, Hickle P *et al.* Tissue-type plasmnogen activator therapy versus primary coronary angioplasty: impact on myocardial tissue perfusion and regional function 1 month after uncomplicated myocardial infarction. *J Am Coll Cardiol* 1998; **31**:338–43.

69. Kircher BE, Topol EJ, O'Neill WW *et al.* Prediction of coronary artery recanalization after intravenous thrombolytic therapy. *Am J Cardiol* 1987; 59:513–15.

70. Topol EJ. Catheter-based reperfusion for acute myocardial infarction. In: *Textbook of interventional cardiology,* 3rd ed. Philadelphia: Saunders 1998.

71. Ellis SG, Van der Werf F, Ribiero-da Silva E, Topol EJ. Present status of rescue coronary angioplasty: current polarization of opinion and randomized trials. *J Am Coll Cardiol* 1992; **19**:681–86.

72. Grines Cl, Marsalese Dl, Brodie B *et al.* Safety and cost-effectiveness of early discharge after primary angioplasty in low risk patients with acute myocardial infarction. *J Am Coll Cardiol.* 1998; **31**:969–72.

73. Zijlstra R, van't Hof AW, Liem AL *et al.* Transferring patients for primary angioplasty: a retrospective analysis of 104 selected high risk patients with acute myocardial infarction. Heart 1997; **78**:333–336.

74. Aguirre FV, Topol EJ, Donohue TJ *et al.* Impact of ionic and non-ionic contrast media on postPTCA ischemic complications: Results from the EPIC trial. *J Am Coll Cardiol* 1995; (Suppl) 901–14.

75. Califf RM, Glycoprotein IibIIa blockade and thrombolytics: Early lessons from the SPEED and GUSTO IV trials. *Am Heart J* 1999; **138** (Suppl. S):S12–S15.

76. Topol, EJ. Toward a new frontier in myocardial reperfusion therapy: Emerging platelet preeminence. *Circulation* 1998; **97**:211–18.

Chapter 21

Coronary Stenting

Aran Maree, David Baron and Paul Roy

History

For more than 20 years, transluminal approaches to improve or restore patency in diseased blood vessels have been challenging medical minds. Andreas Gruentzig is credited with having performed the first percutaneous transluminal coronary angioplasty (PTCA) in 1977.[1] Its widespread application is a testament to the usefulness of this procedure. Yet, despite procedural success rates exceeding 85–90%, some important issues limit the success of balloon angioplasty in the definitive treatment of coronary atheromatous disease. Restenosis may occur in up to 40% of patients after PTCA,[2–4] more often after a suboptimal result. Major ischaemic complications develop in 4–5% percent of elective procedures.[5,6] Attempts to achieve long-term patency by PTCA in chronically totally occluded vessels have yielded less than impressive results,[7,8] with restenosis and reocclusion a common sequel.[7–9]

In 1968, Charles Dotter inserted plastic graft tubes into canine femoral and popliteal arteries.[10] An appalling initial patency rate improved somewhat when stainless steel coils were substituted and heparin was administered concomitantly after implantation. Since the first human implantation of the coronary stent by Jacques Puel in Toulouse, France and Ulrich Sigwart in Lausanne, Switzerland in 1986, coronary stenting has progressed from a series of pioneering registries in the 1980s to an era of randomised trials in the 1990s, to become an accepted and valued tool in the continuing struggle to restore and maintain luminal patency.[11]

The present

The rapid and widespread use of coronary stents can best be understood when one considers the complications of balloon angioplasty that may be avoided by stenting. These problems include plaque fissuring and disruption under radial compression, leading to particulate emboli, unstable vessel surfaces and flap formation, which may be a precursor to vessel occlusion. Furthermore, the tendency of the wall of an elastic vessel to rebound significantly after dilatation is significantly reduced after insertion of a stent. Stents have a low profile, and if pre-mounted on a balloon are as quick to prepare as a balloon alone. The results of stent use are predictable, and procedure time is often dramatically reduced.

Stenting came to be viewed as the natural successor to balloon angioplasty, as it was often employed as a rescue device to treat threatened or acute vessel closure. It greatly simplified percutaneous treatment of the trickier coronary procedures such as venous by-pass conduits, ostial lesions, and chronically occluded arteries. Landmark clinical trials rapidly provided the evidence needed to show that the risk of restenosis was significantly reduced when a stent was implanted electively.

A vast body of data is now becoming available to the interventional cardiologist in support of stents over balloon angioplasty alone in the treatment of coronary disease. The following overview discusses the history, development and appplication of coronary stenting in relation to the various clinical trials and studies undertaken over recent years.

Previous trials

Two landmark trials established coronary stenting as a legitimate alternative to balloon angioplasty. The STRESS trial was a study comparing the **clinical restenosis rates of stents and PTCA in de-novo native coronary lesions.**[12] The trial enrolled 410 patients, who were randomised to the stent or the PTCA arm. They all had symptomatic coronary disease, with lesions > 70% diameter and < 15 mm length, and vessel diameter > 3.0 mm. The primary endpoints in this trial included death, myocardial infarction (MI), coronary artery bypass grafting (CABG) or re-PTCA at 6 months. The immediate results, as measured by residual luminal stenosis after the procedure, were significantly better in the stented population (19± 11% vs. 35 ± 14%, p< 0.001). There was also a lower 6-month restenosis rate in the stent arm than the PTCA arm (31.6% vs. 42.1%p=0.046).[12]

A similar trial in Europe (BENESTENT) showed a non-significant benefit of stenting over angioplasty.[13] In both of these trials, stented patients were treated with oral antico-agulants, and in these patients the incidence of access site bleeding was unacceptably high. Following recognition that oral anticoagulation is not necessary after stent implantation, the BENESTENT II trial comparing coronary **stenting in conjunction with aspirin and ticlopidine versus PTCA**[14] was performed. This trial enrolled patients with un-stable angina and randomised them to either a heparin-coated stent plus aspirin and ticlopidine, or to balloon angioplasty alone. The primary endpoints of the trial were death, MI or target-lesion revascularisation (TLR) at 6-months follow-up. Cost-analysis was per-formed at 12 months. At 6 months the incidence of the combined endpoints in the stented group was 12.8% compared to 19.3% in the PTCA group (p=0.013). This difference was driven fundamentally by the fact that target-lesion revascularisation in the stented arm was only 5.4% when compared with 12.4% in the balloon arm. Angiography at 6 months demonstrated an impressive reduction in restenosis of 16% in the stented arm when com-pared to 31% for PTCA. The cost, however, was still higher in the stented patient than in the angioplasty alone patient, by US$1126. By 12 months, total expenses were similar in the two groups.

More recently, the EPISTENT investigators compared **PTCA plus the new antiplatelet agent abciximab, stent plus placebo and stent plus abciximab** in a randomised trial.[15] With an impressive patient population of 2399 and primary endpoints of death, MI and urgent revascularisation, the trial demonstrated that stenting plus abciximab may be the revascularisation strategy of choice, with this group having an event-rate at 30 days of 5.3% compared to PTCA and abciximab of 6.9%. This should translate into a reduction of 7 deaths, 51 MIs and 30 revascularisation procedures per 1000 pa-tients at 6 months.

Special situations

Small vessels

The STRESS I+II (small vessel sub-study) triallists[16] attempted in a post-hoc analysis to evaluate whether the Palmaz- Schatz stent reduces clinical and angiographic restenosis rates compared with balloon angioplasty in patients with de novo coronary lesions in smaller vessels (< 3.0 mm). These patients all had symptomatic coronary artery disease, > 70% stenoses, lesion length < 15 mm and reference vessel diameter < 3.0 mm. Patients randomised to Palmaz-Schatz stents numbered 163, and 168 were randomised to PTCA. The clinical endpoint was TLR at 1 year; the angiographic endpoint was restenosis, with measurement of the minimal lumen diameter at 6 months. The conclusion of this trial is that elective stenting with the Palmaz-Schatz stent in vessels < 3 mm diameter provides superior clinical and angiographic outcomes when compared to PTCA.

A further study of stenting in even smaller coronary arteries (< 2.5mm) using stents specifically designed for these arteries suggests the safety and immediate superiority of stenting over angioplasty in these small vessels.[17] Data collated in this trial suggest that, although revascularisation rates and combined endpoints of death/MI/revascularisation were converging in both populations when follow-up in excess of 6 months was performed, 81% of stented patients were symptom-free as opposed to 62% of patients with PTCA alone, with an average follow-up time exceeding 12 months.

Multivessel disease

The case for stenting multiple lesions in diffusely diseased arteries has not yet been proven.

Calcified lesions

Calcified coronary arteries have long been a challenge to the interventionalist. Debulking by rotational atherectomy prior to stent implantation has become a popular means of approaching this problem.[18] However, results of trials comparing balloon and stent with debulking and stent are not yet available. Intravascular ultrasound, although adding extra procedural time, may play an important role in the decision to debulk prior to stenting, and in evaluating the adequacy of stent apposition to the vessel wall.

Bifurcation lesions

The complex issue of stenting bifurcation lesions has not yet been satisfactorily resolved. Bifurcation lesions are present in 2–16% of stenoses that are considered for percutaneous intervention. Conventional balloon angioplasty in the treatment of such lesions is associated with an increased rate of complications and reduced success. An assortment of devices including rotational atherectomy, directional atherectomy and various coronary stents have been developed to overcome the challenge posed by such lesions.[19] The two techniques of 'kissing' stents and 'T' stenting have been used by experienced operators.[20,21] Specialised bifurcation stents are being developed and trialled.

Bypass grafts

Another challenge for modern cardiology is that of treating the diseased saphenous venous bypass graft. Approximately 50% of these have significant disease 10 years after surgery.[22]

Repeat bypass surgery is often a difficult or high-risk proposition.[23] Studies have been performed using both self-expanding Wallstents and the Palmaz-Schatz stent. The Saphenous Vein de Novo (SAVED) trial, in which the Palmaz-Schatz stent was used and compared to balloon alone in 220 patients, suggested a benefit in terms of the restenosis risk; it also highlighted a significantly better outcome in the stented group in terms of freedom from death, MI, repeat bypass surgery or target lesion revascularisation.[24] Currently, new self-expanding devices and graft stents are being developed and tested in the hope that these will aid in preventing further disease progression. Further trials are required to assess the long-term outcomes of stenting in saphenous veins and in particular to accurately compare these outcomes with regrafting.

Aorto-ostial lesions

Results of treatment of aorto-ostial lesions with balloon angioplasty alone are often suboptimal due to the composition of the aortic wall, which can be both elastic and very rigid. The immediate results are significantly better with stenting, with a restenosis rate of only 15% in some lesions and up to 60% in aorto-ostial saphenous vein graft lesions.[25,26] The role of rotational atherectomy with subsequent stent placement remains unclear at this time in the absence of randomised study data.

Left main disease

The era is long gone when stenting was acceptable for only uncomplicated double-vessel coronary disease, or with threatened closure after angioplasty. The ongoing ULTIMA study in Japan is studying the outcomes of patients having stents placed in their left main coronary arteries.

Acute myocardial infarction

In The Netherlands a trial was performed comparing primary coronary stenting with primary balloon angioplasty in 222 selected patients with acute myocardial infarction; it demonstrated a significant reduction in both repeat MI and target-lesion revascularisation at 6 months follow-up.[27] Primary success was achieved in 98% of the stent group compared with 96% of the balloon group. Sub-acute closure occurred in none of the stented group as compared to 5.4% of the PTCA group; death occurred in none of the stent

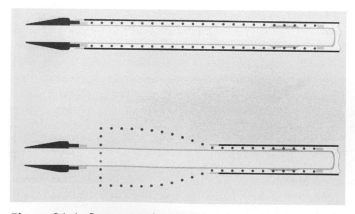

Figure 21.1. *Demonstration of the self-expanding delivery system for the Wallstent, showing how the stent expands* in situ *as the sheath is withdrawn. (Courtesy of Boston Scientific).*

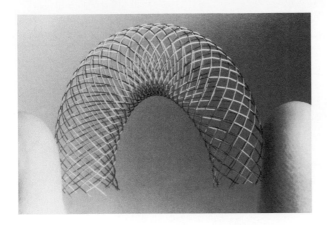

Figure 21.2. *Flexibility of the Wallstent. (Courtesy of Boston Scientific).*

group and 2.1% of the PTCA group. The combined end-point of death/MI or reintervention was significantly lower in the stent group (p=0.03). This and several larger trials provide impressive evidence that stenting is a safe and effective strategy for reperfusing an acutely occluded coronary artery. In centres with the appropriate facilities and expertise, stenting for acute myocardial infarction has become the preferred means of myocardial perfusion.

Preliminary data suggests that stenting can be performed safely and is a good option for patients who are unsuitable for surgical revascularisation. However, the incidence of restenosis and late sudden death remains disturbingly high. Much of the pioneering work in the coronary tree has led to great advances in both the technology used to deliver the devices and the quality of the devices employed, while being parallelled by advances in anti-platelet and anticoagulant regimens. Stents are currently being placed in all branches of the arterial tree, in what might be seen as a natural evolution in patient care.

Some common stents

A number of companies currently design, manufacture and market stents internationally. The requirements of the ideal coronary stent are that it be flexible, trackable, provide good radial support, and be readily visible under fluoroscopy. It is obviously advantageous if the stent design minimises the risk of restenosis, caused by reactive neointimal proliferation. Each individual stent possesses a variety of these characteristics in varying degrees, and choice of stent for an individual case is generally a result of operator experience with a particular design, the known qualities and characteristics of a particular design, and the availability in the laboratory of an appropriately-sized (both diameter and length) stent. There are many different designs of stent including slotted tube, mesh, coil, hybrid, ring, etc. Stents are made from stainless steel, nitinol, tantalum, platinum and other materials.

The self-expanding mesh stent (e.g. Wallstent/Boston Scientific)

The self-expanding wire mesh stent is delivered mounted on a coaxial catheter on which it is constrained by a retractable rolling membrane or sheath (Fig 21.1). The current stent is a cobalt-based alloy with a platinum core. The first human coronary Wallstent was inserted by Puel in Toulouse in 1986.[28] There have been several evolutionary stages in the design of this stent. It is flexible, tracks well and has good radio-opacity (Fig.21-2). Its self-expanding design leads to excellent radial expansion when correctly sized. It is commonly

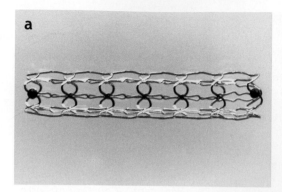

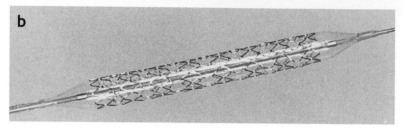

Figure 21.3a. The BeStent, an example of a slotted tube stent. (Courtesy of Medtronic).

Figure 21.3b. The Pura-Vario slotted tube stent, shown in expanded form over an inflated balloon. (Courtesy of Devon Medical).

used in both native coronary vessels and venous bypass grafts. There is a tendency for the stent to shorten upon deployment (less apparent in later models), which requires careful placement and use of markers on the delivery vehicle as a guide to correct positioning. In general it is deployed following balloon angioplasty to the lesion as it is not balloon-mounted. It is frequently employed in the treatment of diseased venous bypass grafts where the risks of balloon angioplasty are high.

The slotted tube stent (e.g. Palmaz-Schatz/Johnson and Johnson, BeStent/Device Technologies, Pura-Vario/Devon Medical, Joflex/Jomed International)

These balloon-expandable stents are either hand-crimped onto the balloon or come ready-mounted (Fig 21.3a, b). The Palmaz-Schatz stent was the stent employed in the landmark STRESS and BENESTENT trials.[13,16] The earlier model, though exerting great radial strength, was very rigid, which often complicated delivery. The later version has a mid-point articulation, consisting of a short bridge between both halves of the stent (PS153 series), permitting easier delivery. With good wall coverage, excellent radial strength and minimal recoil once expanded, it is easy to see why this stent became the work-horse in

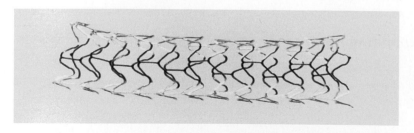

Figure 21.4. The Multilink Stent, showing its characteristic multiple annular links. (Courtesy of Medtronic).

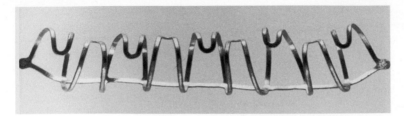

Figure 21.5. The GR II stent, showing its coiled helical configuration. (Courtesy of Medtronic).

many of the earlier trials. The Spiral and Crown designs are both modifications of the earlier PS153 model. The balloon expandable Spiral design is a thicker stent, exerting even greater radial force than the PS153. The Improved Spiral coronary stent is a further modification aimed at increasing the flexibility of the stent, with slightly thinner struts. The Crown design is said to retain the radial force of the original stent while permitting greater flexibility and trackability, without incorporating specific articulating points into the body of the stent. The Mini-Crown, a more flexible version of the Crown stent, was designed specifically for use in arteries < 3 mm diameter. Both the PS153 and coronary Spiral series are available with a heparin coating covalently bonded to the stent.

Hybrid stent (e.g. Multilink/Advanced Cardiovascular Systems)

The Multilink stent is a stainless steel, balloon-expandable, slotted tube and consists of multiple rings with small bridges linking the rings (Fig. 21.4). There are a variety of delivery systems available for this stent. The Multilink RX Duet differs in the shape of the repeating unit, thickness of the strut and the frequency of articulating bridges.

Variants of slotted tube stent (e.g. Jostent Plus and Jostent Flex/Jomed International)

The Jostent Plus and Jostent Flex are both second-generation stainless steel, balloon-expanded slotted-tube stents. The Plus is designed to fit vessels up to 6 mm in diameter and its design incorporates both radial strength and flexibility. The Jostent Flex version has been designed to track into lesions that are awkwardly situated.

Wire stents (e.g. Crossflex/Cordis, a Johnson & Johnson Interventional Systems Co., Wiktor/Medtronic, Gianturco Roubin Stents/Cook Co.)

The Crossflex Stent is a stainless steel balloon-expandable wire stent. The wire is coiled into a helical configuration. The open nature of the design facilitates side branch access, and is often employed at branch points within the coronary tree, where it may be necessary to recross a stented segment and possibly pass another stent into a sidebranch. The Wiktor and Gianturco-Roubin stents (Fig 21.5) are also extremely flexible wire stents that have largely been superceded by the second and third generation slotted-tube stent.

The Nir stent (e.g. Nir and Nir Royal/Scimed Life Systems)

The Nir and Nir Royal are balloon-expandable stainless steel stents (Fig 21.6) that are cut, rolled and welded from a metal sheet. The cellular design of this stent permits relatively easy tracking to a lesion point, allowing differential elongation of various portions of the

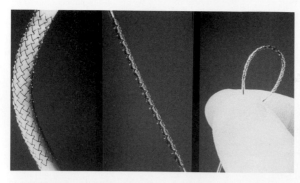

Figure 21.6. *The The Nir stent. Figure at left shows its appearance when deployed, the middle image shows the stent ready-mounted on the balloon prior to use, and the figure at right shows the flexibility of the stent. (Courtesy of Boston Scientific).*

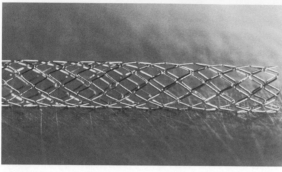

Figure 21.7. *The S670 stent, showing its continuous ring structure formed from single thin rods. (Courtesy of Medtronic).*

stent. The characteristics of this stent include excellent radial strength, with the cellular design minimising tissue prolapse through the struts while also keeping the metal coverage of the tissue to a minimum. There are some further modifications in the second generation of the design to improve the geometry when placed in curved portions of the artery and further increase radial strength at both ends of the stent.

The GFX-2 stent (GFX-2, S670, S540/Medtronic)

The Continuously Connected Element design of the GFX stent is comprised of short 2 mm length sinusoidal elements that are individually formed from stainless steel rings into

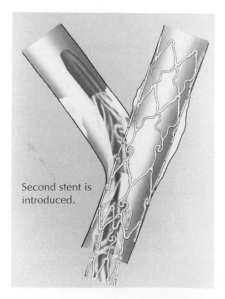

Second stent is introduced.

Figure 21.8. *The Bifurcation stent, showing the large cells that permit access for additional stent deployment at side branches. (Courtesy of Device Technologies Australia).*

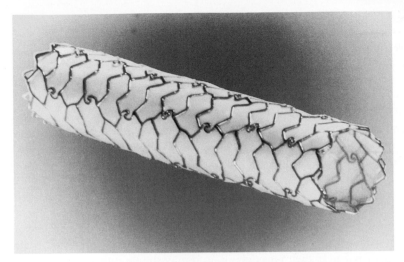

Figure 21.9. The Jostent Coronary Graft stent. This design consists of an ultrathin membrane sandwiched between two thin stents, forming a seal over the internal lining of the artery. (Courtesy of Device Technologies Australia).

stainless steel rods. The individual rings are then shaped into sinusoidal elements, using an ellipto-rectangular strut design and are connected by laser fusion and then polished (Fig. 21.7). The GFX2 has added a further 15% reduction in profile over that of the GFX and has demonstrated itself to be a highly trackable and flexible stent, and is particularly valuable for those difficult-to-reach lesions. Its moderate radio-opacity aids stent placement.

Stents for bifurcation lesions (e.g. Jostent B/Jomed International, Bard Bifurcation Stent/Bard)

Some stents have been specifically designed for bifurcation lesions. These include the Jostent B (Jomed International AB) and the Bard Bifurcation stent. These stents are designed to help overcome the problems associated with manoeuvring straight tubular stents into arteries and trying to place them so as not to jail a sidebranch, or at least to permit access to the side branch (Fig. 21.8). The Jostent B is designed with larger cells at one end of the stent, allowing access through the struts into a side branch. The Bard stent is designed as a true bifurcation stent in a 'Y' configuration and mounted on twin balloons to minimise the risk of prefential expansion of one limb of the bifurcation.

Stents for aneurysmal dilatations, ruptured/perforated coronaries or friable vein grafts

These stents are designed to seal over a defect in the lining of the artery, and the Jostent Coronary Stent Graft (Jomed International) does this by sandwiching an ultrathin layer of graft material between two thin stents (Fig.. 21.9). There is also an internal heparin coating to reduce thrombogenicity on implantation.

Radioactive and coated stents

These are part of the armamentarium currently being assembled to reduce the incidence of stent restenosis, and have only recently come into use (see Chapter 22). Evaluation of their long-term success must therefore wait.

The future

It is difficult to directly compare stents in the absence of randomised trials. However, there is evidence that differences in metal composition, surface area, geometry, surface texture and electronic charge may impact on restenosis rates. The manner of delivery may also affect the degree of injury to the vessel wall, as does low-pressure vs high-pressure balloon inflation, or whether the stent is self-expanding.

Interventional cardiologists may too often be flattered by excellent initial cosmetic results, perhaps at the expense of long-term patency, and will in future have to focus more acutely on emerging data differentiating the various stents and situations in which they may be most successfully employed.

Future generations of stents will incorporate computer-generated features to maximise the positive mechanical attributes of the deployed stent while facilitating deployment. Stent coatings, whether simply chemical-based to inhibit restenosis or carrying genetically-active molecules to modify tissue reaction, may play an important role. Results of current trials on coated stents may soon lead to their introduction into mainstream interventional practice.

References

1   Gruentzig AR, Senning A,Slegenthaler WE. Nonoperative dilatation of coronary artery stenosis: percutaneous transluminal coronary angioplasty. *New Engl J Med* 1979; **301**:61–68.

2   Kaltenbach M, Kober G, Scherer D, Vallbracht C. Recurrence rate after successful coronary angioplasty. *Eur Heart J* 1985; **6**:276–81.

3   Leimgruber PP, Roubin GS, Hollman J *et al.* Restenosis after successful coronary angioplasty in patients with single-vessel disease. *Circulation* 1986:**73**:710–17.

4   Whitworth HB, Pilcher GS, Roubin GS, Gruentzig AR. Do proximal lesions involving the origin of the left anterior descending artery have a higher restenosis rate after coronary angioplasty? *Circulation* 1985:**72**(Suppl III):III-398 (Abstract).

5   Detre K, Holubkov R, Kelsey S *et al.* Percutaneous transluminal angioplasty in 1985–1986 and 1977–1981. The National Heart, Lung and Blood Institute Registry. *New Engl J Med* 1988; **318**:265–70.

6   Bredlau CE, Roubin GS, Leimgruber PP *et al.* In-hospital morbidity and mortalityin patients undergoing elective coronary angioplasty. *Circulation* 1985; **72**: 1044–52.

7   Serruys PW, Umans V, Heyndrickx GR *et al.* Elective PTCA of totally occluded coronary arteries not associated with acute myocardial infarction; short-term and long-term results. *Eur Heart J* 1985; **6**:2–12.

8   Kereiakes DJ, Selmon MR, McAuley BJ *et al.* Angioplasty and total coronary occlusion: Experience in 76 consecutive patients. *J Am Coll Cardiol* 1985; **6**:526–33.

9   Ellis SG, Shaw RE, Gershony G *et al.* Risk factors, time-course and treatment effect for restenosis after successful percutaneous transluminal coronary angioplasty for chronic total occlusion. *Am J Cardiol* 1989; **63**:897–901.

10   Dotter CT. Transluminally placed coil springs and arterial tube grafts: Long-term patency in the canine popliteal artery. *Invest Radiol* 1969; **4**:329–332.

11   Sigwart U, Puel J, Mirkovitch V *et al.* Intravascular stents to prevent occlusion and restenosis after transluminal angioplasty. *New Engl J Med* 1987; **316**:701–06.

12   Fischman DL, Marin BL, Donald SB *et al.* A randomised comparison of coronary stent placement and balloon angioplasty in the treatment of coronary artery disease. *N Engl J Med* 1994; **331**:496–501.

13   Serruys PW, de Jaegere P, Kiemeneij F *et al.*, for the BENESTENT Study group. A comparison of balloon-expandable stent implantation with balloon angioplasty in patients with coronary artery disease. *N Engl J Med* 1994; **331**:489–95.

14   Serruys PW, van Hout B, Bonnier *et al.* For the Benestent Study Group. Randomised comparison of implantation of heparin-coated stents with balloon angioplasty in selected patients with
coronary artery disease (Benestent II). The Lancet 1998; **352**:673–81.

15   The EPISTENT investigators. Randomised placebo-controlled and balloon-angioplasty-controlled trial to assess the safety of coronary stenting with the use of platelet-IIb/IIIa blockade.
Lancet 1998; **352**:87–92.

16   The Stent Restenosis Group. STRESS I+II (small vessel substudy). *J Am Coll Cardiol* 1998;
31:307–11.

17   Muller DWM, Lansky AJ, Kaul V *et al.* Small native coronary vessel stenting. Results from the
Asia-Pacific Minicrown Registry (in preparation).

18   Mintz GS, Dussailant GR, Wong SC *et al.* Rotational atherectomy followed by adjunct stents:
The preferred therapy for calcified lesions in large vessels? (abstract). *Circulation* 1995; **92**(Suppl
I):I–329.

19   Dauerman HL, Higgins PJ, Sparano AM *et al.* Mechanical debulking vs balloon angioplasty
for the treatment of true bifurcation lesions. *J Am Coll Cardiol* 1998; **32**:1845–52.

20   Meier B. Kissing balloon coronary angioplasty. *Am J Cardiol* 1984; **54**:918–920.

21   Carlson TA, Fuarneri EM, Shela KMS *et al.* 'T-stenting': The answer to bifurcation lesions?
(Abstract). *Circulation* 1996; **94**(Suppl I):I–86.

22   Bourassa MG, Enjalbert M, Campeau L, Lesperance J. Progression of atherosclerosis in coronary arteries and bypass grafts: Ten years later. *Am J Cardiol*1984; **53**(suppl C):102–07.

23   Foster ED, Fisher LD, Kaiser GC, Myers WO. Comparison of operative mortality and morbidity for initial and repeat coronary artery bypass grafting: The Coronary Artery Surgery Study
(CASS) Registry experience. *Ann Thorac Surg* 1984; **38**:563–70.

24   Savage MP, Douglas JS, Fischman DL *et al.* A randomised trial of coronary stenting and balloon angioplasty in the treatment of aortocoronary saphenous venous bypass graft disease. *N
Engl J Med* 1997; **337**:740–47.

25   Kobayashi N, Finci L, Ferraro M *et al.* Restenosis after coronary stenting -Clinical and
angiographic predictors in 1906 lesions. *J Am Coll Cardiol* 1999; **33**,2:32A.

26   Kobayashi N, Vaghetti M, Kobayashi Y *et al.* Coronary stenting of ostial lesions: results are
different between arteries. *Circulation* 1998; **98**(Suppl I):I–286.

27   Suryapranata H, van't Hof AW, Hoorntje JC *et al.* Randomised comparison of coronary stenting
with balloon angioplasty in selected patients with acute myocardial infarction. *Circulation* 1998;
92(25):2502–05.

28   Rousseau H, Puel J, Joffre F *et al.* Self-expanding endovascular prosthesis: An experimental
study. *Radiology* 1987; **164**:709–14.

Chapter 22

Percutaneous Coronary Interventions: Alternatives to Balloon Dilatation

David W.M. Muller

There is no doubt that by far the greatest contribution to the welfare of patients undergoing percutaneous vascular interventional procedures in the past two decades has been the development of the endoluminal stent. The improvement in stent profile and tracking is such that stents can be placed in almost any sized epicardial coronary artery with the prospect of a better initial clinical outcome and a reduced need for repeat intervention. Over the past two decades, several other devices have also been developed and evaluated clinically as alternative approaches to the management of subsets of patients requiring coronary interventions. This chapter deals with devices currently in clinical use that have a role in selected patients when used alone or prior to coronary stenting.

Directional atherectomy

The directional atherectomy catheter was developed as a means of removing atheromatous tissue from the coronary artery wall. It was expected that this would optimise the initial improvement in luminal dimensions, reduce the potential for coronary dissection and abrupt closure, and improve the long-term clinical outcome by reducing the incidence of restenosis. The catheter is an over-the-wire system that consists of a metal housing assembly that is open on one side, with an inflatable balloon attached to the external surface of the contralateral side (Fig. 22.1). Within the housing is a cup-shaped cutting tool attached to a rotating shaft. When activated by a hand-held motor drive unit, the cutting blade rotates at 2000 rpm. Tissue is resected by advancing the cutting blade forward while the housing is held in place against the vessel wall by inflation of the balloon to 10–15 psi (0.5–1 atm). The atheromatous tissue is pushed forwards into a cone-shaped collecting chamber in front of the metal housing. After each passage of the cutting blade, the balloon is deflated, the device is rotated through 90°, the balloon is reinflated, and the blade is withdrawn to its starting position. This sequence is repeated 6 to 8 times before the entire device is removed and the nose cone is cleared of the retrieved atheromatous tissue. During a typical passage of the device, 8–10 mg of atheroma may be retrieved from the collecting chamber. If residual disease is apparent by repeat angiography, further resection can be performed to remove as much tissue as possible. Finally, low-pressure balloon inflation with a slightly oversized angioplasty balloon is usually required to optimise the angiographic result.

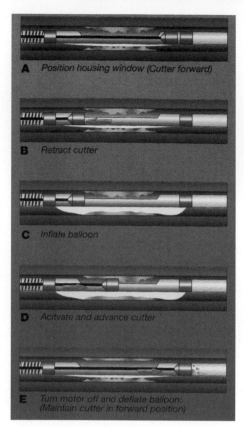

A   Position housing window (Cutter forward)

B   Retract cutter

C   Inflate balloon

D   Acitvate and advance cutter

E   Turn motor off and deflate balloon:
    (Maintain cutter in forward position)

Figure 22.1. The directional atherectomy catheter. After inflation of the balloon, the rotating blade is advanced forwards, excising tissue and pushing it forwards into the collecting chamber at the distal end of the device. (Reproduced with permission courtesy of Mallinckrodt Inc., St Louis, Missouri.)

The major advantage of directional coronary atherectomy (DCA) over conventional balloon angioplasty is that a larger initial lumen can be achieved.[1,2] Tissue resection may also be particularly useful in avoiding side branch closure in bifurcation lesions by minimising plaque redistribution across the origin of the side branch ('snow-plough effect'); it is also one of the most effective treatments for ostial lesions in large arteries. The extent of lumen enlargement may be comparable to that achieved by coronary stenting[3,4] and one study has suggested that aggressive debulking may achieve long-term results that are equal to, or better than, those of coronary stenting.[4] However, use of the device is limited by the fact that it is bulky, relatively inflexible and requires the use of 9.5–10F guiding catheters. The redesigned Flexicut system has a lower profile and greater capacity for tissue resection, but remains relatively inflexible. Randomised trials of directional atherectomy and balloon angioplasty have also failed to show a reduction in restenosis

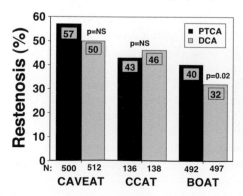

Figure 22.2. Comparison of restenosis rates between patients treated by PTCA and directional atherectomy in the randomized CAVEAT, CCAT and BOAT trials.[1-3]

(Fig. 22.2), need for target lesion revascularisation or improvement in event-free survival even when atherectomy is performed aggressively to optimise the initial angiographic result.[2] Indeed, in one study,[5] the one-year mortality and myocardial infarction rates were higher in patients treated by DCA than in those treated by conventional balloon angioplasty.

In many centres in the United States, directional atherectomy at one time constituted approximately 10% of interventional procedures performed and was considered to be an excellent alternative to coronary stenting. However, the change in anticoagulation protocol for stents and concomitant reduction in access site complications, together with improvements in stent technology, have resulted in a progressive decline in use of the directional atherectomy catheter and an overwhelming preference for coronary stents as the primary therapy for coronary interventions. In some centres, directional atherectomy prior to coronary stenting remains in vogue. Preliminary data have suggested that debulking prior to stenting may further reduce the incidence of restenosis.[6] In a case control study, Bramucci and colleagues compared the outcomes of 100 patients undergoing directional atherectomy and stenting with those of a matched series of patients undergoing stenting without initial debulking.[6] Event-free survival was better in the DCA/stent patients and the restenosis rate was lower (6.8% vs 30.5%, p<0.0001). These results have not yet been confirmed in large randomised trials. Other small studies have not been as positive and suggest comparable results for patients stented with or without initial debulking.[7]

Rotational atherectomy

A second debulking device that has been widely used is the rotational atherectomy catheter. Debulking is achieved by the action of a diamond-encrusted, olive-shaped burr that rotates at speeds of up to 200 000 rpm (Fig. 22.3); the rotation speed of the drive is regulated by an air turbine. As the burr is advanced over a specialised wire into contact with the lesion, the plaque surface is ablated by abrasion, forming microparticulate debris (<5 μ diameter) that passes through the myocardial capillaries into the general circulation. The burrs are available in 0.25 mm increments from 1.25 mm to 2.5 mm for use in coronary arteries. Larger sizes are available for use in peripheral arteries. The very high rotation

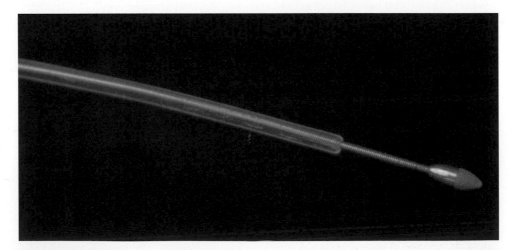

Figure 22.3. The rotational atherectomy catheter (Rotoblator™ Scimed, Boston Scientific Corporation). The diamond-tipped burr rotates at up to 200 000 rpm and abrades fibrocalcific plaques forming a fine slurry of microparticulates.

speed almost eliminates friction between the device and the guidewire, which allows it to be passed readily through tortuous, calcified coronary segments. The heat generated by the high rotation speed is limited by infusion of a saline solution through the catheter sheath.

Although the rotational atherectomy catheter was designed to remove tissue as a means of improving the initial and late outcomes of balloon angioplasty, its greatest value is in the treatment of heavily calcified lesions. Abrasion and tissue ablation occur maximally where atheromatous tissue is densely fibrotic and calcified. The burr has relatively little effect on adjacent normal elastic tissue. The mechanism of action of the device almost certainly includes not only tissue ablation but also release of fibrotic contractures by formation of microfissures, thereby allowing subsequent balloon dilatation of the lesion. Indeed, some lesions cannot be dilated or stented without initial treatment by rotational atherectomy.

The major limitation of rotational atherectomy is the formation of sufficient microparticulate matter to cause sludging of flow in the myocardial microcirculation. 'Slow-flow' or 'no-flow' occurs in up to 10% of patients treated with rotational atherectomy and may cause non-Q wave or Q-wave myocardial infarction. It occurs most commonly after treatment of long, heavily calcified lesions in large coronary arteries. In addition to capillary plugging by microemboli, coronary epicardial or microcirculatory spasm may also play a role.

The frequency of this complication can be reduced by meticulous attention to some technical considerations. First, the initial burr size should be small, particularly in diffusely diseased or heavily calcified arteries. The burr should be engaged with the lesion for relatively short periods (~30 secs) before retraction to allow flushing and distal passage of any particulate debris. The burr should be advanced very slowly with a constant rotation speed. A fall in rotation speed of more than 5000 rpm is associated with an increased risk of vessel wall injury (dissection and heat injury), formation of larger particles and poor distal flow. Various medical cocktails have been used to minimise the risk of poor distal flow. These include use of nitroglycerin (4 mg/L), verapamil (10 mg/L) and heparin (5000 U/L) in the infusion solution.

If no-reflow does occur, it can usually be treated by a combination of intracoronary verapamil (100–1000 mg in increments of 100–300 mg) and nitroglycerin (in incremental doses of 150–300 mg). Manual perfusion by vigorously flushing saline or autologous blood into the coronary artery also seems to improve flow. More refractory cases may require use of adenosine, a glycoprotein IIb/IIIa antagonist, or an intra-aortic balloon pump to improve distal perfusion.

Like directional atherectomy, rotational atherectomy has become a niche device with relatively few clear indications. Randomised comparisons of rotational atherectomy with balloon angioplasty have shown little benefit of debulking over conventional angioplasty, with disappointingly high restenosis rates.[8] Attempts to improve the long-term outcomes of rotational atherectomy by more aggressive debulking using large burrs have not been fruitful. More recently, rotational atherectomy has been proposed as a means of treating in-stent restenosis but data supporting this approach are not strong.[9] Nonetheless, rotational atherectomy prior to angioplasty or stenting still plays a very valuable role in the management of densely fibrotic or calcified lesions. Whether debulking prior to stenting reduces the incidence of restenosis remains to be determined. In one study,[10] the use of aggressive rotational atherectomy prior to stenting (burr:artery ratio >0.80) resulted in a lower restenosis rate than stenting after less aggressive debulking (30.9% vs 50.0%, p<0.05) but this strategy was associated with a higher incidence of procedural complications.

Transluminal extraction atherectomy

Several devices developed for atheroma removal have proven to be most effective in removing thrombotic material and the loose gruel of degenerated saphenous vein grafts. They have been less effective in removing the fibrocalcific disease of native coronary artery disease. The transluminal extraction catheter (TEC) is one such device. It consists of a cone-shaped head with two cutting blades and a central hollow aspiration channel through which excised debris is removed. The cutting head is driven by a battery-operated hand-held motor drive unit and rotates at 750 rpm. Excised tissue is collected in a vacuum bottle connected to the aspiration channel. The devices are available in 0.5 F increments from 5.5 F to 7.5 F and are used over a specialised 0.014 inch wire that has a 0.021 inch ball at its tip to limit the extent of travel of the device.

Like directional and rotational atherectomy catheters, the TEC catheter requires a 10 F guiding catheter to provide adequate support during passage of the device and to allow adequate contrast opacification of the segment being treated. The procedure is limited by the maximum size of the device (7.5 F), with the majority of lesions having a significant residual narrowing that requires adjunctive balloon dilatation and stent implantation. Widespread use of the device has been limited by the fact that distal embolisation and no-reflow occur with similar frequency to that of balloon dilatation and stenting alone, and that in treated saphenous vein grafts, restenosis and late total occlusion occur disappointingly frequently.[11] The device may nonetheless have a role as one of several devices that can facilitate vein graft angioplasty by removing bulky thrombotic or friable atheromatous debris.

Several other catheter systems have been designed to remove arterial obstructions. The X-Sizer™ catheter system (Endicor Medical Inc., Carlsbad, CA, USA) uses a spinning 'helix cutter' to excise and aspirate thrombus and atheromatous debris from diseased coronary arteries. Its action is similar to that of a corkscrew. It is a disposable, single-use, hand-held device and can be used with a variety of catheters and guidewires. It may prove useful in treating in-stent restenosis.

Ultrasonic ablation devices

Therapeutic ultrasound is based on delivery of high-energy, low-frequency ultrasound from an external piezo-electric crystal to the tip of a relatively inflexible catheter. Rapid oscillation of the catheter tip and the sound waves generated by this process cause cyclic cavitation (bubble formation) and implosion in adjacent fluids and tissues. Cavity implosion generates local pressures equivalent to those used in balloon angioplasty. This is believed to be the primary mechanism of action of the device; other mechanisms include a mechanical effect of the device itself and heat generation. *In vitro* studies suggest that ultrasound energy may be used to ablate atheromatous plaque including fibrocalcific disease. However, clinical studies suggest that the greatest value of the device is in dissolution of fresh thrombus. Following ultrasound ablation, the vast majority of the remaining particulate debris is <10 μ in diameter and passes readily through the coronary microcirculation.[12] An additional potential benefit seen in some studies[13] is vasodilatation, plus an increase in epicardial coronary flow and myocardial perfusion.[14]

Relatively few clinical data are currently available to determine the ultimate role of ultrasound ablation devices. Preliminary data suggest that thrombus dissolution prior to angioplasty or stenting in the setting of acute myocardial infarction[15] may reduce the potential for distal thromboembolism and poor flow, thereby providing more complete reperfusion than can be achieved by primary angioplasty and stenting. However, this remains to be proven in larger scale randomised clinical trials.

Laser facilitated angioplasty

Devices designed to deliver laser energy to a catheter tip have been available for use by cardiovascular interventionists for well over a decade. Laser energy is generated by stimulation of a liquid, solid or gaseous medium. This results in excitation of atoms and subsequent release of photons with specific wavelengths ranging from approximately 300 nm to >10 000 nm. The characteristics of the electromagnetic energy generated by these devices depend on its wavelength, pulse repetition rate, and duration of the pulse (pulse width). Excimer lasers produce energy from a gaseous medium (xenon-chlorine) with a wavelength of 308 nm, have a relatively small penetration threshold (30–50 mm), and produce little thermal injury. Solid-state lasers in the mid-infrared range, such as the holmium:YAG laser, have a higher ablation threshold and penetration depth than excimer lasers.

Although the initial enthusiasm for laser-facilitated angioplasty was dampened by disappointing results from randomised clinical trials,[8] improvements in device technology have led to a resurgence in interest in laser energy and its application to several specific patient sub-groups. In particular, the development of a laser guidewire has been of value in the treatment of chronic total occlusions. The Spectranetics excimer laser wire is a steerable 0.018 inch wire that consists of 12 optical fibres with a shapeable tip. In one series, 56% of chronic total occlusions were crossed with this wire after failure of a conventional guidewire.[16] It should be noted, however, that the results of 'conventional' angioplasty for chronic total occlusions have improved considerably since the introduction of wires with hydrophilic coatings. Use of these latter wires may provide comparable success rates to those achieved with laser wires, at considerably lower cost.

Laser-facilitated angioplasty has also been used as treatment for in-stent restenosis. Simple balloon dilatation of the recurrent lesion is associated with a high incidence of a further recurrence, particularly when the lesion is diffuse and involves the full extent of the stented segment. It has been proposed that debulking the neointima inside the stent prior to angioplasty will reduce the likelihood of a further recurrence. Certainly, debulking the in-stent restenosis lesion by laser angioplasty does appear to result in a better initial result with a larger lumen than achieved by balloon dilatation alone.[17] Whether this translates into any significant improvement in long-term clinical outcome is unclear.[18]

There are two additional non-coronary interventional procedures for which laser energy may prove valuable. Extraction of permanent pacemaker leads appears to be greatly facilitated by the use of a purpose-designed laser sheath. This can be passed distally over the pacemaker lead to ablate fibrotic adhesions between the lead and the underlying myocardium, thereby allowing safe removal of the leads, and in many instances obviating the need for surgical extraction.

Transmyocardial laser revascularisation (TMR) and percutaneous endomyocardial revascularisation (PMR) have been advocated as treatments for refractory angina in patients with severe, non-operable coronary artery disease. Initially, CO_2 or holmium:YAG lasers were used to create channels from the epicardial surface, through the ischaemic myocardium to the left ventricular cavity as a means of providing an alternative vascular conduit.[19] More recently, catheters have been designed and tested clinically as a means of applying the same concept percutaneously from the endocardial surface.[20] Several series have reported substantial symptomatic improvements in patients treated in this manner, though few have consistently demonstrated objective evidence of resolution of the under-lying ischaemia. Histological studies have shown that the new channels invariably thrombose rapidly but that this is associated with a local inflammatory response and neovascularisation with formation of small capillary channels.[21,22] Whether this approach has any widespread application or advantage over more biologically appropriate approaches to angiogenesis (such as gene therapy) remains to be seen. At this point, laser-facilitated angioplasty remains an expensive option that may have a role in the treatment of small sub-groups of patients. Further improvement in device technology may, however, increase its applicability not only to endovascular therapies, but also to other cardiovascular inter-ventions.

Distal protection devices

Although sound in principle, debulking of atheromatous lesions with any of the above devices does have some hazard. Embolisation of atheromatous debris may occur during any of these procedures,[23] and probably also occurs frequently during apparently uncom-plicated balloon dilatation and stent procedures.[24,25] Distal embolisation is particularly likely to occur during percutaneous interventions in degenerated vein grafts, in which it commonly causes poor flow, myocardial infarction and profound haemodynamic com-promise. During carotid or vertebral interventions, even minor episodes of distal embolisation may cause profound neurological complications; following renal artery in-terventions, atheroembolism may result in deterioration of already compromised renal function.

Recognition of the clinical importance of distal atheroembolism after vascular inter-ventions has led to the design and development of a number of distal protection devices.[26] Broadly speaking, these devices may be classified as passive filters or systems designed to capture material by arterial occlusion, and to retrieve it by active aspiration. By far the greatest clinical experience has been reported with a proprietary balloon occlusion and retrieval system. The PercuSurge® system (Percusurge Inc., Sunnyvale, CA) (Fig. 22.4) consists of a 0.014 or 0.018 inch steerable wire on a nitinol hypotube.[27,28] Arterial occlu-

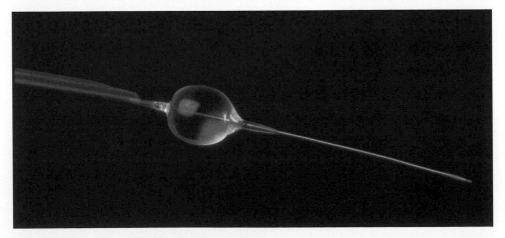

Figure 22.4. The PercuSurge™ distal protection device. Particulate matter, which is captured by a low inflation pressure balloon, can be retrieved by aspiration through a large lumen monorail catheter. Particles up to several millimeters in diameter can be retrieved in this manner.

sion is achieved by inflation of a low-pressure elastomeric balloon. Prior to deflation and removal, a catheter with a 1 mm aspiration port is advanced to a point immediately proximal to the balloon and 50–60 ml of blood containing the captured debris is aspirated. Several small series have been reported[27,28] and suggest that particulate matter typically falls in the 50–200 μ range, although particles in excess of 3 mm in diameter have been retrieved (M. Henry, unpublished data). Randomised studies are not yet available but data from unpublished series suggest that the incidence of distal embolism and poor flow is gratifyingly low when these devices are used. These devices have several potential limitations. These include the potential for the occlusion balloon to cause arterial injury or distal embolism, the risks of end-organ ischaemia during the period of balloon occlusion, and a reduction in precision of stent deployment because contrast angiography cannot be performed with the balloon inflated.

Several passive filters have been designed as alternatives to the balloon occlusion systems. They have the apparent advantages of allowing perfusion during distal protection, and perhaps, of limiting arterial trauma during the time the device is in position. Each system consists of a retractable membrane that has a series of 50, 100, or 200 μ diameter holes. Atheromatous debris has been retrieved from coronary, renal and carotid arteries and from saphenous vein grafts during a variety of interventions (J. Yadav, unpublished data). It has become clear that even routine, apparently uncomplicated coronary balloon angioplasty procedures can lead to embolisation of atheromatous debris. Whether this results in myocardial injury and an adverse long-term outcome remains controversial.[26] It does seem likely, however, that use of these devices will become routine in the percutaneous management of carotid, renal, and saphenous vein graft disease. Further clinical experience will be required before any one system can be recommended as the most effective and most reliable.

Intracoronary radiation

Recurrent narrowing or restenosis has been a major limitation of coronary angioplasty and related interventions. Multiple trials of drug therapies have failed to show any reduction in the incidence of restenosis after balloon angioplasty of uncomplicated lesions.[29] Coronary stenting clearly improves the long-term clinical outcome in these patients but, as the boundaries of eligibility for stenting have been stretched to include long lesions in diffusely diseased arteries, lesions in small calibre arteries, and chronic total occlusions, restenosis has re-emerged as an ongoing limitation of percutaneous coronary interventions. Brachytherapy, or endoluminal radiation therapy, has evolved to become the one approach currently available that appears to have a significant impact on the extent of post-angioplasty and in-stent restenosis. Similar approaches have been used in the past to control keloid scar formation, pterygia, and heterotopic bone formation.

Two primary types of ionising radiation have been used in clinical and experimental trials. Beta sources, such as ^{32}P, ^{90}Sr, ^{90}Y, and ^{188}Re, emit electrons with a broad distribution of energies, typically in the 0.2–2.5 MeV range. Gamma sources, including ^{192}Ir and ^{125}I, produce high-energy photons that have a much greater tissue penetration than the electrons released from beta sources. Both beta and gamma radiation occur naturally and are emitted during the transition of unstable radioisotopes to more stable, lower-energy states. Beta sources have the advantage that the electrons emitted interact strongly with adjacent tissues and therefore act locally, with little penetration to other tissues. Shielding requirements are limited and, since high-activity sources can be used, the time required to deliver the calculated radiation dose to the treated site (dwell time) is short. In contrast, gamma sources deliver photons that interact weakly with tissues, penetrate deeply beyond the treated tissues, and require far more shielding than is provided in conventional catheterisation laboratories to protect staff and other hospital personnel. The lower activity of the gamma emitters used clinically also necessitates long dwell times during which all personnel must leave the catheterisation laboratory.

Although clearly more user-friendly, beta radiation has some limitations. The lower depth of penetration of beta radiation results in the potential for variable circumferential dosing for eccentric lesions or non-centred catheter sources. Beta sources may not be suitable for very large non-coronary arteries or saphenous vein grafts and, since beta radiation is efficiently blocked by metal, may not provide optimal inhibition of neointimal hyperplasia after stent implantation. Some of these limitations may be overcome by selecting delivery modalities other than a central catheter or ribbon. Radioisotope-filled balloons are not limited by centering or distance issues and the use of stents coated with a radiation source may avert the shielding effects of the stent metal. However, unlike other delivery systems, use of isotope-filled balloons exposes the patient and operator to the risk of leakage or radioisotope spill in the event of balloon rupture or during preparation of the balloon. Similarly, as discussed below, early data from clinical trials have shown that radioisotope-coated stents have their own unique limitations.

Endovascular radiation was first shown to inhibit neointimal hyperplasia in the mid-1960s.[30] Several models of restenosis have now been used to examine the efficacy of both beta and gamma radiation. Although there is some variability in the results of published trials, most studies have shown a significant degree of inhibition of intimal hyperplasia at doses of 15–20 Gray (Gy). Importantly, some studies have shown that high dose radiation also causes inhibition of endothelial cell proliferation and an absence of endothelial covering at the treated sites.[31] This suggests the potential for late thrombotic occlusion at the site of angioplasty or stent implantation because of failure of the injured site to heal.

Much of the initial clinical evaluation of endovascular radiation was performed with ^{192}Ir (gamma) radiation sources. The first randomised clinical trial of intracoronary gamma radiation enrolled 55 patients with post-angioplasty or in-stent restenosis.[32] Actively treated patients received between 8 and 30 Gy of gamma radiation delivered from a catheter-based array of radioactive seeds. At follow-up, the angiographic restenosis rate was reduced from 54% in the control group to 17%. One-year event-free survival was 85% in the treated group compared with 52% in the untreated group.[32] Similar magnitudes of benefit have been observed in two other randomised gamma studies, the GAMMA-1[33] and WRIST[34] trials.

Data from several trials suggest that catheter-based beta radiation may be as effective as gamma radiation for prevention of restenosis[35] but no direct comparisons of beta and gamma radiation have yet been performed. The results from observational studies of radioisotope-impregnated stents have been disappointing.[36,37] Stents covered with beta-emitters such as ^{32}P have several obvious advantages, including low toxicity to the operator, a prolonged treatment period, and uniform circumferential delivery without attenuation of the dose by the stent metal. However, there is some evidence that very low dose radiation may promote intimal hyperplasia after arterial injury. This may explain the fact that while follow-up studies have shown relatively little intimal hyperplasia within the stented segment, stenoses of one or both ends of the treated segment, outside the stent, have occurred with far greater frequency than would normally be expected. This appearance has been referred to as the 'candy-wrapper' effect.[36] Whether this effect can be overcome by changes in stent design, or in the distribution of radiation activity along the length of the stent, remains to be determined.

As clinical experience with these devices increases, it is likely that the reported incidence of complications will rise. It has recently become apparent, for example, that thrombotic occlusion may occur 12 months or more after stent implantation, presumably because of incomplete stent endothelialisation. Failure of wound healing may also lead to aneurysm formation. Very long-term follow-up will be required to ensure that endovascular radiation does not cause late vascular fibrosis, myocardial dysfunction or pericardial thickening, each of which has been reported after external beam thoracic radiation for malignant disease. It is clear that use of endovascular radiation is still in its infancy and may be modified greatly over the next few years. Because of ongoing concerns about radiation exposure to patients and staff, it is likely that if an alternate pharmacological or biological solution is identified as a method of preventing restenosis, radiation therapy will almost certainly become obsolete. In the meantime, however, endovascular radiation appears to be the only approach with a high probability of limiting recurrent stenosis in the relatively few patients who would otherwise require coronary bypass grafting because of failure of a percutaneous intervention to maintain long-term coronary patency.

Intravascular ultrasound

The profound technological improvement in catheter, stent and adjunctive device design witnessed over the past two decades has, fortunately, been matched by unparalleled improvements in radiological imaging and on-line computing (Fig. 22.5). Intravascular ultrasound (IVUS) imaging provides an even greater depth of understanding of the extent and morphological characteristics of atherosclerotic lesions. The insights derived from IVUS clearly indicate that coronary cineangiography can no longer be considered the gold standard diagnostic tool for coronary atherosclerotic disease, no matter how good the image quality may be.

The first intravascular ultrasound images were recorded in 1988, using a very bulky (7 F) system.[38] The subsequent decade saw a reduction in catheter size to 2.9 F (<1.0 mm) and an increase in ultrasound frequency to 40MHz. There are currently two distinct methods of generating ultrasound images. Solid-state, or electronic phased-array, systems consist of a series of imaging elements arranged circumferentially at the catheter tip. Each ele-

a   b

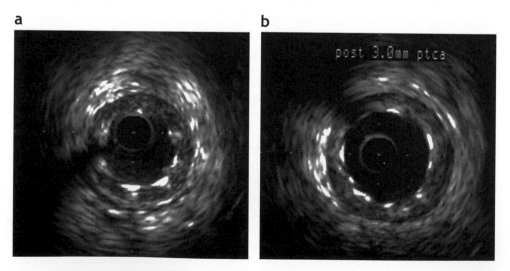

Figure 22.5. *Intravascular ultrasound image showing a metallic stent in situ. The stent in a) is shown to be suboptimally expanded. The stent in b) has been symmetrically expanded and the struts are well apposed to the artery wall.*

ment sends and receives ultrasound images that are then integrated to form a two-dimensional image of the arterial wall perpendicular to the long axis of the catheter. There are no moving parts and preparation of the device is relatively simple. Current systems (Endosonics, Rancho Cordova, CA) incorporate 64 elements and recent improvements have allowed incorporation of Doppler colour flow imaging to provide not only morphological information, but also some physiological data. Until recently, the images obtained from solid-state imaging catheters did not have the quality of those obtained from competing mechanical transducers. However, it has been predicted that the potential for further increases in image quality, and incorporation of additional features such as on-line focusing of the beam to improve far-field resolution, is greater with solid state catheters than with mechanical systems.

The mechanical systems generate ultrasound images from a single rotating transducer element that rotates at 1600–1800 rpm within a guiding sheath. Because image quality is profoundly affected by the presence of even small air bubbles, preparation of the catheter includes meticulous flushing of the sheath; inadequate flushing may mean the catheter provides no useful images. The catheters are available in several configurations. The MicroRail catheter (Boston Scientific, San Jose, CA) is a 3.2 F simple monorail design. The rail segment measures 1.5 cm and the transducer lies approximately 1cm behind the rail opening. The guidewire therefore runs alongside the transducer element and causes an artifactual shadowing that may interfere with image interpretation or quantification. It has the advantage of being a true rapid exchange system that limits the potential for ischaemia during image acquisition. However, the very short rail segment does reduce its tracking in tortuous arteries, and predisposes the system to guidewire buckling and entrapment. An alternative system is the MicroView catheter that has a 2.9 F distal sheath diameter. It has a 30 cm rail segment but the 0.014 inch guidewire must be pulled back approximately 20 cm before the transducer can be advanced into the coronary artery. This has the advantage of having no guidewire artifact in the image, and better tracking, but the absence of the wire may provide poor support and the potential for buckling of the sheath, particularly when aorto-ostial lesions are being investigated. Because removal of the system is a multi-step process (retraction of the transducer, reinsertion of the guidewire, then removal of the guiding sheath), this catheter should be avoided if catheter-related ischaemia is likely to cause significant haemodynamic compromise.

The principal advantage of IVUS over cineangiography is its ability to define the elements of the arterial wall. Contrast angiography provides considerable information about the dimensions of the arterial lumen, including the presence or absence of lesions that encroach on the lumen, the location of sidebranches and, to some extent, the presence of mural calcium or intraluminal thrombus. However, at its best cineangiography provides a very limited image of the extent and morphological characteristics of atherosclerotic lesions. In part this is because the process of atherosclerosis is complex and involves an adaptive process (first described by Glagov and colleagues in 1987).[39] Glagov's histological studies demonstrated that as an atheromatous deposit enlarges, the external elastic lamina that delineates the outer dimension of the artery commonly expands to accommodate the disease (positive remodeling). This observation has been confirmed in *in vivo* intravascular ultrasound studies.[40] Thus, in the early and intermediate stages of atherosclerosis, there may be a considerable build-up of atheroma without encroachment on the lumen. It is only in the later stages of the disease process that luminal narrowing occurs, and it may only be at this point that it becomes apparent angiographically. Occasionally, in more advanced disease and after balloon angioplasty, adventitial scarring may result in contracture of the external elastic lamina, or negative remodeling.[41] These observations have particular relevance for determining the extent and severity of disease and for measuring reference diameters in diffusely diseased arteries.[42] Because ultrasound provides a 360° image of any point along the length of the artery, evaluation of disease severity is not limited by the presence of overlapping side branches, or by incomplete visualisation of highly eccentric stenoses.

Intravascular ultrasound also provides far more information about lesion morphology than conventional cineangiography. Low-density lesions are lipid rich and behave differently from denser lesions in response to balloon dilatation;[43] they may also be the lesions at greatest risk of rupture and progression to acute thrombotic closure. In these arteries, lumen expansion occurs predominantly by axial redistribution of the atheroma, with relatively little expansion of the external elastic elamina.[43] In contrast, high-density lesions are fibrotic or fibrocalcific and do not respond well to balloon dilatation alone. Enlargement of the lumen results almost entirely from expansion of the external dimensions of the artery with or without associated dissection, and elastic recoil is more likely to occur than after angioplasty of low density lesions.[43] Similarly, heavily calcified stenoses respond very poorly to balloon dilatation and stenting, particularly when the calcium is superficial and circumferential. In these cases, rotational atherectomy is required to remove or fracture the calcium prior to balloon dilatation.[44]

In addition to providing two-dimensional images, IVUS offers the potential for volumetric lesion analysis. This requires pullback of the imaging catheter at a regulated speed (0.5 or 1.0 mm/sec), using a customised pullback device. Automated computer algorithms are then used to stack each adjacent individual cross sectional image to give a three-dimensional representation of the arterial lumen and the arterial wall.[45] The volume of the artery wall and associated atheroma or neointima can be determined by subtracting the lumen volume from the total arterial volume. This is particularly useful for serial studies of disease progression or regression, for evaluating the mechanisms of lumen enlargement after coronary interventions,[17,44] and for evaluating the severity of intimal hyperplasia and negative remodelling in restenosis trials.[32] Longitudinal display of an arterial segment is also an excellent way of clarifying the relationships between atheromatous lesions, sidebranches, dissections and implanted stents.

Intravascular ultrasound is now a well established adjunct to cineangiography and plays an invaluable role in evaluating coronary arteries when questions remain after routine angiography. Whether IVUS should be performed routinely before or after percutaneous coronary interventions is still controversial. Several studies have suggested that superior acute angiographic and long-term clinical results can be achieved using IVUS-guided angioplasty[46] or stent implantation.[47] (Fig. 22.5) In the CRUISE trial,[47] for example, patients randomised to IVUS-guided stent implantation had a significantly lower target lesion revascularisation rate than patients in whom stents were implanted without IVUS guidance (8.5% vs 15.3%, p<0.05). However, the imaging catheters are expensive. In many parts of the world, the cost of the imaging catheter is greater than the cost of a stent. Thus, cost effectiveness models performed in the United States showing cost savings if stent implantation can be avoided may not apply elsewhere. Nevertheless, intravascular ultrasound may become critically important if ultrasound-derived predictors of the risk of distal embolisation, non-Q wave myocardial infarction and late sudden cardiac death are described. If that occurs, monographs describing the roles and relative merits of catheters for debulking, imaging, protecting or irradiating atherosclerotic coronary arteries may need to be reviewed.

Measurement of functional flow

The PressureWire™ sensor system (Radi Medical Systems AB, Uppsala, Sweden) is gaining increasing attention as an adjunct to PTCA, particularly for lesions of doubtful severity. The PressureWire measures intracoronary pressure proximal and distal to a lesion to calculate the coronary fractional flow reserve (FFR), as a measure of obstruction to flow across a lesion. The PressureWire sensor can be used as an alternative to IVUS to determine whether a lesion is severe enough to merit intervention, and to assess whether additional revascularisation of a residual lesion is required.

FFR is expressed as the ratio of mean pressure distal to the lesion over mean aortic pressure, according to the formula:

$$FFR = \frac{\text{mean distal pressure}}{\text{mean aortic pressure}}$$

If distal pressure is not much less than aortic pressure, this indicates that there is good coronary flow; the FFR will be high (e.g. 0.85) and the lesion is not clinically significant. If distal pressure is markedly lower than aortic pressure, there is restriction to flow and the FFR will be low (e.g. 0.65), indicating the lesion is clinically significant. There is evidence that the FFR can also be used to predict the clinical event rate following successful balloon angioplasty. A high residual FFR (FFR>0.90) predicts a favourable clinical outcome, particularly in combination with a good angiographic result.[48]

Another device, the Doppler FloWire™ (EndoSonics Inc, Rancho Cordova, CA, USA), measures the flow velocity in the coronary circulation at rest and during hyperaemia. It therefore provides a measure of restriction to flow caused not only by the lesion, but also from defects in the microvasculature of the myocardium. The FloWire™ monitor displays real-time blood flow velocity and measures the coronary flow researve (CFR).[49,50] CFR is defined as the ratio of average peak flow velocity during hyperaemia over the average baseline peak flow velocity:

$$CFR = \frac{\text{average peak blood flow velocity}}{\text{average baseline peak flow velocity}}$$

Hyperaemia is induced by injection of vasodilators such as adenosine after measuring baseline flow. A ratio <3.0 is consistent with an abnormal CFR due to epicardial coronary disease or defects in the microcirculation.

Percutaneous coronary bypass

Yet another novel approach to percutaneous reperfusion therapy involves creating an anastomosis between a coronary artery (the left anterior descending) and its neighbouring vein to create an arterio-venous fistula connecting the two vessels. This technique is designed for treatment of long chronic total occlusions and requires intravascular ultrasound guidance. After passing a wire from the proximal arterial segment through its wall to the adjacent vein, a stent is deployed, allowing the vein segment to act as a natural conduit for blood flow past the site of the occlusion. The two vessels are connected distally via a second stent deployed using a retrograde approach from the coronary sinus. This technique thus becomes a form of percutaneous bypass without surgery, and has proved successful in animal studies. It has only recently been attempted in humans, but its continued application will depend on its long-term success rate.

References

1. Topol EJ, Leya F, Pinkerton C *et al.* A comparison of directional atherectomy with coronary angioplasty in patients with coronary artery disease. *N Engl J Med* 1993; **329**:221–227.
2. Baim DS, Cutlip DE, Sharma SK *et al.* Final results of the Balloon vs Optimal Atherectomy Trial (BOAT). *Circulation* 1998; **97**:322–331.
3. Adelman A, Cohen E, Kimball B *et al.* A comparison of directional atherectomy with balloon angioplasty for lesions of the left anterior descending coronary artery. *N Engl J Med* 1993; **329**:228–233.
4. Tsuchikane E, Sumitsuji S, Awata N *et al.* Final results of the Stent versus directional coronary Atherectomy Randomized Trial. *J Am Coll Cardiol* 1999; **34**:1050–7.
5. Elliott JM, Berdan LG, Holmes DR *et al.* One year follow-up in the Coronary Angioplasty Versus Excisional Atherectomy Trial (CAVEAT-I). *Circulation* 1995; **91**:2158–2166.
6. Bramucci E, Angolini L, Merlini PA *et al.* Adjunctive stent implantation following directional coronary atherectomy in patients with coronary artery disease. *J Am Coll Cardiol* 1998; **32**:1855–60.
7. Gruberg L, Mehran R, Dangas G *et al.* Effect of plaque debulking and stenting on short- and long-term outcomes after revascularization of chronic total occlusions. *J Am Coll Cardiol* 2000; **35**:151–6
8. Reifart N, Vandormael M, Krajcar M *et al.* Randomized comparison of angioplasty of complex coronary lesions at a single center. Excimer laser, Rotational atherectomy, Balloon Angioplasty Comparison. *Circulation* 1997; **96**:91–98.
9. Schiele F, Meneveau N, Vuillemenot A, Bassand J. Rotational atherectomy followed by balloon angioplasty for treatment of intrastent restenosis: a pilot study with quantitative angiography and ultrasound. *Eur Heart J* 1997; **18**:499.
10. Kobayashi Y, De Gregorio J, Kobayashi N *et al.* Lower restenosis rate with stenting following aggressive versus less aggressive rotational atherectomy. *Cathet Cardiovasc Interv* 1999; **64**:406–14.
11. Safian RS, Grines CL, May MA *et al.* Clinical and angiographic results of transluminal extraction coronary atherectomy in saphenous vein bypass grafts. *Circulation* 1994; **89**:302–312.
12. Rosenschein U, Bernstein JJ, Segni E *et al.* Experimental ultrasonic angioplasty: disruption of atherosclerotic plaques and thrombi in vitro and arterial recanalization in vivo. *J Am Coll Cardiol* 1990; **15**:711–717.
13. Fischell TA, Abbas MA, Grant GW, Siegel RJ. Ultrasonic energy: effects on vascular function and integrity. *Circulation* 1991; **84**:1783–1795.
14. Muller DWM, Moncur J, Rosenschein U, Nicklas J. Ultrasound thrombolysis: ablated thrombus does not impede microcirculatory flow or impair regional left ventricular wall motion. *Aust NZ J Med* 1998; **28**:128.
15. Rosenschein U, Roth A, Rassin T *et al.* Analysis of coronary ultrasound thrombolysis endpoints in acute myocardial infarction (ACUTE trial). Results of the feasibility phase. *Circulation* 1997; **95**:1411–6.
16. Hamburger JN, Gijsbers GHM, Ozaki Y *et al.* Recanalization of chronic total occlusions using a laser guidewire: a pilot study. *J Am Coll Cardiol* 1997; **30**:649–656.
17. Mehran R, Mintz GS, Satler LF, *et al.* Treatment of in-stent restenosis with excimer laser coronary angioplasty: mechanisms and results compared to PTCA alone. *Circulation* 1997; **96**:2183–2189.
18. Mehran R, Dangas G, Mintz GS *et al.* In-stent restenosis: 'The Great Equalizer' – disappointing clinical outcomes with all interventional strategies. *J Am Coll Cardiol* 1999; **33**:63A
19. Allen KB, Dowling RD, Fudge TL *et al.* Comparison of transmyocardial revascularization with medical therapy in patients with refractory angina. *N Engl J Med* 1999; **341**:1029–36.
20. Lauer B, Junghans U, Stahl F *et al.* Catheter-based percutaneous myocardial laser revascularisation in patients with end-stage coronary artery disease. *J Am Coll Cardiol* 1999; **34**:1663–70.
21. Gassler N, Wintzer Ho, Stubbe HM. Transmyocardial laser revascularization: histologic features in human nonresponder myocardium. *Circulation* 1997; **95**:371–375.

22. Chu V, Kuang JQ, McGinn A *et al*. Angiogenic response induced by mechanical transmyocardial revascularization. *J Thorac Cardiovasc Surg* 1999; **118**:849–56.

23. Abbo KM, Dooris M, Glazier S *et al*. Features and outcome of no-reflow after percutaneous coronary intervention. *Am J Cardiol* 1995; **75**:778–782.

24. Ravkilde J, Nissen H, Mickley H *et al*. Cardiac troponin T and CK-MB mass release after visually successful percutaneous transluminal coronary angioplasty in stable angina pectoris. *Am Heart J* 1994; **127**:13–20.

25. Tardiff BE, Califf RM, Tcheng JE *et al*. Clinical outcomes after detection of elevated cardiac enzymes in patients undergoing percutaneous intervention. IMPACT-II Investigators. Integrilin (eptifibatide) to Minimize Platelet Aggregation and Coronary Thrombosis-II. *J Am Coll Cardiol* 1999; **33**:88–96.

26. Topol EJ, Yadav JS. Recognition of the importance of embolization in atherosclerotic vascular disease. *Circulation* 2000; **101**:570–580.

27. Webb JG, Carere RG, Virmani R *et al*. Retrieval and analysis of particulate debris after saphenous vein graft intervention. *J Am Coll Cardiol* 1999; **34**:468–75.

28. Carlino M, De Gregorio J, Di Mario C *et al*. Prevention of distal embolization during saphenous vein graft lesion angioplasty: experience with a new temporary occlusion and aspiration system. *Circulation* 1999; **99**:3221–3223.

29. Popma JJ, Califf RM, Topol EJ. Clinical trials of restenosis after coronary angioplasty. *Circulation* 1991; **84**:1426–36.

30. Friedman M, Felton L, Byers S. The antiatherogenic effects of Ir-192 upon the cholesterol-fed rabbit. *J Clin Invest* 1964; **43**:185–192.

31. Carter AJ, Laird JR, Nailey LR *et al*. Effects of endovascular radiation from a beta-emitting stent in a porcine coronary restenosis model. A dose-response study. *Circulation* 1996; **94**:2364–8.

32. Teirstein PS, Massullo V, Jani S *et al*. Catheter-based radiotherapy to inhibit restenosis after coronary stenting. *N Engl J Med* 1997; 336:1697–703.

33. Leon MB. GAMMA-I trial. Presented at the American Heart Association Annual Scientific Sessions, Atlanta, November 1999.

34. Leon MB. WRIST trial. Presented at the American Heart Association Annual Scientific Sessions, Atlanta, November 1999.

35. King SB 3rd, Williams DO, Chougule P *et al*. Endovascular beta-radiation to reduce restenosis after coronary balloon angioplasty: results of the beta energy restenosis trial (BERT). *Circulation* 1998; **97**:2025–30.

36. Albiero R, Adamian M, Kobayashi N *et al*. Short- and intermediate-term results of (32)P radioactive beta-emitting stent implantation in patients with coronary artery disease: the Milan Dose-response study. *Circulation* 2000; **101**:18–26.

37. Wardeh AJ, Kay IP, Sabate M, *et al*. Beta-particle-emitting radioactive stent implantation. A safety and feasibility study. *Circulation* 1999; 100:1684–9.

38. Yock PG, Johnson EL, Linker DT. Intravascular ultrasound: Development and clinical potential. Am J Card Imaging 1988; **2**:185–193.

39. Glagov S, Weisenberg E, Zarins CK *et al*. Compensatory enlargement of human atherosclerotic coronary arteries. *N Engl J Med* 1987; **316**:1371–1375.

40. Tanaglia AN, Kisslo KB, *et al*. In vivo validation of compensatory enlargement of atherosclerotic coronary arteries. *Am J Cardiol* 1993; 71:6655–668.

41. Mintz GS, Kent KM, Pichard AD, *et al*. Contribution of inadequate remodeling to the development of focal coronary artery stenoses: An Intravascular ultrasound study. *Circulation* 1997; **95**:1791–1798.

42. Mintz GS, Painter JA, Pichard AD, *et al*. Atherosclerosis in angiographically 'normal' coronary artery reference segments: An intravascular ultrasound study with clinical correlations. *J Am Coll Cardiol* 1995; **25**:1479–1485.

43. Cao N, Werns SW, Moscucci M, Bates ER, Muller DWM. Relationship between quantitatively determined lesion density and mechanism of coronary balloon dilatation. *Circulation* 1995; **92**:I–401.

44.   Kovach JA, Mintz GS, Pichard AD *et al*. Sequential intravascular ultrasound characterization of the mechanisms of rotational atherectomy and adjunct balloon angioplasty. *J Am Coll Cardiol* 1993; **22**:1024–1032.

45.   Roelandt JR, Di Mario C, Pandian NG *et al*. Three-dimensional reconstruction of intracoronary ultrasound images: Rationale, approaches, problems, and directions. *Circulation* 1994; **90**:1044–1055.

46.   Stone GW, Hodgson JM, St Goar FG *et al*. Improved procedural results of coronary angioplasty with intravascular ultrasound-guided balloon sizing: The CLOUT pilot trial. *Circulation* 1997; **95**:2044–2052.

47.   Fitzgerald P. CRUISE trial. Presented at the American Heart Association Annual Scientific Sessions, Atlanta, November 1999.

48.   Bech GJ, Pijls NH, De Bruyne *et al*. Usefulness of refractory flow researve to predict outcome after balloon angioplasty. *Circulation* 1999; **99**(7):883–888.

49.   Cohen DJ. In-hospital and 6-month follow-up costs of universal vs provisonal stenting: Results from the DESTINI trial. *Circulation Scientific Sessions Abstracts* 1998; **98**(17):I–499.

50.   Schwarzacher SP, Uren NG, Ward MR, *et al*. Determinants of coronary remodelling in transplant coronary disease: A simultaneous intravascular ultrasound and Doppler flow study. *Circulation* 2000; **101**(12):1384–1389.

Chapter 23

Percutaneous Non-coronary Interventions

David W.M. Muller

The remarkable progress made in the design and development of devices for percutaneous coronary interventions has been paralleled by bioengineering triumphs that allow the treatment of a range of congenital heart disorders. These procedures include closure of atrial and ventricular septal defects, patent ductus arteriosus and foramen ovale, and aorto-coronary fistulae. Balloon dilatation of valvular stenoses and stenting of aortic coarctation are now routinely performed. Improvements in guidewire and stent technology have also greatly facilitated the treatment of peripheral vascular disease and have improved the results of percutaneous management of carotid artery disease. This chapter deals with some of the newer non-coronary procedures that are now commonly performed in adult cardiac catheterisation laboratories.

Closure of septal defects

The percutaneous management of congenital atrial and ventricular septal defects has been the subject of investigative effort for more than a decade. Some of the early prototypes were difficult to position and deploy, could not be retrieved once deployed, and had design defects that, in several instances, led to their recall. Of the devices currently available, the Amplatzer™ septal occlusion device (AGA Medical Corporation, Golden Valley, MN, USA) appears to be the most robust, most readily placed and retrieved, and is the device of choice at many major institutions.

Atrial septal defect (ASD)

Atrial septal defects may occur in the region of the foramen ovale (ostium secundum defects), at the junction of the superior vena cava and right atrium (sinus venosus defects), or as part of an endocardial cushion defect (ostium primum defect). The ostium secundum atrial septal defect is the most common congenital defect encountered in adults. It accounts for approximately 7% of all congenital heart disease and for 30–40% of all patients presenting with a congenital defect in adult life. Atrial septal defects occur more frequently in women than in men, with a female to male ratio of 1.5–2.0:1.[1] Sinus venosus defects are commonly associated with anomalous drainage of the right upper and lower pulmonary veins into the right atrium. Ostium primum defects may be associated with other developmental defects of the endocardial cushion (the fibrous structure that forms the tricuspid and mitral valve annulus), such as a cleft mitral valve and a membranous ventricular septal defect. Ostium primum and sinus venosus defects are not suitable for percutaneous closure since the accompanying abnormalities usually require surgical correction.

Isolated atrial septal defects are commonly asymptomatic during the first three decades of life. Most often, they are diagnosed following a routine physical examination, a routine chest x-ray, or an echocardiogram for atypical symptoms. Approximately 70% of patients with an atrial septal defect are symptomatic by the fifth decade, and the morbidity and mortality of the condition rise quickly during the sixth decade of life. Almost 50% have at least mild pulmonary hypertension by the age of 40 years. Those few patients who develop severe pulmonary hypertension, with or without shunt reversal (Eisenmenger's syndrome), usually do so within several years of birth. When symptoms do occur, they usually consist of exertional fatigue, breathlessness, and palpitations. Ultimately, longstanding right ventricular volume overload and pulmonary hypertension may result in right heart failure, atrial arrhythmias, and stroke due to atrial thrombus formation or, less commonly, to paradoxical embolism.

The functional significance of an atrial septal defect is determined in the cardiac catheterisation laboratory by oximetry studies (see Chapter 17) and calculation of the pulmonary to systemic flow ratio (Qp/Qs). The conventional criterion for closure of an ASD is a Qp/Qs ratio of 1.5:1. However, closure is now often recommended if there is echocardiographic evidence of right ventricular volume overload, regardless of the calculated shunt ratio. Surgical closure requires cardiopulmonary bypass, a right atriotomy, and primary closure or closure using a pericardial or synthetic patch. Although the mortality risk for otherwise healthy young patients is very low, the risk is higher in older patients with co-morbidities; the morbidity, cost, and inconvenience are considerable for patients of any age.

Several devices have been designed for percutaneous treatment of septal defects.[2–7] The Amplatzer septal occlusion device is a self-expanding, self-centering double disc made from 0.004 to 0.005 inch Nitinol™ (Fig. 23.1).[5,7] The left atrial disc is 7 mm larger in diameter than the waist diameter, and the right atrial disc is 5 mm larger than the waist. Each disc has a central, thin polyester membrane that contributes to the early closure of the defect and promotes endothelialisation. Devices are available in 1mm increments, with central waist sizes ranging from 4 mm to 38 mm. The device size is selected according to the size of the defect, with a central waist size 1–2mm larger than the measured size of the

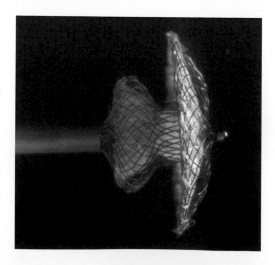

Figure 23.1. The Amplatzer atrial septal occlusion device shown with delivery sheath immediately prior to deployment.

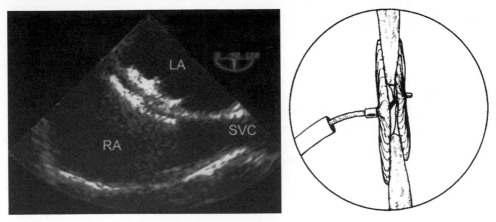

Figure 23.2. Transoesophageal echocardiogram showing the Amplatzer septal occlusion device in situ, and its diagramatic appearance when deployed. (Courtesy of AGA Medical corporation, Golden Valley, MN, USA.)

defect. Devices up to 20 mm can be deployed through an 8 F sheath; those between 20 and 26 mm require a 9 F sheath, those between 26 and 30 mm can be deployed through a 10 F sheath, and larger sizes require a 12 F delivery sheath.

Placement of atrial septal occlusion devices is most reliably performed using transoesophageal echocardiographic guidance. Direct measurement of the defect by echocardiography underestimates the true size, but more accurate estimates can be made using a customised sizing balloon. Once the device has been deployed, correct positioning is confirmed by fluoroscopy and echocardiographic criteria before the delivery cable is unscrewed, leaving the device *in situ* (Fig. 23.2). Post-operative care is as for coronary stenting and most patients can be discharged from hospital on the first post-operative day. Animal studies have shown that endothelialisation of the metal struts is usually complete within 3–4 months.[7] Daily antiplatelet therapy and antibiotic prophylaxis for invasive procedures should be given for 6 months to minimize the risks of thrombus formation and infective endocarditis.

Worldwide experience with the Amplatzer device now includes more than 4000 patients. Complications have been infrequent. Atrial septal defect closure has been attempted in 41 patients to date at St Vincents Hospital, Sydney. The mean shunt ratio was 2.2:1 and device sizes ranged from 14 to 38 mm, with a median size of 25 mm. All but two were successfully deployed, with an average fluoroscopy time of 14.7 minutes. The only complications encountered were transient atrial fibrillation in two patients, and cardiac tamponade requiring pericardial drainage in one patient. Small residual left-to-right shunts were documented in five patients. Follow-up echocardiography in these patients showed a progressive decrease in size of the shunt over 6–12 months. Perhaps the most likely late complication expected is atrial arrhythmias. New palpitations have been reported by two patients in our series, one of whom has had documented non-sustained atrial fibrillation. Late atrial fibrillation or flutter has been reported in 50–60% of patients after surgical closure of ASDs.[8] A similar number may also develop late rhythm disturbances after percutaneous closure with the Amplatzer device.

Patent foramen ovale

A similar device to the Amplatzer ASD occluder has been designed for closure of patent foramen ovale (PFO) in patients with a history consistent with paradoxical embolism.

After birth, the left-sided septum primum and the right-sided septum secundum, which overlap to form the atrial septum, usually fuse and prevent flow between the left and right atria. However, in 20% or more of the adult population the foramen remains patent.[9] This is usually of no haemodynamic consequence. However, under certain circumstances, right-to-left shunting may occur. For example, during the inspiration that follows straining or the Valsalva manouevre, a fall in intrathoracic pressure causes a rapid increase in venous blood return, a rise in right atrial pressure relative to left atrial pressure, and right atrial distension. If transient right-to-left shunting occurs, small thrombi may cross from the venous to the arterial circulation, causing transient cerebral ischaemia or cerebral infarction, or infarction of other organ systems.

Paradoxical embolism through a patent foramen ovale is almost always a diagnosis of exclusion. It is unusual to be able to make a definitive diagnosis, although thrombi straddling the atrial septum have occasionally been seen on transoesophageal echocardiographic and post-mortem studies.[11,12] Approximately 40% of strokes in the adult population are cryptogenic i.e. no intracranial, carotid or cardiovascular cause can be found. In this group of patients, the incidence of patent foramen ovale is considerably higher (>50%) than in the general population, particularly in patients younger than 40 years.[13] Most of these individuals do not have a history of deep venous thrombosis or pulmonary embolism, and few have a history or laboratory evidence of an underlying thrombotic disorder. Recurrent stroke may occur in spite of anticoagulation therapy, particularly if the PFO is associated with an atrial septal aneurysm.[14] Because of this risk of recurrence, and the risks associated with lifelong anticoagulant therapy, percutaneous closure of patent foramen ovale should be considered for patients who have had an unequivocal neurological event and in whom no other cardiac or vascular cause can be found.[6,15]

The Amplatzer PFO device is similar in design to the ASD occlusion device, with several modifications.[6,15] The PFO device has a larger right atrial disc (26 mm) than left atrial disc (18 mm) and has a long, narrow waist (Fig. 23.2). The only technical difficulty in using this or any of the other devices designed for PFOs is in ensuring that the catheter used to cross the septum passes through the foramen rather than through the membrane adjacent to the foramen. In the latter case, the device may be deployed too high and fail to close the defect. As in ASD closures, transoesophageal echocardiography is valuable for ensuring correct positioning of the device and complete closure of the foramen, but the procedure can be performed under fluoroscopic guidance. Once the septum has been crossed appropriately, deployment of the device is straightforward with sequential release of the left and right atrial discs on either side of the atrial septum.

Ventricular septal defect (VSD)

Defects of the ventricular septum are among the most common congenital cardiac anomalies seen clinically. Subpulmonary or 'supracristal' defects lie above a muscular ridge in the right ventricular outflow tract called the crista supraventricularis. Defects below the crista may be in the region of the membranous septum ('membranous' VSDs) or in the muscular portion of the septum ('muscular' VSDs). Membranous VSDs are the most common form; muscular VSDs are commonly multiple. Like atrial septal defects, VSDs are generally well tolerated though severe pulmonary hypertension and shunt reversal (Eisenmenger's syndrome) may occur. Many patients with congenital VSDs do not require treatment, since spontaneous closure often occurs during the first decade of life. However, defects that are still present at 8–10 years of age are unlikely to close spontaneously and should be closed if a functionally significant left-to-right shunt is detected. Conventional treatment is surgical closure, which is generally well tolerated. However, surgical closure is associated with significant morbidity and mortality, especially if multiple muscular defects are present.[16]

The Amplatzer muscular ventricular septal closure device is similar in concept to the ASD device but has a thicker waist and symmetrical right and left ventricular discs. Devices designed specifically for membranous VSDs are not yet generally available but are being evolved in early clinical trials. Balloon sizing is usually not required for VSD closure, as transoesophageal echocardiography is more reliable in this situation than for sizing ASDs. Muscular defects may be closed using either a venous or an arterial approach. They are most readily crossed from the left ventricular side. In children, in whom use of large calibre sheaths in the femoral artery may lead to significant vascular injury, it is safest to pass a wire from the arterial side and to retrieve it through the femoral or internal jugular vein using a snare. The device can then be deployed from the right ventricular side without risk of arterial injury.[17] In adults, delivery from the arterial (left ventricular) side can be performed if long delivery sheaths are available. This may also be necessary in children if the delivery sheath kinks when used from the right ventricular side. Closure of VSDs is technically more challenging than closure of atrial defects, with longer fluoroscopy and procedure times. However, preliminary results seem to be favourable, with a low incidence of complications and a high closure rate.[17] Like many complex procedures, results are likely to be best in experienced hands.

Patent ductus arteriosus

The same technology that has been used for atrial and ventricular septal defects has been used for closure of patent ductus arteriosus defects. The ductus arteriosus connects the pulmonary artery to the descending aorta at the level of the origin of the subclavian artery. During foetal life, venous blood is shunted from the pulmonary artery through the ductus to the arterial circulation, bypassing the developing pulmonary circulation. After birth, the ductus usually closes to form the ligamentum arteriosum. In children in whom the ductus remains patent, a left to right shunt develops after birth with oxygenated blood passing from the aorta to the pulmonary artery. Severe pulmonary hypertension may occur and cause shunt reversal and Eisenmenger's syndrome.

Closure of the ductus may be accomplished surgically or by using thrombogenic coils. A specifically designed Amplatzer device can also be used for large defects.[18] The champagne cork-shaped device can usually be deployed from the pulmonary arterial side. Occasionally, it may be necessary to cross the defect with an exchange wire from the aortic side and to then snare it from the femoral or internal jugular vein. Once the delivery sheath has been passed across the defect from the pulmonary artery to the aorta, the disc of the device is deployed in the aorta, then the whole system is pulled back until it is wedged in the ductus. Occlusion of the ductus is confirmed by aortography before the cable is detached. Clinical experience with the device is limited, but preliminary data suggest this is a very viable and convenient alternative to surgical closure.

Peripheral vascular interventions

As coronary stent technology has advanced in recent years, application of the principles of coronary angioplasty and stenting to the management of peripheral vascular disease has become widespread. In particular, endovascular stenting of carotid, renal and iliofemoral disease has become accepted as an alternative to surgical therapy. Increasingly, since widespread vascular disease is commonly present in patients with coronary artery disease, risk factor management in patients with peripheral vascular disease, and selection

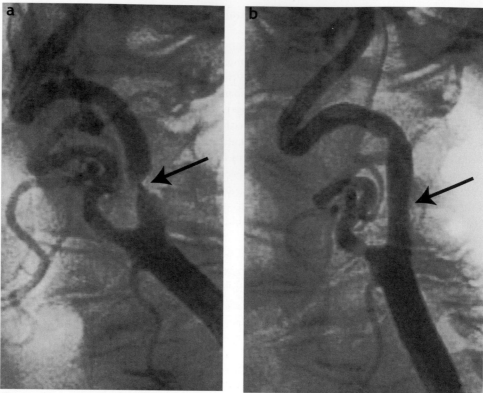

Figure 23.3. Carotid angiography pre (a) and post-stenting (b) after deployment of a 10x30mm Wallstent across the origin of the external carotid artery.

of appropriate revascularisation strategies, are becoming the domain of interventional cardiologists.

Carotid angioplasty and stenting

Atherosclerotic carotid artery disease involving the origins of the internal carotid artery and the distal common carotid artery is a frequent clinical problem associated with a significant risk of debilitating stroke. Several recent studies have indicated that in symptomatic, medically treated patients with haemodynamically significant carotid stenoses, the risk of ensuing stroke is substantial.[19-21] In one study, in patients treated with antiplatelet therapy alone, the 2-year cumulative stroke rate was 26%.[21] The same trial showed a reduction in morbidity and mortality for patients treated by surgical endarterectomy in whom the 2-year cumulative risk of ipsilateral stroke was only 9%.[21] Surgical complications of endarterectomy are relatively infrequent, with a combined risk of death or stroke in symptomatic patients of 5.6% reported in one recent review of the published literature.[22] The role of carotid endarterectomy for asymptomatic patients remains somewhat debatable, with one study showing a modest reduction in adverse outcomes in surgically treated patients with lesions greater than 60%.[23]

Carotid artery stenting has been proposed as an alternative to carotid endarterectomy in selected patients (Fig. 23.3). Although surgical therapy is associated with low morbidity and mortality in the majority of patients, certain groups are known to be at increased risk of adverse outcomes. These include patients with distal disease, high carotid bifurcations, aorto-ostial disease, post-radiation scarring, and restenosis following previous endarterectomy. Although many procedures are now performed surgically under local anaesthetic, even this is considered an increased hazard to patients with concomitant severe coronary artery disease and poor cardiovascular reserve. In these patients, carotid stenting offers an attractive alternative to surgery.

Patients with symptomatic stenoses ≥60% diameter stenosis and those with high-grade asymptomatic stenoses are potential candidates for stenting. The following classification of indications has been proposed. It must be recognised, however, that these indications are evolving and may change as further data become available.[24]

Class A lesions are those for which surgery is difficult and high-risk. There is little controversy about the role of stenting in these patients. Class A lesions include: (i) distal lesions (both atherosclerotic and those secondary to fibromuscular dysplasia); (ii) those distal to high bifurcations that require manipulation of the mandible for adequate surgical exposure; (iii) lesions arising after previous cervical radiation therapy, and (iv) patients with common carotid or aorto-ostial lesions.

Class B lesions are those for which surgery carries higher morbidity and mortality than usual, and stenting is an attractive alternative. These include patients with severe cardiopulmonary disorders precluding general anaesthesia or a prolonged supine surgical procedure, patients with a history of prior carotid endarterectomy, and those with an evolving stroke.

Class C lesions are those for which either surgery or stenting may be the approach of choice depending on the expertise of the surgeon and interventionist. These include lesions that meet NASCET[21] and ACAS[23] trial eligibility criteria. Patients are not considered eligible for carotid stenting if angiography shows (i) a bulky, mobile or pedunculated thrombus; (ii) severe tortuosity, calcification or disease of the proximal aortic arch vessels, or (iii) severe iliofemoral disease precluding femoral arterial access (brachial access may be possible).

Carotid artery dilatation and stenting can, in general, be performed using conventional coronary angioplasty equipment.[25,26] After femoral arterial and venous access is obtained, a diagnostic right Judkins catheter or a cerebral angiography catheter (most frequently an HN2 catheter) is advanced into the common carotid artery and is used to perform selective baseline carotid and vertebral angiography. The number of angiograms should be kept to a minimum, but should include projections that display the carotid bifurcation and others that show the distribution of the intracranial vessels. Extreme care must be taken at all times to prevent embolisation of air or thrombus. Following angiography, 5000–10 000 units heparin are given to achieve a target ACT of 200–250 secs. The diagnostic catheter is then exchanged for a guiding catheter or sheath over a 0.035" guide wire or, if the carotic origin is highly angulated, over a 0.038" extra stiff Amplatz exchange wire with its distal tip placed in the external carotid artery. The guiding catheter or sheath should be advanced to within 2–3 cm of the carotid bifurcation.

The lesion in the internal carotid artery is then crossed using a 0.014 inch or 0.018 inch coronary guide wire and is pre-dilated with a low-profile coronary angioplasty balloon (usually 4.0 x 40 mm). Several types of stent design have been used. In general, self-expanding stents should be chosen over balloon-expandable stents because of the potential of the latter for crush injury. The Wallstent is currently the most frequently used device for carotid stenting. An appropriate size is selected, using the diameter of the common carotid. The size chosen should be such that the maximal expanded diameter of the stent is at least 1mm greater than the widest segment of the artery stented. The stent is advanced over the coronary guide wire and deployed across the lesion in the internal

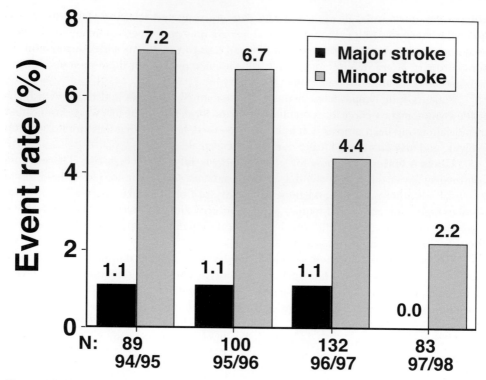

Figure 23.4. *Learning curve effect of carotid stenting in a single centre. The major stroke rate was low at each of the time periods examined but the minor complication rate fell substantially over the 4 year study period. Data adapted from reference 30.*

carotid artery, commonly extending back into the common carotid artery across the origin of the external carotid artery. Flow in the external carotid may become compromised, particularly if its ostium is severely diseased. This is rarely a cause for concern but, if necessary, the origin of the external carotid artery can be dilated through the side of the Wallstent. Occasionally, if flow in the external carotid remains suboptimal, jaw claudication may ensue. This is usually a self-limiting complication.

Following stent placement, it is usually necessary to dilate the stent to optimise its expansion. Appropriately sized balloons are selected for the internal carotid artery and for the external carotid artery. It should be noted that balloon expansion at the level of the carotid sinus is often associated with vagal responses that may include severe bradycardia and profound hypotension. This can be managed using intravenous atropine, temporary cardiac pacing and, if necessary, aramine or a dopamine infusion. Occasionally, hypertension may occur. This usually responds to intravenous or sublingual nitroglycerine. If cerebral embolism occurs, the stenting procedure should be completed and optimal stent expansion obtained before any attempt is made to treat the embolic event. The options available for management of distal embolisation include mechanical disruption by balloon angioplasty, systemic administration of a glycoprotein IIb/IIIa antagonist such as abciximab, and infusion of a calcium antagonist, urokinase, or heparin. This complication is likely to become less frequent as use of distal protection devices becomes commonplace.[27] (See Chapter 22.)

Following carotid stenting, patients should be treated with aspirin 300 mg/day and clopidogrel 75 mg/day for 4 weeks according to usual stent protocols. Patients with uncomplicated procedures and without haemodynamic compromise can be transferred to the general ward or short stay ward for post-operative care. Ideally, all patients should be seen by a consultant neurologist as soon as possible after the procedure and prior to discharge. In the absence of complications, patients may be discharged the following morning.

Although some observational series of carotid stenting have reported high complication rates,[28] the majority have suggested that these procedures can be performed in high-risk patients with complication rates that are similar to surgical revascularisation.[25,26,29] In one study, for example, the 30-day minor stroke rate was 6.2% and the major stroke rate was 0.7%. A substantial learning curve effect has been reported by Iyer[30] and colleagues. Although the incidence of major stroke remained approximately 1% across the study period, the incidence of minor stroke fell from 7.2% in the first annual cohort of 89 patients (1994/95) to 2.2% in the 83 patients treated in 1997/98[30] (Fig 23.4). On the basis of these data, it seems reasonable to offer balloon dilatation and stenting to patients with carotid disease and absolute or relative contraindications to surgical endarterectomy. Whether carotid stenting should be offered to patients at low risk for surgery remains to be determined by careful scrutiny of data from ongoing randomised clinical trials.[31]

References

1. Kaplan S. Natural and postoperative history across age groups. *Cardiol Clin* 1993; **11**:543–556.
2. Ende DJ, Chopra PS, Rao PS. Transcatheter closure of atrial septal defect of patent foramen ovale with the buttoned device for prevention of recurrence of paradoxical embolism. *Am J Cardiol* 1996; **78**:233–236.
3. Bridges ND, Hellenbrand W, Latson L *et al.* Transcatheter closure of patent foramen ovale after presumed paradoxical embolism. *Circulation* 1992; **86**:1902–1908.
4. Rome JJ, Keane JF, Perry SB, Spevak PJ, Lock JE. Double umbrella closure of atrial defects. Initial clinical applications. *Circulation* 1990; **82**:751–758.
5. Thanopoulos BV, Laskari CV, Tsaosis GS *et al.* Closure of atrial septal defects with the Amplatzer Occlusion Device: preliminary results. *J Am Coll Cardiol* 1998; **31**:1110–1116.
6. Windecker S, Meier B. Percutaneous patent foramen ovale (PFO) closure: it can be done but should it? *Cathet Cardiovasc Intervent* 1999; **47**:377–380.
7. Sharafuddin MJA, Gu X, Titus J *et al.* Transvenous closure of secundum atrial septal defects: preliminary results with a new self-expanding nitinol prosthesis in a swine model. *Circulation* 1997; **95**:2162–2168.
8. Konstantinides S, Geibel A, Olschewski M *et al.* A comparison of medical and surgical therapy for atrial septal defect in adults. *N Engl J Med* 1995; **333**:469–473.
9. Hagen PT, Scholz DG, Edwards WD. Incidence and size of patent foramen ovale during the first 10 decades of life: an autopsy study of 965 normal hearts. *Mayo Clin Proc* 1984; **59**:17–20.
10. Lynch JJ, Schuchard GH, Gross CM, Warn LS. Prevalence of right-to-left atrial shunting in a healthy population: detection by Valsalva manoeuver contrast echocardiography. *Am J Cardiol* 1984; **53**:1478–1480.
11. Johnson BI. Paradoxical embolism. *J Clin Pathol* 1951; 4:316–332.
12. Nellesen U, Daniel WG, Matheis G *et al.* Impending paradoxical embolism from atrial thrombus: correct diagnosis by trans oesophageal echocardiography and prevention by surgery. *Am J Cardiol* 1985; **5**:1002–1004.
13. Webster MWI, Chancellor AM, Smith HJ *et al.* Patent foramen ovale in young stroke patients. *Lancet* 1988; **2**:11–12.
14. Mugge A, Daniel WG, Angerman C *et al.* Atrial septal aneurysm in adult patients: a multicenter study using transthoracic and transoesophageal echocardiography. *Circulation* 1995; **91**:2785–2792.
15. Han Y-M, Gu X, Titus JL, Rickera C, Bass JL, Urness M, Amplatz K. New self-expanding patent foramen ovale occlusion device. *Cathet Cardiovasc Intervent* 1999; **47**:370–376.

16. Kitagawa T, Durham LA, Mosca RS, Bove EL. Techniques and results in the management of multiple ventricular septal defects. *J Thorac Cardiovasc Surg* 1998; **115**:848–56.

17. Hijazi ZM, Hakim F, Al-Fadley F, Abdelhamid J, Cao Q-L. Transcatheter closure of single muscular ventricular septal defects using the Amplatzer muscular VSD occluder: initial results and technical considerations. *Cathet Cardiovasc Intervent* 2000. In press.

18. Masura J, Walsh KP, Thanopoulos B *et al.* Catheter closure of moderate to large-sized patent ductus arteriosus using the new Amplatzer duct occluder: immediate and short-term results. *J Am Coll Cardiol* 1998; **31**:878–82.

19. Mayberg MR, Wilson SE, Yatsu F *et al.* Carotid endarterectomy and prevention of cerebral ischaemia in symptomatic carotid stenosis. *JAMA.* 1991; **266**:3289–2394.

20. European Carotid Surgery Trialists Collaborative Group. MRC European Carotid Surgery Trial: interim results for symptomatic patients with severe (70-90%) or mild (0-29%) stenosis. *Lancet.* 1991; **337**:1235–1243.

21. North American Symptomatic Carotid Endarterectomy Trial Collaboration. Beneficial effect of carotid endarterectomy in symptomatic patients with high grade carotid stenosis. *N Engl J Med.* 1991; **235**:445–453.

22. Rothwell PW, Slattery J, Warlow CP. A systematic review of the risks of stroke and death due to endarterectomy for symptomatic carotid stenosis. *Stroke.* 1996; 27:260–265.

23. Executive Committee for the Asymptomatic Carotid Atherosclerosis Study. Endarterectomy for asymptomatic carotid artery stenosis. *JAMA.* 1995; **273**:1421–1428.

24. Bettman MA, Katzen BT, Whisnant J *et al.* Carotid stenting and angioplasty. A statement for healthcare professionals from the Councils on Cardiovascular Radiology, Stroke, Cardio-thoracic and Vascular Surgery, Epidemiology and Prevention, and Clinical Cardiology, American Heart Association. *Circulation* 1998; **97**:121–123.

25. Iyer JS, Roubin GS, Yadav JS *et al.* Elective stenting of the extracranial carotid arteries. *Circulation* 1997; **95**:376–381.

26. Yadav JS, Roubin GS, King P, Iyer S, Vitek J. Angioplasty and stenting for restenosis after carotid endarterectomy: initial experience. *Stroke* 1996; **27**:2075–2079.

27. Theron JG, Payelle GG, Coshun O, Huet HF, Guimareaus L. Carotid artery stenosis: treatment with protected balloon angioplasty and stent placement. *Radiology* 1996; **201**:627–636.

28. Naylor AR, Bolia A, Abbott RJ *et al.* Randomised study of carotid angioplasty and stenting versus carotid endarterectomy: a stopped trial. *J Vasc Surg* 1998; **28**:326–34.

29. Mathur A, Roubin GS, Iyer SS *et al.* Predictors of stroke complicating carotid artery stenting. *Circulation* 1998; **97**:1239–45.

30. Iyer SS, Roubin G, Vitek J *et al.* Four year experience with carotid stenting. J Am Coll Cardiol 1999; **33**:21A

31. Major ongoing stroke trials: carotid and vertebral artery transluminal angioplasty study (CAVATAS). *Stroke* 1996; **27**:358.

Chapter 24

Mitral Valvuloplasty

Paul Roy

P ercutaneous transvenous mitral valvuloplasty (PTMV) was first introduced into clinical practice by Inoue *et al.* in 1984[1] and is now a safe and effective therapy that replaces the need for surgery in many patients with symptomatic mitral stenosis. Worldwide, more than 20 000 patients have had successful mitral dilatation using this method, with a procedural success rate greater than 95%. Operator experience is a determining factor in this outcome, with the highest success rates reported by Inoue and Hung.[2]

Mitral stenosis

In normal adults the mitral valve orifice is 4–6 cm². When the orifice is reduced to approximately 2 cm² (which is considered mild mitral stenosis) blood flow from the left atrium to the left ventricle occurs only if propelled by an abnormal pressure gradient. When the mitral valve opening is reduced to 1 cm² (which is considered severe mitral stenosis) a left atrial pressure of approximately 25 mmHg is required to maintain a normal cardiac output. This elevated left atrial pressure in turn raises pulmonary venous and capillary pressures, reducing pulmonary compliance and causing exertional dyspnoea.

Patient selection

Once the symptomatic patient has been assessed clinically, careful selection is required to ensure that the valve is suitable for this procedure. Commissural splitting is the dominant mechanism by which mitral valve area is increased by the balloon,[3] therefore the extent of fusion, fibrosis or calcification of one or both commissures is a major determinant of the outcome of mitral valvotomy. Patients with pliable valves without severe sub-valvular lesions are ideal candidates, whereas patients with poorly mobile mitral leaflets, severely fused commissures and significant sub-valvular lesions may obtain less than optimal results and are at higher risk of developing mitral regurgitation.[4]

Echocardiography

Echocardiography allows careful analysis of mitral valve morphologies. Echocardiographic scoring systems based on qualitative assessment of leaflet and sub-valvular morphology[4,5] were devised to predict the outcome of mitral valvotomy. The specific importance of commissural morphology was for some time neglected, but Inoue considered this an important determinant. Echocardiographic studies have confirmed the importance of commissural morphology[5] to the extent that, before undertaking mitral balloon valvuloplasty, more reliance is now placed on echocardiographic evaluation of commissural morphology than on other echo-scoring mechanisms.

The procedure is not usually performed if there is more than trivial to mild mitral regurgitation. Presence of thrombus in the left atrial appendage is a relative contraindication. Patients with atrial fibrillation are usually subjected to a transoesophageal echo-doppler study prior to the procedure to ensure that there is no left atrial thrombus likely to become dislodged. As the atrial septum is punctured during the procedure, any thrombus in the left atrium can easily be dispersed into the circulation. This may be caused either by the transeptal needle if thrombus is on the atrial septum, or by the wire or balloon should either of these enter into the left atrial appendage. If thrombus is present, the patient should be treated with warfarin for two to three months, then reassessed by transoesophageal echo before the procedure is undertaken.

Generally, symptoms do not occur until the orifice of the mitral valve is less than 1.5 cm^2 but disabling symptoms do sometimes occur in patients performing heavy physical work with a mitral orifice larger than 1.5 cm^2. In patients whose valve morphology is not ideal for balloon dilatation, associated illnesses prohibiting open heart surgery may nonetheless favour the balloon method. Occasionally, during pregnancy, pulmonary oedema may result from severe mitral stenosis. In this situation the balloon procedure can be performed as an ideal alternative to surgery. With a pregnant patient it is preferable to wait until after five months, when the impact of any x-ray irradiation on the foetus is minimal.

The procedure

Patients are admitted to hospital on the day of the procedure, having had a transoesophageal echocardiogram and assessment prior to admission.

Echo doppler is usually performed in the catheterisation laboratory at the same time as the mitral procedure. A 6F pigtail catheter is passed to the left ventricle via a right femoral artery percutaneous puncture. The purpose of this catheter is to measure left ventricular pressure for estimation of the mitral gradient. It also permits the operator to see exactly where the aorta lies in order to avoid damage during transeptal puncture. Right heart catheterisation is then performed via a sheath from the right femoral vein, and a pigtail catheter is used to perform a right atrial angiogram before commencing.

The next part of the procedure, perforating the inter-atrial septum, is the most delicate and one where an inexperienced operator is most likely to encounter serious difficulty, as it requires experience to safely perform a transeptal puncture. The two major problems inherent in this technique are cardiac perforation and puncture of an inappropriate atrial septal site. The former may lead to the serious complications of cardiac tamponade and the latter leads to difficulties in subsequently trying to manoeuvre the Inoue balloon catheter across the mitral orifice. For anyone beginning this technique, reference 6 is highly recommended.

A simple method is used by Inoue to locate the site of transseptal puncture, the *foramen ovale*: by applying a slightly complicated formula, examining flow of contrast from the right atrium through the pulmonary circulation into the left atrium indicates approximately where the *foramen ovale* is situated on the atrial septum. First, a Brockenbrough needle is passed via the venous sheath into the right atrium and the tip is placed against the selected puncture site. Normally, at the point of needle puncture a distinct pulsation can be felt, particularly when left atrial pressure is high. When the operator is satisfied with the intended puncture site, the needle is advanced 1 cm across the septum and blood is withdrawn. Measurement of left atrial pressure at this point confirms that the catheter is in the appropriate site. A small amount of pure contrast is also injected, further confirming the left atrial position of the needle tip. Should it transpire that the needle tip is in the aorta or the pericardium, generally no problem will result provided the needle only is advanced at this stage. It is therefore important at this point not to push the catheter over the needle point until the operator is certain of the position of the needle tip.

Precautionary measurement of right atrial pressure on entry into the right atrium allows the operator to observe any subsequent rise in right atrial pressure that could indicate tamponade from an inappropriate puncture.

If no blood is aspirated when the needle is first passed through the chosen site, this indicates that the needle has either dissected the high septum or is caught in a thickened septum. Staining of the septum with injection of a small amount of contrast easily distinguishes the two.

When the high septum is dissected, myocardial staining spreads in a vertical fashion. In this situation the needle needs to be withdrawn and septal puncture made at a lower site.

When the needle is caught in the thickened septum, the stain takes a more horizontal orientation. If this occurs, it requires some experience to decide whether to persist in this area or attempt puncture at another site. It is not possible to differentiate dissection of the high septum from entrapment of the needle in a thick septum by pressure monitoring alone.

Heparin is usually given at a dose of 5000 units at the commencement of the procedure, with a further 5000 units once septal puncture is safely performed. While this may appear excessive in the small female patient, it removes the risk that can result if a lengthy delay occurs in trying to cross the mitral orifice with the Inoue catheter. If this occurs, extra heparin is required.

Once septal puncture has been safely performed, the long guiding stilette of the Inoue apparatus is passed into the left atrium. The stilette is an ingenious needle with a long, soft curved tip that sits safely in the left atrium, but with a very rigid distal end of the shaft allowing passage of the Inoue balloon into the left atrium.

The Inoue balloon

The Inoue balloon has a 12F polyvinyl tube shaft with a co-axial double lumen. The inner lumen of the catheter permits pressure measurement and blood sampling and insertion of metal tube, guide wire or stilette. The outer lumen connects proximally with a two-way stopcock used to connect the catheter to an inflation/deflation syringe and a vent, distally mounted with a balloon at the end of the shaft.

The balloon is made of double layers of latex tubing and can be transformed into various shapes from its natural form to serve different functions. The balloon is stiffened and slenderised when the rubber balloon is stretched by inserting a metal tube. In this shape, the size of the hole used to enter the left atrium is minimised as the balloon is passed across the atrial septum. Once in the left atrium the stretching metal tube is withdrawn and the balloon assumes a more semi-circular shape. Usually at this point a recording of the pressure gradient across the mitral valve is made using the lumen of the Inoue balloon to measure left atrial pressure and the pigtail balloon in the left ventricle to measure left ventricular pressure (Fig. 24.1).

Now the balloon is ready to be passed across the mitral valve. A slightly differently shaped wire is then inserted into the Inoue balloon. This wire allows various manoeuvres to be made to attempt to cross the mitral valve with the Inoue balloon. Before commenc-

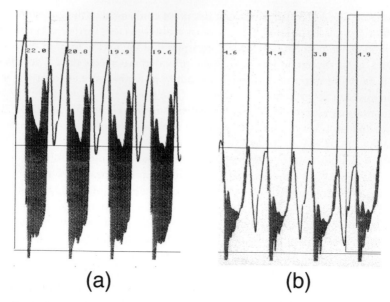

(a)   (b)

Figure 24.1. Simultaneous left ventricular and left atrial pressure tracings in a patient with severe mitral stenosis before and after mitral balloon valvuloplasty. Mean gradient across the mitral vale (shaded area) was 20.9 mmHg before the procedure (a) and 4.6 mmHg after (b).

ing this part of the procedure, the distal section of the Inoue balloon is inflated to prevent the balloon slipping back across the atrial septal puncture. Difficulties are sometimes encountered trying to cross the mitral valve. Occasionally a slippery black guide wire through the Inoue lumen allows easier crossing and, very occasionally, use of the Mullins sheath has been described to cross a difficult valve.

Balloon inflation

The Inoue balloon has an ingenious feature called differential compliance, which allows the more distal half of the balloon to inflate first when dye is injected into the balloon.

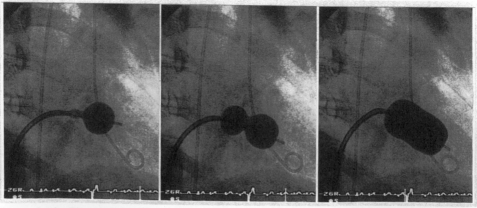

Figure 24.2. The three stages of Inoue balloon inflation. The first inflation dilates the distal end of the balloon, allowing positioning against the mitral orifice. The second inflation dilates the proximal end, locking the waist across the mitral valve. Commissural splitting occurs with the third inflation, which dilates the waist.

Once the distal half of the balloon is inflated, the balloon is pulled back against the mitral valve orifice and the proximal half of the balloon is then inflated (Fig. 24.2). Usually an obvious constriction is seen as a waist in the middle of the balloon where the balloon sits across the mitral valve. This serves to locate the balloon snugly across the valve. Further inflation dilates the waist. It is this third inflation that splits the commissures and dilates the mitral opening.

Balloon size is chosen according to the patient's height. There is a set formula for this, which is obtained from the manufacturer's information in the balloon kit.

Following the first inflation it is important to re-measure the pressure gradient across the valve (Fig. 24.1). If the gradient has fallen to less than 5 mmHg this would generally be considered a satisfactory result, although reduction of the original gradient by 50% is acceptable and provides symptomatic relief. It is important at this stage to monitor the 'v' wave in the left atrial trace, which gives a measure of any increasing degree of mitral regurgitation. It may be necessary to repeat the inflation and slowly increase the size of the Inoue balloon until an adequate result is obtained. At first sign of any rise in the 'v' wave, no further dilatation should be made, otherwise severe mitral regurgitation may occur due to oversplitting of the commissures. Cardiac output and valve area measurements are not necessarily performed at this time, as they are routinely assessed echocardiographically after the procedure.

Balloon removal

Once a satisfactory result is achieved, before removing the Inoue balloon catheter from the left atrium, a stretching metal tube needs to be carefully reinserted to slenderise the balloon for withdrawal across the atrial septum from the femoral vein. A 9F sheath is usually inserted over the guide wire after removal of the Inoue balloon, which allows the patient to be immediately removed from the catheter table. Compression of the femoral artery and vein is done in the recovery area.

Prospective randomised clinical trials comparing valvuloplasty and surgical closed mitral commissurotomy have shown no difference in early results or late clinical follow-up, assessed by calculation of mitral valve area during cardiac catheterisation at 8 months and at 3.5 years following the procedures.[7] Thus PTMV is now providing results that are comparable with those obtained by surgical closed valvotomy, with low morbidity and mortality. In most countries, cost of the procedure is a fraction of that of surgical treatment and hospital stay is reduced to 24 hours. Prior to the Inoue design, mitral valvuloplasty was undertaken with double balloon techniques that were quite cumbersome. It is a genuine tribute to Kanji Inoue that the methodology has been simplified to such an extent by his ingenious device.

References

1. Inoue K, Owaki T, Nakamura T *et al*. Clinical application of transvenous mitral commissurotomy by a new balloon catheter. *J Thorac Cardiovasc Surg* 1984;**87**:394–402.
2. Inoue K, Hung JS. Percutaneous transvenous mitral commissurotomy: The Far East experience. In: Topol ES (ed). *Textbook of Interventional Cardiology*. Philadelphia: WB Saunders 1990, pp 887–99.
3. Bassand JP, Schiele F, Bernard Y *et al*. The double-balloon and Inoue techniques in percutaneous mitral valvuloplasty. Comparative results in a series of 232 cases. *J Am Coll Cardiol* 1991;**18**(4):982–9.
4. Wilkins GT, Weyman AE, Abascal VM *et al*. Percutaneous balloon dilatation of the mitral

valve: an analysis of echocardiographic variables related to outcome and the mechanism of dilation. *Br Heart J* 1988;**4**:299–308.

5.   Fatkin D, Roy PR. Percutaneous balloon mitral valvotomy with the Inboue single-balloon catheter: commissural morphology as a determinant of outcome. *J Am Coll Cardiol* 1993;**21**(2):390–97.

6.   Inoue K, Hung JS, Chen TO. Mitral stenosis: Inoue balloon catheter technique. In: Chen TO (ed). *Percutaneous Balloon Valvuloplasty.* New York: Igaku-Shoin 1992, pp 237–79.

7.   Turi ZG, Reyes VP, Soma R *et al.* Percutaneous balloon versus surgical closed commissurotomy for mitral stenosis. A prospective, randomized trial. *Circulation* 1991;**83**:1179–85.

Chapter 25

The Electrophysiology Laboratory

Dennis L. Kuchar and Charles W. Thorburn

In order for the heart to pump efficiently, an electrical wiring system is present in the heart to coordinate its activity. An electrical impulse normally originates in the upper-most part of the heart (SA node) and then travels through the AV node, down toward the apex of the heart. When this orderly flow of current is disturbed, an arrhythmia re-sults. This is usually manifested as a bradycardia (<50 bpm) or a tachycardia (>100 bpm). By placing electrical wires or catheters into the heart and performing a stimulation study, the normal or abnormal electrical condition of the heart can be assessed.

The normal heart

The heart constantly pumps blood to deliver oxygen and nutrients to the body. It is com-prised of four chambers, two on the right side and two on the left. The upper chambers on each side, the atria, receive and collect blood. The lower chambers, the ventricles, pump blood. All four chambers work in synchrony to move blood through the body. Rhythmic cardiac contractions depend on the electrical system to conduct electrical impulses through-out the heart. The electrical impulse normally begins in the sino-atrial (SA) node (Fig. 25.1), setting the pace for the heartbeat. The impulse spreads through the atria, causing a contraction, thereby forcing blood into the ventricles. From the atria, the impulse reaches the atrioventricular (AV) node, where each electrical impulse slows down before it passes through to the ventricles. Except at the AV node, the atrium is normally electrically insu-lated from the ventricle by fibrous tissue. Through a specialised muscle fibre system, the impulse is distributed throughout both ventricles, causing ventricular contraction. This normal conduction is normal sinus rhythm. The rhythm is regular and the heart beats 60–100 times per minute.

Diagnosis of arrhythmia

Patients with heart rhythm disturbances are studied and treated in the electrophysiology (EP) laboratory. If an arrhythmia is suspected, one or more of the following diagnostic tests may be performed to determine the source of the symptoms. Therapeutic proce-dures performed in the electrophysiology laboratory include transcatheter radiofrequency ablations, implantations of permanent pacemakers and defibrillators, overdrive pacing and cardioversions.

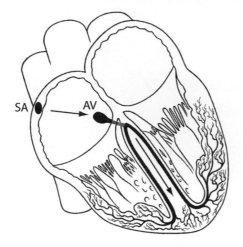

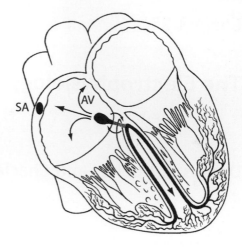

Figure 25.1. Normal conduction pathway of electrical excitation from the sino-atrial (SA) node via the atrio-ventricular (AV) node to the ventricles.

Figure 25.2. Depiction of the recirculation pathway connecting atria and ventricles in AV nodal re-entrant tachycardia.

An abnormal heart rhythm is a change in either the speed or the pattern of the heartbeat. The heart may beat too slowly, too rapidly or irregularly. A heart which beats too fast or too slow can cause lightheadedness or dizziness, palpitations (skipping, fluttering or pounding in the chest) fatigue, chest pressure or pain, shortness of breath, fainting spells, or sudden death.

Sometimes there are no symptoms at all. Left untreated, certain abnormal heart rhythms can cause death, but some arrhythmias are common and not associated with any untoward conditions, so-called benign arrhythmias. One of the goals of evaluation is to sort out the serious from the benign forms of heartbeat disturbances.

Invasive electrophysiology studies (EPS) involve the recording of spontaneous and pacing-induced intracardiac electrical activation patterns for study in a controlled environment. The aim is to investigate the electrical aspects of abnormal heart function for diagnostic, therapeutic and/or prognostic purposes. EPS may be performed:

1. To establish the site of origin and the mechanism of a tachycardia or bradycardia (e.g. the cause of a cardiac arrest or to assess a documented arrhythmia in which the diagnosis may not be apparent from the surface electrocardiogram (ECG).
2. To guide in the treatment of arrhythmias (e.g. drug therapy or other interventions such as implantation of defibrillators, radiofrequency ablation, surgery).
3. To assess the likelihood of future arrhythmic events.

The premature heartbeat

A premature heartbeat comes too soon and interrupts the regular rhythm of the heart. Premature beats may originate in the atrium (premature atrial contraction or PAC) or in the ventricles (premature ventricular contraction or PVC), producing a sensation that the heart is 'skipping' or 'flip-flopping.' Although premature beats are more common in people with heart disease, almost everyone experiences a 'skipped' beat once in a while. This may result from smoking, fatigue, alcohol, caffeine, other stimulants, or may have no apparent cause. Usually, single premature beats require no treatment, but occasionally they may be frequent or troublesome.

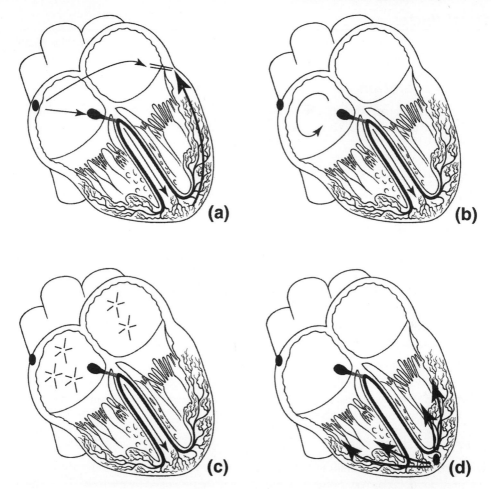

Figure 25.3. Illustration of various electrical mechanisms that cause (a) Wolf-Parkinson-White syndrome, showing the extra pathway connecting atria and ventricles; (b) atrial flutter, with an abnormal circuit around the tricuspid annulus; (c) atrial fibrillation, with irregular atrial activation; and (d) ventricular tachycardia, with an abnormal ventricular ectopic focus.

Fast heart rhythms

Problems with electrical signals can make the heart beat too fast. Below are some common types of fast heart rhythms.

AV node re-entrant tachycardia (AVNRT)

With AVNRT, an extra pathway lies in or near the AV node (Fig. 25.2). Signals travelling through the AV node may get trapped in this pathway. The trapped signals make the heart beat faster.

Wolff-Parkinson-White (WPW) syndrome

With WPW, an extra pathway connects the ventricles and the atria (Fig. 25.3a). Signals passing through the ventricles may travel along this extra pathway back to the atria. The signals from the extra pathway make the heart beat faster. The ECG has a short P–R interval and a 'delta curve' sloping upwards on the R wave.

Atrial flutter

With atrial flutter there is an abnormal circuit around the tricuspid annulus (Fig. 25.3b). Signals loop around and around inside this circuit.

Atrial fibrillation

With atrial fibrillation, the atria have many circuits that lead to very rapid and uneven activation of the atria (Fig. 25.3c), which may subsequently stop contracting and begin to quiver.

Ventricular tachycardia

This is commonly the cause of arrhythmia in patients with prior myocardial infarction. Patients may present with syncope or cardiac arrest. In many cases this arrhythmia can be induced by programmed stimulation of the ventricles. It is caused by an ectopic focus in the ventricle overriding the normal pacemaker (Fig. 25.3d).

Electrophysiologic evaluation of cardiac conduction and rhythm

Holter monitor

The Holter monitor is a small, portable machine that is worn to make a 24-hour continuous recording of electrical impulses during normal daily activities. The machine detects arrhythmias that may not show up in an ECG. It is necessary to maintain a diary of all activities and symptoms while wearing the monitor.

Exercise stress test

The exercise stress (treadmill) test enables physicians to record cardiac electrical activity that may not occur at rest. Some arrhythmias may be provoked by exercise.

Event recorder

The event recorder (transtelephonic monitoring) is a digital recorder with a memory chip capable of recording an electrocardiac event for a few minutes. When the patient feels an arrhythmia, the recorder on the chest can be activated to record the event. This can then be transmitted via telephone to a monitoring station so a record of the episode can be analysed.

The electrophysiology study

The EP study is conducted to:

1. provoke and examine an arrhythmia under controlled conditions;
2. acquire more accurate, detailed information than with any other diagnostic test;
3. choose the most effective treatment;
4. in many cases, provide treatment (i.e. catheter ablation) during the same session.

During the study, special electrode catheters are inserted into veins and are guided into the heart. These catheters sense electrical impulses and may also be used to stimulate different areas of the heart. Sites that are causing serious arrhythmias can be localised and, if appropriate, ablated.

The tilt table test

Vasovagal syncope (neurocardiogenic syndrome or vasodepressor syncope) is a relatively common syndrome seen in young people, more commonly in women. The clinical setting is usually related to standing for a prolonged period in a crowded environment, e.g. inside a bus, train or underground railway system or following situations such as fright, a dentist's chair or the sight of blood. The patient may feel dizzy, shortness of breath, a 'black screen' may occur in front of the eyes and may then collapse with a brief period of loss of consciousness. It may be preceded by an awareness of a faster heartbeat and nausea and sweatiness. This is usually a benign situation and the patient awakens in seconds to minutes. If the patient is examined during that time, hypotension and bradycardia will usually be evident. A vasovagal episode is the most common cause of syncope in otherwise healthy young persons. Investigation is mainly to exclude other causes of syncope (e.g. arrhythmias, drugs, epilepsy).

The underlying mechanism of this syndrome is still unknown. It may be due to hypersensitivity and over-reaction of the autonomic nervous system that produce slowing of the heart rate and/or low blood pressure. A cardiovascular cause of syncope can be identified in most patients by electrophysiological studies or the head-up tilt test. Tilt testing with or without isoprenaline can provoke hypotension and bradycardia in patients with neurocardiogenic mechanisms of syncope.

Treatment includes beta-blockers, disopyramide, fluoxetine, mineralocorticoids or even permanent pacemaker insertion for those with severe cardioinhibitory effect (profound bradycardia or asystole during attack). It must be emphasised, however, that syncope can be a sign of more sinister heart disease, particularly in patients with structural heart disease. These patients should be considered for investigation with electrophysiological testing.

Procedure

No hospital admission is required for tilt tests, which may be conducted on an outpatient basis. Bookings are made with the procedure room nurse. The patient is assessed in the flat position for 5 minutes before being tilted at 60° for 45 minutes or until onset of syncope. If syncope occurs, blood pressure is recorded and the patient is returned to the horizontal position. If no syncope occurs after 45 minutes, isoprenaline infusion at 1 mg/min is given and increased until heart rate is 120% of baseline. This is continued for 15 minutes or until the patient becomes syncopal.

Therapeutic interventions

Catheter ablation

This is a new technique designed to cure certain types of tachycardia. From ECG tracings, it may be possible to identify patients who are suitable for this technique. There are two broad types of tachycardia that may be suitable for treatment. These are supraventricular tachycardia (SVT) and ventricular tachycardia (VT).

SVT comprises abnormal heart rhythms that either originate in the atria, causing the heart to beat rapidly (may be regular or irregular beating), or may arise because of an abnormal extra connection between the atrium and ventricle, leading to a short circuit in the heart. SVT may be due to a bypass tract or to a double circuit in the central electrical junction in the heart, the AV node. Other types of SVT amenable to ablation include atrial fibrillation, atrial tachycardia and flutter. Sites of ablation may be the abnormal pathway or the normal electrical system itself. If the normal electrical system is the target, a permanent pacemaker may also be required.

VT is an abnormal rapid beating of the ventricles and may result from scarring in the heart from a heart attack, or it may be seen in young people with structurally normal hearts. A small area in the ventricle is the usual target for ablation in these cases. The ablation procedure is very similar to the electrophysiological study. The EP study makes it possible to study heart rhythm disturbances under controlled conditions. By using special insulated catheters, the heart rhythm disturbance can be identified and a decision made on whether to proceed with the ablation procedure.

Preparation

The patient is required to fast for at least 6 hours before the study so that the stomach remains empty. A light sedative tablet is ordered just prior to the study.

Procedure

The EP study and ablation are performed in a dedicated laboratory. The patient is awake during the procedure, but lightly sedated. Once in the laboratory, the patient is attached to monitoring equipment by way of adhesive electrodes on the chest and arms, an automatic blood pressure cuff on the arm and a finger cuff to monitor oxygen level in the blood. Next, the groin (and in many cases, the neck) is cleaned with an antiseptic solution and sterile towels are placed over the body. Local anaesthetic is then injected into these areas and the catheters are inserted into the heart. While this is happening, the patient may be aware of some extra or missed heartbeats, or the tachycardia may occur. This is caused by the catheters inside the heart and the doctor will be able to terminate this, with restoration of the normal heartbeat, once the catheters are in place. Various areas in the heart are stimulated to obtain the information necessary to determine the mechanism of the tachycardia. It is then possible to decide if ablation is feasible. The ablation involves passage of a specialised catheter via either the artery or vein in the groin into the heart. Certain types of tachycardia require passage of the catheter into the left ventricle or into the right atrium and ventricle. Once the abnormal circuit is located, one or more applications of cautery are made through this catheter. The patient does not usually feel any pain, but some patients have described a mild discomfort lasting only for a few seconds. After the cautery has been applied, the electrical system in the heart is retested to ensure that the tachycardia circuit has been eliminated (ablated). If a satisfactory result has been achieved, the catheters are removed and the patient is returned to the ward. Pressure is then applied to the neck and groin sites for several minutes. If the ablation catheter was inserted via an artery, pressure may be applied for up to 30 minutes and a sandbag may be left on the groin for the next few hours. The patient needs to stay in bed for 4 hours after the procedure and remains connected to the ECG monitor for the next 24 hours.

Risk of complications

There is a small risk of complications associated with the procedure. This ranges from minor discomfort and bruising associated with the sites of catheter insertion to a risk of heart damage. There is a small risk of damaging the 'normal' electrical system in the heart, particularly if the area of ablation (the abnormal circuit) is located close to the normal electrical system. If this occurs, a permanent pacemaker may be required to restore normal heart action. In some situations, intentional ablation of the normal electrical system is the goal for successful control of some tachycardias such as atrial fibrillation. In addition, perforation of the heart by the catheter and damage to internal structures of the heart is always a potential risk with catheter procedures. Such risk is estimated at less than 1 in every 100 cases, based on world experience. In cases where the ablation catheter is inserted into the left ventricle via the arterial system, there is a small risk of a clot forming on the catheter during the procedure and becoming dislodged into the circulation. In order to minimise this risk, an anticoagulant drug is routinely given during the procedure and aspirin is taken generally for 1 month after the procedure. The decision to proceed with catheter ablation, therefore, must be made after the risks and benefits of the procedure have been considered and discussed between patient and doctor.

His bundle ablation

His bundle ablation (HBA) is a procedure used to stop AV conduction in atrial fibrillation, flutter (when flutter ablation is not indicated) or tachycardia. A permanent pacemaker (PPM) must be inserted. A ventricular pacing catheter and an ablation catheter are inserted via the femoral vein. The ablation catheter is positioned on the His bundle and the conductive tissue is destroyed by application of radiofrequency energy so the abnormal atrial rhythm is not conducted through to the ventricles.

Permanent pacemaker implantation

The presence of symptoms remains the most common indication for pacemaker treatment. Symptomatic bradycardia is the term used to identify clinical manifestations associated with a heart rate that does not allow cardiac output to meet physiologic demands. The aim of the procedure is to ensure optimal heart rate in a heart with a conduction deficit. Duration of the implant is 1–2 hours depending on the number of leads and difficulty of access. Local anaesthetic (usually Marcain 0.4%) is administered at the site. It is an aseptic procedure, in which the medical practitioner scrubs, gowns and gloves. Cutdown cannulation of the cephalic vein and/or percutaneous cannulation of the subclavian vein provides access to the right atrium and ventricle. Pacing leads are then inserted into the heart via this access and the lead parameters measured via the alligator leads and the pacing system analyser (PSA). The pacing device is then connected to the lead(s), inserted into a pre-pectoral pocket, and the wound closed. A drain may be required, particularly if the patient has been anti-coagulated. Antibiotic prophylaxis is given routinely, usually a cephalosporin, occasionally with gentamycin cover. If the patient is allergic to penicillin, a skin test for drug reaction is performed with the cephalosporin. Cardioversion may (rarely) be required to continue the procedure (e.g. in the event of VF or VT).

Internal cardioverter defibrillator (ICD) implantation

The ICD maybe used in patients with prior cardiac arrest or ventricular tachycardia. It is used when medications fail to control the arrhythmia or when the patient is at high risk of sudden death. The antitachycardia pacemaker is an important adjunct to ICD therapy for patients with frequent episodes of well-tolerated VT. Some devices have the facility to perform antitachycardia pacing as well as delivering shocks, others are shock-only.

Procedure

Duration of the implant is 1–2 hours depending on difficulty of access, positioning the leads to get satisfactory parameters, and testing of the device. Local anaesthetic is administered at the site. It is an aseptic procedure, in which medical staff scrub, gown and don sterile gloves. Cutdown cannulation of the cephalic vein and/or percutaneous cannulation of the subclavian vein provides access to the heart. The pacing/sensing lead also delivers the shock. It is inserted into the right ventricular apex via the cephalic or subclavian vein, and the lead parameters are measured via the alligator leads and the PSA. An 'Active Can' is implanted and the device delivers a shock between the lead and the generator can. If defibrillation thresholds are high, however, a second lead may be inserted via the subclavian vein into the superior vena cava. Alternatively, some new leads have a second pole incorporated into the 'shocking' lead, which is positioned in the vena cava. The ICD is then connected to the leads and tested. It is inserted into a pre-pectoral pocket, and the wound is closed. An anaesthetist delivers a general anaesthetic before any shocks are delivered. Antibiotic prophylaxis, usually a cephalosporin, is given routinely, with occasional gentamycin cover also. If the patient is allergic to penicillin, a skin test for drug reaction is performed with the cephalosporin. Back-up transthoracic cardioversion may be required.

Cardiac resynchronisation for heart failure

Patients with dilated cardiomyopathy and end-stage heart failure may now be treated with a new procedure called atrial synchronised biventricular pacing (ASBP). These patients may develop inter- and intra-ventricular conduction delays (IVCD) which can have serious haemodynamic consequences. Coordinated biventricular activation and contraction by means of ASBP is currently being evaluated as potential therapy to correct haemodynamic derangement in these patients. With IVCD left ventricular contraction is delayed, but atrial contraction is not, leading to ventricular dyssynchrony. ASBP results in improved left ventricular stroke volume by simultaneously activating both left and right ventricles, thereby increasing ventricular filling time, improving the ejection fraction and increasing left ventricular stroke volume. Clinical trials currently in progress may, if successful, provide a simple and effective means of improving overall ventricular function and quality of life for patients with terminal heart failure.

Further reading

Podrid PJ, Kowey PR (eds). *Cardiac arrhythmia: mechanisms, diagnosis and management*. Baltimore: Williams and Wilkins 1995.

Jackman WM, Wang X, Friday KJ *et al*. Catheter ablation of accessory atrioventricular pathway by radiofrequency current. *N Eng J Med* 1991; **324**:1605–11.

Barold SS, Mujica J (eds). *New perspectives in cardiac pacing*, 2nd ed. Mt Kisco: Futura 1991.

Mirowski M, Mower MM, Langer A *et al*. A chronically implanted system for automatic defibrillation in active conscious dogs: experimental treatment for sudden death from VF. *Circulation* 1978; **58**:90–94.

Kuchar DL, Thorburn CW, Sammel NL. Signal-averaged ECG for evaluation of recurrent syncope. *Am J Cardiol* 1986; **58**:949–53.

Grubb BP, Gererd G, Roush K *et al*. Cerebral vasoconstriction during head-up tilt-induced vasovagal syncope. A paradoxic and unexpected response. *Circulation* 1991; **84**:1157–64.

Chapter 26

Right Heart Catheterisation and Haemodynamic Evaluation of the Heart Transplant Patient

Ruth Arnold, Anne Keogh and Peter Macdonald

The first human heart transplant was performed in 1967 but the procedure did not gain widespread acceptance until the 1980s, when the advent of more effective immunosuppression (cyclosporin) and improvements in surgical technique led to a marked improvement in graft and patient survival. Cardiac transplantation now plays a significant role in the management of patients with advanced cardiac failure. However, as donor availability is very limited, potential recipients must be carefully selected. Haemodynamic measurement and optimisation are fundamental in matching donor and recipient and in minimising postoperative right ventricular dysfunction. Cardiac catheterisation is of vital importance in the management of patients after transplantation, in monitoring for rejection and in surveillance for transplant coronary disease.

Recipient selection

Assessment for transplantation requires consideration of the following:

1. Patients with New York Heart Association (NYHA) Class III and IV heart failure and poor quality of life, with expected survival less than 85% at 1 year (i.e. less than the survival with transplantation) should be considered.
2. Intercurrent illness:
   - Malignancy or any other condition that may decrease life expectancy must be excluded. Routine screening for occult malignancy is undertaken in patients over 50 years.
   - Renal impairment, with creatinine level ≥0.20 mmol is a relative contraindication, although in some cases a combined heart-kidney transplant may be considered.
   - Diabetes with extensive micro- or macro-vascular disease is a contraindication.
3. Conditions which usually recur in the transplanted heart should be excluded (e.g. amyloid and haemochromatosis).
4. Psychological assessment. Patients must be compliant with medication and lifestyle modification prior to transplantation.
5. Although the upper age limit is not set, few transplant recipients are over 60 years old. This is due mainly to the high prevalence of co-morbid conditions that prevent successful rehabilitation in the post-transplant period. Limited donor availability is also a factor. Assessment of each potential recipient on an individual basis is necessary.
6. The likelihood of successful rehabilitation.

7.   Obesity (Body Mass Index BMI >25) reduces survival after transplantation. Attempts to lose weight must be demonstrated.

Prognosis

Improvements in medical therapy for heart failure—in particular ACE inhibitors, beta blockers and spironolactone—have benefited many patients, not only by decreasing mortality but by improving symptoms. Every attempt is made to optimise medical therapy before resorting to transplantation. Patients with ischaemic left ventricular dysfunction should be evaluated for reversible ischaemia and suitability for revascularisation. Larger patients of common blood group (O) are less likely to attain a donor and may be considered for left ventricular assist device implantation.

The current survival rate following cardiac transplantation is 85% at 1 year and 78% at 5 years. This compares favourably with medical treatment of Class IV heart failure.

Markers of poor prognosis in heart failure include:

1.   NYHA functional Class IV.
2.   Lack of haemodynamic improvement in response to oral or intravenous therapy; low cardiac index, high pulmonary artery wedge pressure unresponsive to medication.[1]
3.   Maximal oxygen consumption less than 14 ml/kg/min.[2]
4.   Hyponatraemia.
5.   Ventricular tachycardia.

Right heart catheterisation in pre-transplant assessment

Right heart catheterisation is essential in the assessment of prognosis and suitability for transplantation and is generally performed using a right internal jugular approach. A routine procedure takes 15–20 minutes and can be performed on outpatients. No fasting is required. This gives the most true determination of functional pressures. Anticoagulation does not need to be interrupted.

Right internal jugular cannulation

The patient is positioned supine without a pillow on the fluoroscopy table, with the head turned to the left and the neck slightly extended. The operator can then identify the tri-

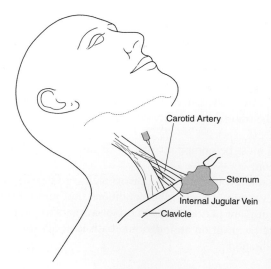

Figure 26.1. Illustration depicting anatomical landmarks for internal jugular cannulation.

angle formed by the two heads (sternal and clavicular) of the sternocleidomastoid muscle and the clavicle (Fig. 26.1). The anatomical landmarks can be made more prominent by asking the patient to lift the head slightly off the bed, or turn the head to the left against resistance.

If the jugular pulsation can be seen, it can be cannulated. Local anaesthetic is injected at a point approximately two fingerbreadths above the clavicle in the middle of the triangle. A 22 guage needle is used to locate the jugular vein, advancing at an angle approximately 40° from vertical and 20° right. The vein is usually located at a depth of 1–2.5 cm below the skin. If the vein is not located, the same approach is repeated with more lateral angulation, and if this is also unsuccessful, a medial approach can be used. Medial angulation must be approached with caution, as the carotid artery lies deep and medial to the internal jugular vein. If venous pressure is low, a head-down tilt, elevation of the legs or valsalva manoeuvre may help increase venous return and make jugular cannulation easier.

Once the vein has been located, a puncture can be made by following the same angle with the 18 guage needle, through which a J guide-wire is advanced into the right atrium. A small nick is then made in the skin at the entry point, using a scalpel blade. The needle is then removed and a 9 F sheath inserted over the guidewire. A Swan-Ganz thermodilution catheter is inserted via the sheath. Catheter passage is made easier with fluoroscopic or echocardiographic guidance, particularly in patients with right ventricular enlargement, tricuspid regurgitation or pulmonary hypertension. Figure 26.2 illustrates examples of pressure tracings and Swan-Ganz catheter placement.

The following measurements are recorded during right heart catheterisation:

Right atrial pressure
Right ventricular pressure
Pulmonary artery pressure (PAP); systole, diastole and mean
Pulmonary artery wedge pressure (PAWP)
Cardiac output (CO) using thermodilution or Fick method
Cardiac index (CI) is calculated to compensate for body surface area
TPG (transpulmonary gradient) is calculated (TPG = mean PAP–PAWP)
PVR (pulmonary vascular resistance) = TPG/CO

Table 26.1 indicates the expected range of cardiovascular pressures measured by Swan-Ganz catheterisation for disease-free and pretransplant patients.

Table 26.1. Comparison of intracardiac pressures (mmHg) in normal and pre-transplant patients.

	Normal patient			Pre-transplant patient*		
	M	S	D	M	S	D
RA	0-8			0-25		
RV		15-30	0-8			
PA	15-30	5-16	10-22		70	50
PAWP	5-15			25-40		
CI	2.5-4			1.5-2.5		

KEY: (RA = right atrium, RV = right ventricle, PA = pulmonary artery, PAWP = pulmonary artery wedge pressure, CI = cardiac index).

Values for pre-transplant patients (*) reflect typical values seen in patients with dilated cardiomyopathy and can change substantially with treatment optimisation. Patients with restrictive aetiology may show different haemodynamic values. Elevated PA values must be reversible for transplantation to proceed.

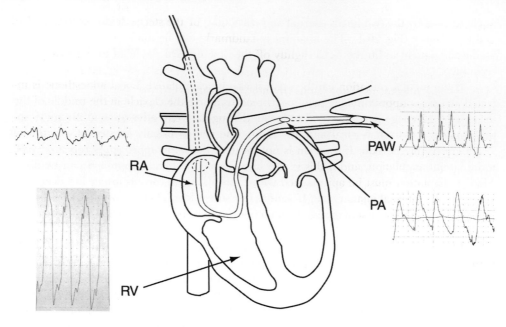

Figure 26.2. Illustration of pressure tracings taken with a Swan-Ganz catheter and its anatomical placement in the pulmonary artery. PAW=pulmonary artery wedge; PA=pulmonary artery; RV=right ventricle; RA=right atrium.

Table 26.2 provides a list of derived haemodynamic variables used to evaluate haemodynamic stability of patients for transplantation.

Pulmonary vascular resistance and transpulmonary gradient (TPG) are vital components of the pre-transplant assessment. In patients with a TPG over 10 mmHg an intravenous vasodilator challenge should be given, as described below, to determine the degree of reversibility of the gradient. Pulmonary resistance is usually reversible to some degree, if not acutely, sometimes responding gradually, over months, to changes in long-term therapy. A fixed TPG >12 mmHg, or PVR >4.0 to 4.5 is associated with reduced

Table 26.2. Derived haemodynamic variables

Variable	Formula	Normal Range
Cardiac index	$\dfrac{\text{CO (L/min)}}{\text{Body surface area (m}^2\text{)}}$	2.8–4.2 L.min.m²
Total peripheral resistance	$\dfrac{\text{(MPA–CVP) x 80}}{\text{CO (L/min)}}$	1200–1500 Dynes.sec.cm⁻⁵
Pulmonary vascular resistance	$\dfrac{\text{(MPA–PAWP) x 80}}{\text{CO (L/min)}}$	100–300 Dynes.sec.cm⁻⁵
Transpulmonary gradient (TPG)	MPA–PAWP	0–10 mmHg

KEY: CO = cardiac output; MPA = mean pulmonary artery pressure; CVP = central venous pressure; PAWP = pulmonary artery wedge pressure.

survival post transplantation from right heart failure, as the donor heart may not adapt sufficiently to pump against abnormally elevated pulmonary pressures.

Patients with elevated fixed transpulmonary gradients in the range of 12–18 mmHg can be considered for orthotopic transplantation (replacement of the existing heart with a donor heart) if the donor has a substantial weight advantage over the recipient. Early right ventricular dysfunction tends to remodel over the first 7–14 days after transplantation as the donor right ventricle adapts to the elevated pulmonary resistance and the resistance drops with improved left ventricular function. In patients with markedly elevated and fixed PVR >18mmHg, heterotopic transplantation, where a donor heart is grafted in parallel with the existing heart, or heart lung transplantation can be considered. Successful conventional orthotopic transplantation is generally not possible in this group.

Patients need regular evaluation whilst on the transplant waiting list. Current practice is to perform right heart catheterisation 6-monthly for those with TPG >10 and annually for those with TPG ≤10.

Vasodilator challenge protocols

Vasodilators currently used are glyceryl trinitrate (GTN) IV, sodium nitroprusside (SNP), intravenous prostacyclin and inhaled nitric oxide.

Glyceryl trinitrate

The concentration is 50 mg glyceryl trinitrate in 100 ml 5% dextrose. Intravenous infusion starting at 10 ml/h and increased by 10 ml/h at intervals of 15 minutes up to 50 ml/h. Monitor systemic blood pressure at 2-minute intervals. If TPG fails to fall below 10, consider challenge with an alternative agent. Patients taking regular nitrate should be challenged with an alternative agent (e.g. sodium nitroprusside, prostacyclin or nitric oxide).

Sodium nitroprusside (SNP)

The concentration is 50 mg SNP in 100 ml 5% dextrose. Start infusion at 10 ml/h and increase by 10 ml/h every 15 minutes up to 40 ml/h. Monitor blood pressure every 2 minutes.

Inhaled nitric oxide (NO)

Inhalation starts at 5–10 ppm and haemodynamic measurements are repeated after 5 minutes.

Prostacyclin (PgI2)

Dilute 0.5 mg prostacyclin powder in 50 ml. Dilute this 50 ml solution in 250 ml normal saline. This gives a solution of 500 mg in 300 ml. Infusion rate based on 70 kg patient:

2 ng/kg/min = 6 ml/h
4 ng/kg/min = 12 ml/h
6 ng/kg/min = 18 ml/h
8 ng/kg/min = 24 ml/h

Start at 2 ng/kg/min and work up by 2 ng/kg/min at 15-minute intervals.

Side effects including systemic hypotension, headaches, nausea, vomiting, facial flushing, abdominal pain, teeth and jaw ache and bradycardia, are often experienced at around 6 ng/kg/min.

Risks associated with right heart catheterisation

The risks of right heart catheterisation are those associated with central venous line placement, such as pneumothorax. The other main risk is induction of atrial or ventricular arrhythmias. Atrial arrhythmias induced by the catheter tip may be transient or sustained. If atrial flutter is sustained, it may be possible to restore sinus rhythm with atrial overdrive pacing. Haematomas may occur at the site of sheath insertion, as many patients are taking warfarin. Temporary hoarseness can occur if local anaesthetic is injected into the recurrent laryngeal nerve.

Rate of complications:

Haematoma	1 in 200
Pneumothorax	1 in 500
Serious arrhythmia	1 in 1000

Right heart catheterisation in pulmonary hypertension

Right heart catheterisation is useful in primary pulmonary hypertension in establishing:

i)   the diagnosis;
ii)   prognosis: poor with raised RA pressure, low CI and high pulmonary artery pressure;
iii) optimal tolerated dose of vasodilator, oral or intravenous prostacyclin;
iv)   responsiveness of the pulmonary circulation to vasodilator therapy.

Vasoconstriction contributes to elevation of pulmonary pressures in all patients with pulmonary hypertension at some stage in their disease. Responsiveness to vasodilators may eventually be lost as intimal fibrosis and medial hypertrophy become established.

Haemodynamic testing with a vasodilator challenge can provide information about prognosis and about the safety of chronic oral vasodilator therapy. Patients who are responsive to vasodilator challenge (responders, defined as having a 25% fall in pulmonary artery pressure during haemodynamic testing) have a better prognosis than non-responders.

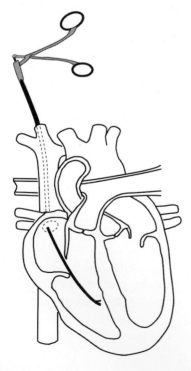

Figure 26.3. Positioning and use of a bioptome (drawing courtesy of R. Hawkins).

There is no selective oral or intravenous pulmonary vasodilator available. The greatest vasodilator effect is produced with inhaled nitric oxide plus prostacyclin. For haemodynamic testing both have the benefit of a short half-life. Inhaled therapies probably affect systemic resistance less than intravenous therapies.

Diagnostic endomyocardial biopsy

The role of endomyocardial biopsy in achieving a diagnosis in cardiomyopathy is limited.[3] This is due to the limited evidence of benefit for immunosuppressant therapy in myocarditis when it is demonstrated, inter-observer differences between reporting pathologists, and the high number of biopsies that show non-specific myopathic changes.[4] The procedure is not without risk, particularly if the ventricle is thin-walled. Perforation and tamponade can occur in up to 1 in 2000 cases, requiring immediate surgical decompression and sometimes oversew, in theatre.

Diagnostic biopsy should be considered in patients with recent (<3 months) onset cardiomyopathy in the absence of significant coronary disease or where there is evidence of a systemic process such as fever or high erethrocyte sedimentation rate (ESR) with disproportionately thick left ventricular wall, or in patients with suspected specific infiltrative cardiomyopathies such as amyloidosis, haemochromatosis or sarcoidosis.

Post-transplant surveillance

Endomyocardial biopsy

Right ventricular biopsy is performed at regular intervals after transplantation to monitor for cellular rejection. Access for biopsy is usually via a right internal jugular approach, but can be performed from the left internal jugular, the subclavian or femoral veins.

Once a 9F venous sheath has been inserted, a bioptome is advanced under fluoroscopic guidance to the right atrium. Using counterclockwise rotation, the bioptome is passed across the tricuspid valve towards the interventricular septum. When the bioptome makes contact with the myocardium, ventricular ectopic beats are seen on the monitor and resistance can be felt by the operator. The bioptome is then withdrawn slightly, the jaws are opened, readvanced to contact the myocardium and the forceps are closed (Fig. 26.3). The bioptome is then withrawn and the piece of tissue removed. Five or six pieces of myocardium of 1–2 mm diameter are necessary for adequate sampling.

Complications of endomyocardial biopsy include atrial and ventricular arrhythmias, perforation, pneumothorax, tissue embolus and damage to the tricuspid valve. The overall complication rate is approximately 1%, with the incidence of perforation with tamponade less than 0.05%. If atrial flutter is induced and sustained, a pacing electrode can be introduced via the sheath and sinus rhythm restored with overdrive atrial pacing.

Tricuspid regurgitation is a very frequent finding in transplant patients, seen in up to 80% of cases, and may in part be related to valve trauma during biopsies.

Transplant coronary disease

Transplant coronary artery disease is the major factor contributing to morbidity and mortality in patients surviving beyond the first year after transplantation. Classical angina may be experienced in up to 50% of patients as the transplanted heart reinnervates. In patients who remain denervated, ischaemia can be silent. Hence in most transplant units routine surveillance by coronary angiography is performed annually or biennially in males, who are most at risk.

There are important morphological differences between coronary artery disease in transplanted versus native hearts. Intimal lesions post transplantation tend in 75%, to be uniform, diffuse, distal and circumferential rather than the eccentric plaques seen in non-transplanted coronaries.[5] Eccentric proximal plaques may be seen in 25% of patients post transplantation, partly from donor coronary artery disease.

Coronary angiography is relatively insensitive in detecting early disease and can be misleading when disease is diffuse, as a uniformly small vessel is seen angiographically. Intracoronary ultrasonography (ICUS) has much greater sensitivity.[6] Pathological vessel wall changes can be demonstrated in over 70% of patients studied with ICUS more than 12 months post transplantation, with coronary angiography detecting abnormalities in only 32%.[7] Intracoronary ultrasonography has the limitation of being unable to sample distally, and structural changes seen may not reflect coronary flow reserve.

Where focal coronary lesions are present, revascularisation with angioplasty and stenting or bypass surgery can be successful in selected patients. Good primary success rates are reported for percutaneous transluminal coronary angioplasty (PTCA) in focal lesions. Nevertheless, a higher rate of restenosis is reported in transplant patients.[8,9]

Bypass surgery has been performed successfully in patients with proximal multi-vessel transplant coronary disease. Care must be taken in patient selection, as high operative mortality is reported in patients with significant distal disease. Some patients may be suited to retransplantation if they are otherwise suitable for re-listing.[8]

References

1. Levine TB, Levine AB, Goldberg AD *et al*. Reversal of end-stage heart failure is predicted by long-term therapeutic response rather than initial hemodynamic and neurohormonal profile. *J Heart Lung Transplant* 1996; **15**:297–303.
2. Mancini DM, Eisen H, Kussmaul W *et al*. Value of peak exercise oxygen consumption for optimal timing of cardiac transplantation in ambulatory patients with heart failure. *Circulation* 1991; **83**:778–86.
3. Mason JW. Endomyocardial biopsy and the causes of dilated cardiomyopathy. (Editorial comment) *J Am Coll Cardiol* 1994; **23**(3):591–2.
4. Kasper EK, Agema WRP, Hutchins GM *et al*. The causes of dilated cardiomyopathy: A clinicopathologic review of 673 consecutive patients. *J Am Coll Cardiol* 1994; **23**(3):586–90.
5. Arbustini E, Roberts WC. Morphological observations in the epicardial coronary arteries and their surroundings late after cardiac transplantation (allograft vascular disease). *Am J Cardiol* 1996; **78**:814–20.
6. Quinn RR, Pflugfelder PW, Goring M *et al*. Threshold plaque burden for angiographic detection of cardiac allograft vasculopathy: Assessment by 3 dimensional intracoronary ultrasound imaging. (Abstract) *J Heart Lung Transplant* 1998; **17**(1):50.
7. Klauss V, Ackermann K, Spes CH *et al*. Coronary plaque morphologic characteristics early and late after heart transplantation: In vivo analysis with intravascular ultrasonography. *Am Heart J*.1997; **133**(1):29–35.
8. Musci M, Loebe M, Wellnhofer E *et al*. Coronary angioplasty, bypass surgery, and retransplantation in cardiac transplant patients with graft coronary disease. *Thorac Cardiovasc Surg* 1998; **46**(5):268–74.
9. Parry A, Roberts M, Parameshwar J *et al*. The management of post-cardiac transplantation coronary artery disease. *Eur J Cardio-thorac Surg* 1996; **10**(7):528–32.

Chapter 27

Cardiac Surgery

David S. Winlaw and Michael K. Wilson

Introduction

The current practice of cardiac surgery is dependent upon accurate diagnosis of specific cardiac problems and the sophisticated application of cardiopulmonary bypass and myocardial protection techniques. These permit anatomical repair or replacement of the structural problem, and have been made possible by giant leaps in the understanding of haemostasis, anticoagulation, membrane oxygenation, cardiopulmonary circulatory physiology and a detailed knowledge of functional cardiac anatomy.

The fundamental principles of cardiac surgery were largely established during the 1960s. Refinements in surgical technique, evolution of cardiopulmonary bypass from bubble oxygenators to membrane oxygenation, and the vastly improved understanding of physiology have lowered the operative mortality from around 30% to less than 1%.

Developments in cardiology have proceeded at a similar pace, with improvements in pharmacology, the advent of angioplasty and stenting, and development of valvuloplasty balloons and devices for closing septal defects. This means that optimal patient management requires a balance between the risks and benefits of medical management with those of interventional cardiology and open heart surgery.

Coronary bypass surgery

The three major indications for coronary re-vascularisation are:

i) **symptomatic**, to relieve angina;
ii) **prognostic**, to prevent myocardial infarction or death;
iii) **combined indications,** e.g. open heart surgery with co-existent coronary artery disease.

Symptomatic indications for myocardial revascularisation may be urgent, as in acute myocardial infarction; semi-urgent, as in unstable angina; or elective, as in stable angina pectoris. Prognostic indications for coronary bypass surgery related to coronary anatomy as displayed by angiography have traditionally been either triple vessel disease or left main coronary artery disease. Symptomatic double vessel disease or single vessel disease that is unsuitable for angioplasty is an acceptable indication for surgery.

Proximal left anterior descending (LAD) artery stenosis, particularly in association with a large first or second diagonal branch, may be better treated by bypass surgery using the left internal mammary artery (LIMA), particularly with the advent of beating heart surgery, as this may offer patency rates of better than 90% at 10–20 years. Restenosis rates

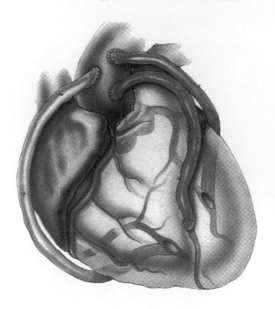

Figure 27.1. Coronary artery surgery with saphenous vein. (From Khonsari S. in Cardiac surgery, 2nd ed. With permission, Lippincott Williams and Wilkins)

of up to 20% after angioplasty and stenting, and the risk of losing a large area of myocardium from an acute occlusion need to be balanced against the morbidity of a bypass operation.

Operative strategy

The goal of bypass surgery is complete myocardial revascularisation, bypassing all vessels with greater than 50% stenosis (75% cross-sectional area loss). Graft patency is maximal when large vessels (>1.5 mm diameter) with high-grade proximal stenoses are grafted. Ten to twenty per cent of coronary bypass operations are re-operations for recurrent disease,

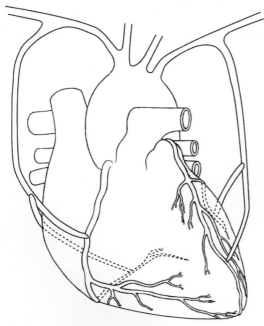

Figure 27.2. Coronary artery bypass grafting with bilateral pedicle internal mammary artery grafts to left anterior descending and right coronary arteries, with 'y' grafts to left circumflex and distal right coronary arteries respectively.

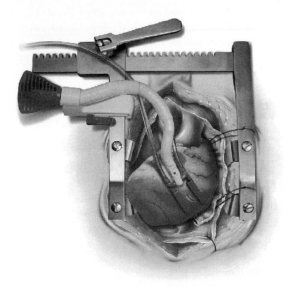

Figure 27.3. The Octopus II Tissue Stabiliser. (Courtesy Medtronic Inc).

usually in the vein grafts used as conduit, or for progression of native disease in the coronary circulation. A pedicle graft of LIMA to LAD has been statistically show to protect against the need for re-operation and death because of its improved long-term patency rate. Existing bypass grafts should be handled carefully during the case to prevent distal atheroembolism, and patent diseased grafts should be replaced.

Coronary artery surgery is generally performed with an arrested heart through a sternotomy, with perfusion supplied by the cardiopulmonary bypass machine. Figure 27.1 demonstrates completed triple coronary artery surgery with saphenous vein grafts performed in this manner. Bilateral mammary grafts may be used and a graft (such as radial artery or saphenous vein) based on the mammary artery itself may be grafted to the circumflex coronary artery or other branches in a 'Y' configuration as shown in Fig. 27.2. Cardiopulmonary bypass provides ideal operating conditions, but is associated with vari-

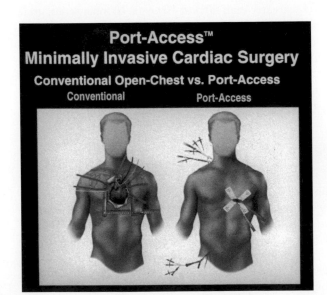

Figure 27.4. Minimally invasive coronary artery surgery using a left anterior small thoracotomy (LAST), also known as MIDCAB (minimally invasive direct coronary artery bypass). For LAD and diagonal grafts using the MIDCAB approach, peripheral bypass is an option (as shown here), but is not usually required.

able lung and neurologic injury. These effects are mild and generally short lived. More recently, surgeons have attempted to reduce the invasiveness of this traditional surgery by altering the site of incision and using stabilisation devices to keep the coronary artery still during the distal anastomosis. Stabilisation devices such as the Medtronic Octopus (Fig. 27.3) are emerging as the principal means of so-called 'off-pump' coronary artery grafting (OPCAB), and multi-graft operations are possible without cardiopulmonary bypass in selected cases. The MIDCAB or LAST technique may be used for isolated grafting of the LAD/diagonal system (Fig. 27.4). These less invasive techniques use pedicled arterial grafting (bilateral IMA) as a means of improving graft patency and reducing manipulation of the ascending aorta, also possibly reducing perioperative stroke.

Operative mortality and morbidity

Overall mortality for cardiac surgery is 3–5%; for a low-risk case it is less than 1%. Five-year survival is 88%, and 10-year survival is 75%. A mammary artery graft (to LAD) favourably affects initial graft patency and mid- to long-term survival. Up to 25% of all deaths after coronary bypass grafting (CAG) are unrelated to ischaemic heart disease. The perioperative infarction rate is 2–5% and freedom from infarction is greater than 95% at five years. Severely impaired cardiac function may be improved where there is stunned, hibernating or dysfunctional ischaemic cardiac muscle that can be revascularised. Extensive scarring and dilatation with end-diastolic ventricular dimensions greater than 7cm is generally associated with a poor result from surgery.

The incidence of major stroke is 1–2% and is raised by increasing age, prior stroke or cerebrovascular aneurysm (CVA) and extensive peripheral vascular disease. Up to 75% of patients may have subtle neurologic deficits in the postoperative period. Severe renal impairment with creatinine levels of 150 μmol/L or more is likely to complicate postoperative recovery and necessitate short- or long-term dialysis. Similarly, respiratory failure is more common when the forced expiratory volume (FEV-1) is less than 50% predicted normal. Permanent haemodialysis is associated with worse graft patency and decreased 5-year survival (50–70%).

Conduit patency rates

Patency of a LIMA graft to the LAD is greater than 90% at 10 years. In some series, graft patency is similar at 20 years. Reversed saphenous vein graft patency has a progressive decline of patency from 70–80 % at 5 years, to around 50% at 10 years, and 20–30% at 20 years. Long-term radial artery graft patency rates are not yet available, but it is believed they will be an improvement over saphenous vein grafts. There has, however, been a significant rate of early graft occlusion. Gastroepiploeic arterial grafts have patency rates of 80–90% at 5–10 years. Freedom from angina is expected to be >90% at one year and 60% at 10 years.

Blood testing for emergency surgery

Emergency transfer of a patient from the catheterisation laboratory for urgent bypass surgery is a rare but realistic possibility. Amid the urgency of stabilising and preparing the patient for transfer, it is necessary to organise a profile of pathology testing prior to surgery. Most commonly ordered tests include (i) a full blood count, (ii) coagulation studies, (iii) renal function and liver function tests, (iv) electrolyte levels and (v) blood group identification for future cross-match.

The full blood count determines (i) haemoglobin level for the patient's ability to transport oxygen, (ii) white cell count for ability to combat infection or foreign bodies and

(iii) platelet count for ability to stem bleeding. Coagulation studies should include both INR and APTT to fully assess both arms of the coagulation cascade (see Chapter 12).

Immunohaematology (Blood Bank) testing usually consists of a 'group and hold' request, which permits cross-matching of packed cells. If necessary, group specific platelets and fresh frozen plasma (FFP) can then be quickly prepared.

Renal function tests (serum urea and creatinine) assess baseline renal function. Exacerbation of renal dysfunction is not uncommon in patients with existing renal disease and may disturb bioavailability of drug metabolites excreted by the kidneys. Similarly, liver function tests assess the patient's ability to metabolise and clear drugs from the liver. Sodium, potassium, calcium and magnesium levels assess the potential for arrhythmia arising from an electrolyte imbalance. Serum glucose levels demonstrate glucose metabolism or diabetic control.

Common postoperative complications

Arrhythmia

The incidence of significant rhythm disturbance is 20–30% for post-bypass patients. It is necessary to determine the nature and effect of the arrhythmia, e.g. fast vs. slow, atrial vs. ventricular, and the degree of haemodynamic compromise. Evaluation of the clinical significance of the arrhythmia includes measurement of heart rate (HR), blood pressure (BP), filling pressures, electrocardiogram (ECG), and serum potassium, magnesium and creatinine levels. Management includes electrolyte replacement, administration of pharmaceuticals (sotolol, amiodarone, digoxin) and cardioversion.

Atrial fibrillation (AF)

AF may be treated with sotolol 40–80 mg bd for patients with new-onset AF and normal ventricular function, with no asthma or other contraindications for sotolol. For patients with impaired ventricular function, or in whom sotolol is contraindicated, amiodarone should be used. An initial dose of 150–300 mg is given over 30 minutes, and either an oral loading regimen of 200–400 mg three times a day is commenced, or an infusion of 900 mg is commenced over 24 hours. The dose of amiodarone is reviewed daily, and decreased appropriately. Ideally the patient should be discharged on a single daily dose of amiodarone. Patients in chronic AF are usually on digoxin and this should continue post operation. Digoxin may be used with amiodarone if further rate control is required. However, amiodarone will increase the digoxin levels and the risk of digoxin toxicity. Digoxin is also a good agent for AF in association with rheumatic valve disease and impaired ventricular function.

Contraindications to Sotolol

History of bronchial asthma or severe chronic airways limitation (CAL)
Patients with clinical heart failure
Ventricular rate <80 bpm or systolic BP<90 mmHg
Documented history of significant bradyarrhythmias
History of drug-induced *torsade de pointes*
Renal impairment.

Hypokalemia

After cardiac surgery, potassium should be maintained in the upper normal range (4.5–5.0). This decreases the incidence of postoperative AF. A potassium level less than 4.0

mmol/L should be treated by oral or intravenous potassium supplementation (e.g. 2–4 g Slow-K orally). Patients on Lasix may require regular potassium supplements. Patients with renal failure are prone to hyperkalemia and care should be exercised with any supplementation.

Magnesium

Hypomagnesaemia (Mg <0.7 mmol/L) should be treated by oral or intravenous magnesium supplements. Increasing Mg levels are thought to protect against ventricular arrhythmias, ectopy and atrial fibrillation.

Anticoagulation

Patients in AF receive subcutaneous heparin, typically 5000 units thrice daily. In some cases, such as patients with large left atria and poor cardiac function, systemic anticoagulation with IV heparin may be required. The need for anticoagulation before DC cardioversion is controversial becuase of the potential risk of stroke (from thromboembolism) at the time of electrical reversion. For patients with good ventricular function and postoperative AF despite pharmacological treatment, early cardioversion without systemic heparinisation has been considered safe.

Cardiac failure

In general, patients with documented congestive cardiac failure should be commenced on afterload reduction postoperatively. An ACE inhibitor should be added to their usual medications. The dose should be increased gradually from days 1 to 2 onwards, titrated according to their systemic blood pressure (BP) and renal function. Increased doses of diuretic are often required.

Hypertension

Hypertension is common post operation and requires adequate control. The patient's usual medications can be restarted or increased. Patients who have had aortic surgery, valve repair or transplantation need particularly vigilant BP control. Short-acting agents for immediate control are hydralazine, sublingual nifedipine and topical nitrates. Maintenance anti-hypertensive medication can be increased and includes beta-blockers, ACE inhibitors, calcium channel blockers and diuretics. Severe hypertension places the patient at risk of convulsions or aortic rupture and should be controlled in intensive care with short-acting agents such as esmolol, sodium nitroprusside or diazoxide.

Hypotension

Hypotension is ominous and may result from preload, afterload or muscle pump imbalances. Investigation includes particular attention to hydration (central venous pressure, peripheral oedema, fluid balance and weight), cardiac function, new ischaemia, new murmurs (mitral dysfunction) and evidence of sepsis or arrhythmias. Pericardial tamponade occurs relatively infrequently but may present insidiously with decreased urine output, increasing creatinine level and borderline haemodynamics. Cardiac echocardiography should be considered early in the series of investigations in any cardiac patient whose clinical condition has worsened unexpectedly, or whose pericardial silhouette is enlarged on chest x-ray.

Atelectasis

Atelectasis (alveolar collapse) is extremely common and is treated by mobilisation and chest physiotherapy. Persistent collapse may require continuous positive airway pressure (CPAP), mini-tracheostomy or re-intubation. Infection should be considered early and treated with intravenous antibiotics.

Decreased urine output

A fall in urine output may be due to pre-renal, renal, or post-renal factors. Pre-renal factors include hypovolaemia and low cardiac output. Renal factors include pre-existing renal disease, and nephrotoxicity due to drug side effects and acute tubular necrosis secondary to prolonged hypotension. Ureteric and urethral obstruction should also be considered. Pre-renal causes can be treated by fluid replacement with blood, colloid or normal saline. In the presence of fluid overload, hypotension requires inotropic support, preferably with low-dose dopamine, which also increases renal perfusion. Intravenous diuretic therapy should be administered once the fluid balance has been optimised. In-dwelling catheters should also be checked for evidence of obstruction.

Venous thrombosis

Venous thrombosis should be treated with a heparin infusion in accordance with current heparin policy. Patients already on warfarin with a therapeutic international normalised ratio (INR) may not need additional treatment.

Cardiac valve surgery

Overview

When valve replacement was first recognised as safe and effective in the 1960s, rheumatic valvular disease was the commonest indication for surgery; now congenital and degenerative pathology account for the majority of referrals. Referral for valve repair and replace-

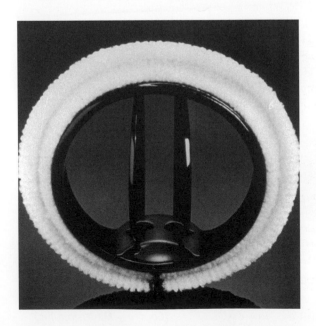

Figure 27.5. St Jude Bileaflet Valve. (Courtesy St Jude Inc).

ment is now made earlier in the natural history of the disease because timely correction may prevent irreversible decline in ventricular function and improve life expectancy.

Several problems remain, such as the complications of long-term anticoagulation, deterioration of bio-prostheses over time, and the small risk associated with surgery itself. This section details the options available for surgical correction and how management is individualised.

Choice of valve

Valve performance is judged using the following parameters:

1. Freedom from structural valve deterioration, or how well the valve copes with haemodynamic stresses and the rate of 'wear and tear'.
2. Haemodynamic performance: This describes any device-related obstruction to flow and regurgitation across the valve.
3. Requirement for anticoagulation: Mechanical valves require lifelong anticoagulation, bioprostheses (tissue valves) and homografts do not.
4. Thromboembolic and bleeding complications: This term describes morbidity and mortality from stroke, peripheral emboli and bleeding complications for a typical population, usually measured in events per patient year.
5. Susceptibility to infection: Biological materials may be more resistant to infection than mechanical valves.

The ideal valve would function indefinitely, mimic the haemodynamics of a normal human valve, not require anticoagulation and be resistant to infection. These characteristics are not found in any single valve replacement device. For individual patients, a risk-benefit analysis is made weighing the benefits of a durable valve against the inconvenience of anticoagulation with warfarin. In other patients, the risk of re-operation for a failing bioprosthesis is weighed against the risks of anticoagulation. Patients requiring anticoagulation for other reasons, commonly atrial fibrillation, generally receive mechanical valves.

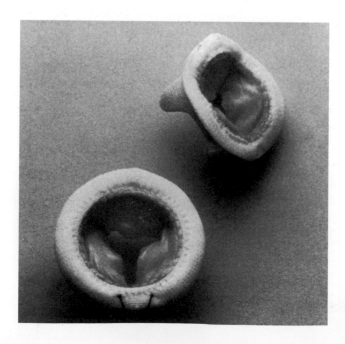

Figure 27.6. Mosaic bioprosthetic Valve. (Courtesy Medtronic Inc).

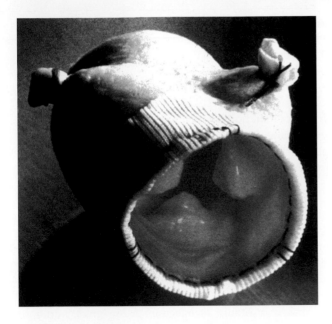

Figure 27.7. Freestyle stentless bioprosthetic aortic valve. (Courtesy Medtronic Inc).

Patients frequently have strong feelings about what sort of valve should be implanted because of lifestyle factors (frequent travel, sport), geographic isolation from medical services, or dislike of regular medication, all of which make effective and safe anticoagulation difficult.

Mechanical valves

Although they are very durable, mechanical valves require warfarin therapy for life. The housing in which the valve mechanism sits is partially obstructive to flow, generating a small pressure gradient across the valve, particularly in small-sized prostheses. Most mechanical valves allow a small amount of regurgitation to wash the hinge mechanism. This clears the leaflet pivot points and reduces the likelihood of thromboembolism. Mechanical valves, including the commonly used St Jude device (Fig. 27.5), consist of a sewing ring and a bi-leaflet-hinged valve made of pyrolite carbon. The sewing ring is used to secure the prosthesis in position. There is no metal in this new generation of valves, unlike their predecessors, although the term 'metal valve' persists. The modern bi-leaflet valves (St Jude Medical and Carbomedics) as well as the Medtronic-Hall tilting disc valve, have good haemodynamic characteristics with minimal obstruction to flow. Ball-and-cage valves, such as the Starr-Edwards device are more bulky and less favorable haemodynamically, yet are still very durable. In most circumstances, a mechanical valve will last more than 30 years given effective anticoagulation and freedom from infection.

Bioprosthetic valves

These devices do not require anticoagulation, but may only last 8–15 years. Biological surfaces, including those from the pig, have low thrombogenicity in high-flow situations. Most bioprosthetic valves are made of porcine valve leaflets, suspended from a dacron-covered scaffold or stent (Baxter Carpentier-Edwards and Medtronic Intact and Mosaic valves) (Fig. 27.6). Pig pericardium may also be used in these so-called 'stented porcine bioprostheses'. Most institutions use warfarin for six weeks postoperatively, until the valve and its sewing ring become endothelialised and resistant to thrombus formation. Wear and tear causes failure of complete coaption, causing regurgitation. This may occur in

5–10 years for a young active patient. In the elderly, the typical lifespan of prosthetic valves is 10–15 years. For this reason their use is generally limited to patients over 70. For patients with a small aortic annulus, small bioprostheses may be unacceptably obstructive to flow.

Newer bioprostheses are available without the stent housing from which the valve leaflets are suspended. These so called 'stentless bioprostheses' include the Medtronic Freestyle (Fig. 27.7), the St Jude Medical and the CryoLife O'Brien valves. These valves have significantly better haemodynamics than both stented bioprostheses and mechanical valves. Their insertion is more technically demanding and involves a longer operation. Their long-term freedom from structural valve deterioration is not yet known. It is possible that new anti-calcification treatments used on these valves may further improve their durability.

Human heart valves

Obtained from organ donors or cadavers, human heart valves provide an alternative form of replacement. These 'homografts' or 'human allografts' do not require anticoagulation and have good durability and haemodynamics. Valves are preserved by freezing and are stored in a valve bank prior to use. They require special expertise to implant and, as with other donor organs, are always in short supply. They are in demand for the treatment of complicated endocarditis because of their resistance to infection. A low-grade immunological response is mounted against the valve, which may contribute to its failure in 15–20 years.

Ross procedure

Another approach to aortic replacement in the young (<45 years) and active has been developed. The 'Ross Procedure' involves removal of the diseased aortic valve, and replacement with the patient's own pulmonary valve as an autograft. A pulmonary homograft is then used in the pulmonary position. This has several advantages in that the pulmonary valve functions and lasts very well in the aortic position. A homograft in the low-pressure pulmonary position is thought to last longer than in the aortic position, where it is exposed to systemic pressure and greater 'wear and tear'. Furthermore, pulmonary regurgitation is better tolerated than aortic regurgitation. It is a technically demanding operation and is dependent on homograft availability. Excellent freedom from structural valve deterioration is achieved (>15 years) although the pulmonary homograft may require replacement.

Repair vs replacement

Valve repair involves tailoring the valve and its supporting structures to remedy stenosis or regurgitation. The mitral valve is better suited to repair than the aortic valve, which is rarely repairable. Common pathologies such as mitral valve prolapse and myxomatous degeneration of mitral valve leaflets cause leaflet redundancy and annular dilatation, which are amenable to repair. These may be corrected by excising portions of valve leaflet and using a ring to reduce annular size. Pathology involving the anterior leaflet is less suitable for repair compared to isolated posterior leaflet pathology. Bileaflet prolapse is difficult to repair and usually requires valve replacement.

In the mitral position, a good repair is better than a replacement, as long-term anticoagulation is not required, valve function is near normal, and further deterioration is unlikely. Maintaining the chordal attachments between papillary muscle and valve leaflet is important in the long-term preservation of ventricular function.

Timing of surgery

There is an optimal time for elective surgery in the natural history of valvular heart disease. The cardiovascular system can compensate for quite significant disease over time, a good example of which is the left ventricular hypertrophy occurring in patients with aortic stenosis. Beyond this point, irreversible changes may occur, exemplified by ventricular dysfunction in patients with gross ventricular dilatation resulting from aortic regurgitation. Valve surgery should be performed at a point when exposure to operative risk and possible anti-coagulation thereafter are warranted because of developing symptoms or echocardiographic findings. The patient's age, co-existing illnesses and lifestyle factors will affect this timing.

Women of childbearing age are usually offered a tissue valve, either a homograft or a Ross (pulmonary autograft) procedure because of the risk of birth defects with maternal warfarin therapy. Valve replacement may need to be performed before pregnancy because of the demand pregnancy places on the cardiovascular system. For those with a mechanical valve who are planning pregnancy, low molecular weight heparin is used instead of warfarin therapy.

Common pathologies, indications for operation and surgical solutions

Aortic valve disease

Indications for aortic valve replacement for aortic stenosis (AS) include symptomatic disease (syncope, angina, congestive heart failure), haemodynamically severe AS as measured by echocardiography and cardiac catheterisation (gradient ≥ 50 mmHg or aortic valve area <0.75 cm^2) and progression of left ventricular (LV) hypertrophy or decline in LV function in patients with asymptomatic AS. Patients with poor LV function and severe AS may not generate high gradients, and valve area is a better guide to severity of AS. Operation for aortic regurgitation (AR) is indicated in all patients with significant LV dysfunction and LV dilation as assessed by echocardiography (left ventricular end-diastolic dimension > 60-65 mm), or LV systolic dimension >55 mm.

Aortic valve surgery is frequently required in conditions that affect the ascending aorta, such as aortic dissection and aneurysmal dilatation. In aortic dissection, the aortic valve is frequently deformed by blood tracking between the layers of the aortic wall, causing aortic regurgitation. Aneurysmal dilatation, such as that caused by Marfan's disease, causes aortic regurgitation as a result of annular dilatation.

Aortic stenosis in the elderly

Calcification of an otherwise normal tri-leaflet valve is a frequent cause of aortic stenosis in the elderly. The heaped-up deposits of calcium restrict leaflet movement and sometimes penetrate the conduction system, giving heart block. These patients are generally more than 65 years of age and have significant left ventricular hypertrophy. Coronary artery disease may co-exist. Seventy years of age is a commonly used cut-off point for use of mechanical valves, after which a bioprosthesis is unlikely to require replacement within a normal life expectancy. A stentless xenograft may be an option in an otherwise fit person, as superior haemodynamics and regression of left ventricular hypertrophy are achieved. If warfarin were required for other reasons, such as chronic atrial fibrillation, then a

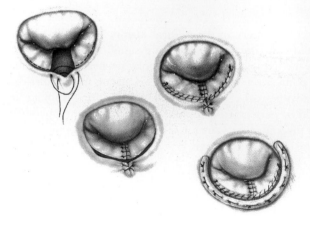

Figure 27.8. Mitral valve repair with quadrangular resection of posterior mitral leaflet and annuloplasty ring. (From Khonsari S. in Cardiac surgery, 2nd ed. With permission, Lippincott Williams and Wilkins).

mechanical valve would be used because of its better haemodynamics. Elderly symptomatic patients with aortic stenosis but in otherwise good health have been shown to benefit from valve replacement even into their eighties. Despite advanced age, replacement can be performed with an acceptable risk considering the improvement in functional status.

Aortic stenosis in the young and middle aged

This is usually due to a congenitally abnormal valve. It is often bicuspid, or functionally bicuspid with fusion of two of the normal three leaflets. This abnormal valve becomes calcified early in life, causing stenosis or mixed stenosis and regurgitation. In young people who are active and/or of childbearing potential, warfarin cannot be used because of its limitations on lifestyle and teratogenic risk. A biological valve may then be used, either as

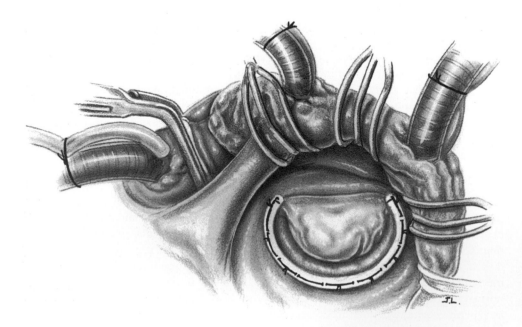

Figure 27.9. Mitral annuloplasty with Cosgrove-Edwards annuloplasty ring. (Courtesy Baxter Healthcare Pty Ltd Australia).

a Ross-pulmonary autograft procedure, or as an aortic homograft. In both cases, a second operation is inevitable within 10–20 years, by which time a mechanical valve may be acceptable. Stented bioprostheses are unsuitable because of their rapid structural deterioration in active people, particularly in the mitral position.

Endocarditis

When an operation is required for this condition it is treated with a tissue replacement, either a homograft or unstented xenograft. Where vegetations are limited to the valve leaflets (which are excised) and the annulus is not involved, a mechanical prosthesis may be used. Tissue valves are preferred because they are considered to be less susceptible to persisting infection. Abscess formation sometimes involves the aortic root, anterior leaflet of the mitral valve, septal structures and conduction tissue. These patients require extensive surgical reconstruction and may need urgent operation to control sepsis since the abscess cavities are not well penetrated by antibiotics.

Mitral valve disease

Indications for mitral valve surgery depend on the presentation. Patients who present in shock with acute severe mitral regurgitation due to ruptured chordae or ischaemic rupture of a papillary muscle require urgent operation. Patients with chronic mitral regurgitation should undergo operation before volume overload causes significant LV dysfunction. Unlike aortic valve disease, significant improvements in LV function are uncommon following valve replacement. Patients with mitral stenosis generally undergo mitral valve replacement when the mitral valve area is below 1 cm², or 1.5 cm² when mixed stenosis and regurgitation exist. Significant symptoms such as episodic pulmonary oedema prompt surgery, despite larger valve orifices.

Rheumatic mitral disease

Until the 1970s rheumatic mitral disease was common, and remains a common illness in the developing world. When stenosis predominates, percutaneous balloon valvuloplasty (see Chapter 24) may be successful in splitting the fused valvular commissures. This is the modern equivalent of closed mitral valvotomy performed through a left thoracotomy, without use of cardiopulmonary bypass. A risk of all blind valvotomies is the creation of mitral regurgitation when the valve does not split along the commissures. To avoid this, open commissurotomy may be performed via sternotomy using cardiopulmonary bypass. Where mixed stenosis and regurgitation co-exist, scarring and shortening of the leaflets and subvalvar apparatus usually necessitate valve replacement. Mechanical valves are mostly used because of their superior haemodynamics, and because warfarin treatment is required for atrial fibrillation, which frequently co-exists. Bioprostheses may be used in the treatment of mitral valve disease in the very elderly with contraindications to warfarin.

Myxomatous or 'floppy' mitral valves causing regurgitation

As discussed earlier, these valves may be repaired. This involves resection of the abnormal portion of the valve, and parts not supported by chordae. Better long-term results may be achieved when an annuloplasty ring is used, resizing the annulus and preventing loss of coaption from further annular dilation (Fig. 27.8). In this group, the benefits of repair over replacement are well proven, not only because warfarin can be avoided but also because LV function is better preserved with repair. Valve repair is also suitable for patients with ruptured chordae.

Chronic ischaemic mitral regurgitation

This is due to wall motion abnormalities and papillary muscle dysfunction caused by coronary insufficiency. Annular dilation is secondary to volume overload and worsens regurgitation. When the subvalvular apparatus is intact, regurgitation may be treated by reduction annuloplasty, using a ring or band (Fig. 27.9), at the same time as coronary artery bypass grafts are performed. Valve preservation with possible improvement in LV function generally makes repair a better solution than replacement.

Prosthetic valve endocarditis: Treatment and prevention

Prosthetic valve endocarditis (PVE) occurs when microorganisms settle on the foreign surfaces of the valve. It is a serious complication because medical treatment for PVE is less successful than for native valves, and re-do valve replacement is frequently required. The incidence of PVE is around 0.5–1% per patient year, and is said to be less common in xenografted than mechanical valves. Freedom from PVE at 10 years following the primary operation is more than 95% for all types of valves.

Antibiotic prophylaxis should be given to all patients with prosthetic valves undergoing even minor procedures, in accordance with local protocols. One such protocol for dental, oral, respiratory tract and oesophageal procedures may be a single 2g dose of amoxicillin given orally one hour before the procedure. In those allergic to penicillins, clindamycin 600 mg or vancomycin is administered. The same doses may be given IV if oral administration is not possible. For genitourinary and gastrointestinal procedures (excluding oesophageal) ampicillin 2g IV and gentamicin 1.5 mg/kg IV should be given, or vancomycin 1g IV in penicillin-allergic patients. Where skin incisions or percutaneous puncture are involved, staphylococcal prophylaxis should be given, using a first-generation cephalosporin such as cefazolin 500 mg q8h for 24 hours. Where medically resistant *Staphalococcus aureus* (MRSA) is prevalent, vancomycin should be used as gram positive cover.

Postoperative management of anticoagulation

The importance of anticoagulation must be reinforced to all patients requiring warfarin therapy. It is often a cause of patient concern, resulting in poor compliance. Dietary and monitoring advice must be understood before discharge. It is likely that home testing kits using finger-prick blood samples, in the way a diabetic tests blood sugar level, will be widely available in the next 5 years. The following information is intended as a guide to typical practice.

Mechanical valves

Subcutaneous heparin (5000 units tds) is commenced, usually in the evening on the day of operation. Warfarin is started in the evening of the first postoperative day. Heparin is ceased when the INR is 2.0 or more.

The following are guidelines only, and require individualisation:

Aortic valve replacement with mechanical bi-leaflet device:	INR 2.0–3.0
Mitral valve replacement in sinus rhythm and normal sized left atrium:	INR 2.5–3.5
Mitral valve replacement in AF or with enlarged left atrium:	INR 3.0–3.5

Stented xenograft (standard tissue valve)

Subcutaneous heparin 5000 tds until warfarin therapeutic.
Warfarin, INR 2–3 for 6 weeks. (Some surgeons may choose aspirin only.)

Aortic homograft or Ross procedure

Subcutaneous heparin 5000 tds for 4 days.

Unstented xenograft

Subcutaneous heparin 5000 tds for 4 days.
Aspirin 150 mg daily for 3 months (some surgeons may choose warfarin for 6 weeks)

Mitral valve repair

Subcutaneous heparin 5000 tds until INR therapeutic.
Warfarin, INR 2–3, for 6 weeks if annuloplasty ring used.

Results and complications of valve surgery

Thirty-day mortality for aortic valve replacement is approximately 3–5%. Mitral valve repair can be accomplished with a 0.5–2% early mortality and freedom from re-operation at five years of 85%. Mitral valve replacement incorporates a much higher-risk group of patients, for whom the 30-day mortality is in the vicinity of 5–8%. Individual patients may be quoted a higher or lower risk on the basis of youth or advanced age and the presence of other problems such as coronary disease, impaired left ventricular function or pulmonary hypertension.

The usual risks of cardiac surgery and cardiopulmonary bypass exist, including bleeding and wound infection. Risk of stroke is higher than that of routine coronary surgery, because it is 'open' heart surgery. There is the possibility of particulate and air embolism causing stroke, occurring at a rate of 2–3%. Injury to the conduction system requiring a permanent pacemaker is uncommon, but may occur particularly with aortic valve replacement, even more particularly when severe annular calcification is present. Pacemaker requirement is less than 2% for most valvular surgery.

Conclusion

With the development of effective percutaneous therapies, in particular coronary stenting, the indications for cardiac surgery are changing. Increasingly, patients with impaired left ventricular function, relatively poor distal vessels and multisystem disease such as diabetes are being shown to benefit from surgical intervention. For others, such as those with isolated LAD disease, surgery offers a lasting solution, reducing the need for anti-anginal medication. Reductions in perioperative risk mandate early repair of valve lesions causing mitral regurgitation, and replacement of the aortic valve.

In this era, discussions between cardiologist and cardiac surgeon permit the individualisation of treatment and optimal patient outcomes.

Further Reading

Edmunds LH Jr (ed). *Cardiac surgery in the adult.* New York: McGraw Hill 1997.
American Heart Association: www.americanheart.org/Scientific/statements/
Khonsari S. *Cardiac surgery - Safeguards and pitfalls in operative technique.* Philadelphia: Lippincott-Raven 1997.

Chapter 28

Angiogenesis and Gene Therapy

Peter R. Vale, Douglas W. Losordo and Jeffrey M. Isner

Summary

Ischaemic muscle represents a promising target for gene therapy with naked plasmid DNA. Striated and cardiac muscles have been shown to take up and express naked plasmid DNA as well as transgenes incorporated into viral vectors. Moreover, previous studies have shown that the transfection efficiency of intramuscular gene transfer is augmented more than five-fold when the injected muscle is ischaemic.

Intramuscular (IM) transfection of genes encoding angiogenic cytokines, particularly those that are naturally secreted by intact cells, is designed to promote the development of supplemental collateral blood vessels that will constitute endogenous bypass conduits around occluded native arteries: a strategy termed 'therapeutic angiogenesis.' In the case of critical limb and myocardial ischaemia, this strategy may constitute an alternative means of treatment for patients in whom contemporary therapies (anti-anginal medications, angioplasty, bypass surgery) have previously failed or are not feasible.

Pre-clinical and human studies suggest that site-specific IM gene transfer of naked plasmid DNA encoding for vascular endothelial growth factor ($phVEGF_{165}$) may promote therapeutic angiogenesis in critical limb ischaemia and more recently in myocardial ischaemia as well. A phase 1, dose-escalating, open-label clinical study was undertaken to determine the safety and bioactivity of direct myocardial gene transfer of naked plasmid DNA encoding for VEGF as sole therapy for patients with symptomatic myocardial ischaemia. Initial results demonstrated that safe and successful transfection can be achieved with a favourable clinical effect. This is supported by objective evidence of improved myocardial perfusion.

Alternatively, early reports from pre-clinical studies suggest that catheter-based myocardial gene transfer is feasible and can be safely and reliably performed. The availability of a catheter-based system for reliable percutaneous myocardial gene delivery coupled to an electromechanical mapping system would obviate the current need for operative thoracotomy, allow the incorporation of a clinical placebo group and permit detailed testing of cardiovascular gene therapy designed to target impaired myocardial function.

Angiogenesis

The establishment and maintenance of a vascular supply is an absolute requirement for growth of normal or neoplastic tissue. Two process are responsible for the formation of simple, endothelium-lined, capillary-like tubes: **Vasculogenesis** is the *de novo in-situ* differentiation of endothelial cells (ECs) from mesodermal precursors in the embryo by association of angioblasts; their subsequent reorganisation into a primary capillary plexus is restricted to early embryogenesis. **Angiogenesis** is the formation of new blood vessels by a process of sprouting from pre-existing vessels, and is characterised and modulated by interactions between stimulators and inhibitors of angiogenesis. This process results from an increase in endothelial mitogens and membrane receptors found in response to angiogenic stimuli such as hypoxia, ischaemia, mechanical stretch and inflammation. Angiogenesis can be both physiological and pathological. The former includes processes such as wound healing and the female reproductive cycle, whereas the latter includes tumor growth, rheumatoid arthritis and diabetic retinopathy.

Folkman and colleagues[1] established that ECs may migrate, proliferate and remodel in response to certain growth factors, and in so doing form new sprouts from parent vessels. This constitutes angiogenesis. A series of polypeptide growth factors has subsequently been purified, sequenced, and demonstrated to be responsible for natural as well as pathologic angiogenesis. It is now clear that bone-marrow-derived endothelial progenitor cells (EPCs) contribute to such neovascular networks as well.[2]

Mechanisms of angiogenesis

The full paradigm for angiogenesis[3] has been suggested to begin with 'activation' of ECs by a local angiogenic stimulus within a parent vessel, causing local vasodilatation, increased vascular permeability and accumulation of extra-vascular fibrin. This is followed by disruption of the basement membrane and subsequent migration of ECs into the interstitial space, possibly in the direction of an ischaemic stimulus. Concomitant and/or subsequent EC proliferation, intracellular-vacuolar lumen formation, pericyte 'capping' and production of a basement membrane complete the developmental sequence.

During angiogenesis, migration precedes proliferation by approximately 24 hours.[4] In contrast to *in vivo* inflammatory models, angiogenesis that develops in response to experimental vascular obstruction, i.e. collateral vessel development, has been shown by several investigators to involve proliferation of not only ECs, but also vascular smooth muscle cells (VSMC). Several important principles were elucidated by these studies:

1. Evidence of EC proliferation is nearly absent in normal arteries,[5] a finding consistent with an estimated EC turnover time of 'thousands of days' in quiescent microvasculature. Even a relatively low percentage of EC proliferation observed in response to arterial occlusion or exogenous growth factors may therefore represent considerable enhancement of EC proliferative activity, and is sufficient to provide the basis for new blood vessel formation.

2. EC proliferation that contributes to naturally occurring collateral development in the setting of vascular occlusion varies from <1% to 6% in various animal models.[6,7]

3. Proliferation of SMCs, the additional requisite cell type for the formation of larger blood vessels, is an implicit component of angiogenesis, regardless of animal species or circulatory site.

4. Proliferative activity (for SMCs as well as ECs) is highest at the level of the smallest-diameter collateral vessels, the so-called midzone collateral segments.

5. While evidence of EC and SMC proliferation alone does not necessarily distinguish new vessel development from an increase in the size of pre-existing vessels, adjunctive data regarding increased capillary density[8] support the notion that proliferative activity does in fact reflect true angiogenesis.

Post-natal vasculogenesis

In the embryonic yolk sac, vasculogenesis involves growth and fusion of multiple blood islands that ultimately give rise to the yolk sac capillary network. After the onset of blood circulation, this network differentiates into an arteriovenous system.[9] Hematopoietic stem cells (HSCs), destined to generate circulating blood cells, are situated in the centre of the blood island. Endothelial progenitor cells (EPCs), or angioblasts, principally responsible for the vessels themselves, are located at the periphery. In addition, HSCs and EPCs share certain antigenic determinants, including Flk-1, Tie-2, Sca-1 and CD-34. These progenitor cells are consequently considered to be derived from a common precursor, putatively termed a hemangioblast.[10]

Postnatal neovascularisation has been previously considered to result exclusively from the proliferation, migration, and remodelling of fully differentiated ECs derived from pre-existing blood vessels, i.e. angiogenesis. The formation of blood vessels from endothelial progenitor cells (EPCs) or angioblasts (i.e. vasculogenesis) has been considered restricted to embryogenesis (Fig. 28.1). Our laboratory reasoned, however, that use of HSCs derived from peripheral blood in lieu of bone marrow to provide sustained hematopoietic recovery constituted inferential evidence for circulating stem cells. Circulating CD34 antigen-positive EPCs were recently isolated from adult species and shown to differentiate along an endothelial cell lineage *in vitro*.[11] EPCs administered systemically to animals with operatively induced hind-limb ischaemia were found to incorporate into foci of neovascularisation in ischaemic muscles of the affected hindlimb. These findings, together with other recent studies[12] have been interpreted as evidence for postnatal 'vasculogenesis'.

EC activation status is determined by a balance between positive and negative regulators, controlled by paracrine signals from angiogenic growth factors such as vascular endothelial growth factor (VEGF), fibroblast growth factor (FGF) and angiopoietins 1 & 2. These growth factors regulate angiogenesis by their ability to act as mitogens for EC, either directly or indirectly by inducing the production of direct-acting regulators by inflammatory and

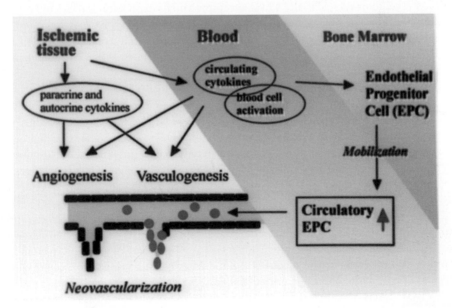

Figure 28.1. Key mechanisms related to angiogenesis.

other non-endothelial cells. These factors or cytokines bind to and modulate the activity of transmembrane receptor tyrosine kinases (RTKs). VEGF binds to two such receptors on endothelial cells (*vide infra*). Angiopoietin 1 & 2 bind to another RTK called Tie 2, producing two opposing effects on this process. Basic FGF is believed to bind to independent RTKs on the cell surface.

Two major factors have been used to induce therapeutic angiogenesis in clinically relevant animal models: 1) Vascular endothelial growth factor (VEGF) and 2) Fibroblast growth factor (FGF).

Vascular endothelial growth factor

Four human VEGF genes have been identified to date: VEGF-1, VEGF-2, VEGF-3, and PIGF. Each is encoded by a different gene, and is localised to a different chromosome, but all share considerable homology. The proteins expressed from these genes are found in many tissues and are enriched in cardiac and skeletal muscle. However, there is considerable divergence of bioactivity that is most likely due to different affinities to the three known endothelial-specific fms-like tyrosine kinases VEGFR-1 (Flt-1), VEGFR-2 (Flk-1/KDR) and VEGFR-3. Flt-1 generates signals that organise the assembly of endothelial cells into tubes and functional vessels while Flk-1/KDR is responsible for endothelial cell proliferation and migration. Hypoxia induces formation of VEGF by endothelial cells and leads to up-regulation of the VEGF receptors.[13]

The initially described vascular endothelial growth factor, VEGF, also known as vascular permeability factor (VPF), and renamed VEGF-A or VEGF-1, is a high-affinity ligand for VEGFR-1 and VEGFR-2, which are expressed specifically on endothelial cells. VEGF-C or VEGF-2[14] and VEGF-B or VEGF-3,[15] have been recently isolated and shown to be abundantly expressed in highly vascularised tissues such as heart and skeletal muscle. VEGF-C/VEGF-2 was shown to bind another recently identified endothelium-specific receptor tyrosine kinase, VEGFR-3 (Flt-4); in addition, VEGF-C binds to VEGFR-2 but not to VEGFR-1.[14] The Flt-4 receptor is related to the VEGF receptors and its expression is restricted mainly to lymphatic endothelia during development. The receptors for VEGF-B have not been characterised to date. The fourth member of the VEGF family, placenta growth factor (PIGF),[16] appears restricted *in vivo* to placenta and certain tumors. It binds with high affinity to VEGFR-1 but not to VEGFR-2 or VEGFR-3.

VEGFs, like other angiogenic growth factors (e.g. FGF), have the ability to stimulate migration and growth of endothelial cells (ECs). However, two features distinguish VEGF from other heparin-binding, angiogenic growth factors. First, VEGF contains a typical signal sequence that, unlike bFGF, allows it to be secreted by intact cells.[17] Second, its high-affinity binding sites are present on ECs, but not other cell types; consequently, the mitogenic effects of VEGF (in contrast to acidic and basic FGF, both of which are known to be mitogenic for smooth muscle cells and fibroblasts as well as endothelial cells) are limited to endothelial cells.[18,19]

The role of VEGF-1 has been studied extensively *in vivo* and *in vitro* (*vide infra*) and has been established as critical for development[20,21] and maintenance[22,23] of the normal vasculature, as well as for therapeutic[24-26] and tumor-induced[27] angiogenesis. VEGF-1 has recently been shown to be expressed in the media of human arteries and veins,[28] consistent with the proposed role of maintaining integrity of the vascular endothelium.

VEGF-1 and VEGF-2 are homologous proteins. While the VEGF-2 precursor is a much longer polypeptide than the VEGF-1 precursor, both proteins undergo post-translational processing and, in their mature forms, exist primarily as homodimers with a monomer size of about 20 kD. The central homology domains of VEGF-1 and VEGF-2 are 32% identical and 48% similar at the amino acid level, and both contain the 8-cysteine residues and the 13-amino acid signature sequence characteristic of the VEGF family of growth factors.

Data regarding the bioactivity of VEGF-2 is limited. Initial evidence for the growth-promoting effects of VEGF-2 were limited to findings that constitutive overexpression of VEGF-2 in the skin of transgenic mice resulted in lymphatic, but not vascular, endothelial proliferation and vessel enlargement.[29] In contrast, VEGF-1 regulates angiogenesis but does not promote lymphangiogenesis. More recently, VEGF-2 was shown to stimulate migration of capillary endothelial cells *in vitro*, suggesting that its effects may extend beyond the lymphatic system, where Flt-4 is expressed. Recent work from our laboratory demonstrated that recombinant VEGF-1 and VEGF-2 have similar biologic activities.[30] Specifically, *in vitro*, VEGF-2 exhibits a dose-dependent mitogenic and chaemotactic effect on ECs, particularly those of the microvasculature, and increases vascular permeability. VEGF-2 has also been shown to stimulate release of nitric oxide from ECs, an important pathway in current concepts of angiogenesis and vascular remodelling.[31] Witzenbichler *et al.* (1998) used a rabbit hind-limb ischaemia model to test the potential of VEGF-2 to promote angiogenesis *in vivo*. VEGF-2, administered as plasmid DNA or recombinant protein, was shown to enhance vascular permeability and promote angiogenesis, as evidenced by increased hindlimb blood pressure ratio, increased Doppler-derived iliac flow, enhanced neovascularity by angiography and increased capillary density at necropsy.[32]

Fibroblast growth factor

FGF is a family of nine factors, namely basic FGF, acidic FGF, and FGF 3-9. Acidic FGF (aFGF or FGF-1) and basic FGF (bFGF or FGF-2) are the most extensively characterised members of the large FGF family. Basic FGF is an 18 kD single chain peptide of 154 amino acids with both angiogenic and mitogenic potential and is found predominantly in the myocardium. Acidic FGF is a 16 kD cationic polypeptide chain made up of 140 amino acids and possesses a 55% sequence homology with bFGF.

FGFs are non-secreted growth factors lacking a signal peptide sequence. Extracellular release of FGF is caused by cell death or damage. FGFs are not endothelial cell-specific, and enhance proliferation of ECs as well as a variety of cells including vascular smooth muscle cells. They bind heparin with high affinity and bind either high-affinity receptors with tyrosine kinase activity or low-affinity/high-capacity receptors in association with heparan sulphate proteoglycans. At least 4 high-affinity FGF receptors have been identified and their cDNAs cloned.

A series of animal experiments has demonstrated that FGF improves myocardial perfusion and function in both acute and chronic ischaemia. This improvement was as a result of angiographically documented and histologically identifiable sprouting of capillary network from the original coronary vessels. After a reasonable exclusion of the tumor-proliferating action of these growth factors, clinical studies have begun.

Gene transfer

Gene therapy is introduction of genetic material into somatic cells of an organism with the aim of achieving high levels of sustained gene expression without provoking adverse host reactions. Arterial gene therapy requires techniques to introduce (transfect) a foreign gene (transgene) into arterial wall cells that may be used to replace or palliate a defective gene or to express a protein with a therapeutic effect. When transferred into vascular cells at a specific site, the transgene is expressed locally, resulting in prolonged and progressive production of the recombinant protein encoded by the transgene at that specific site; local production of the transgene product translates into meaningful biological effects and, ultimately, therapeutic benefit. To achieve expression of foreign DNA, the transferred gene should enter the cell, escape degradation by lysosomal enzymes, cross the nuclear membrane, escape degradation by endonucleases, and eventually be expressed. Each of these steps represents a potential limitation to the efficacy of gene transfer, which make spontaneous transfer and expression of foreign DNA into eukaryotic cells a rare phenomenon.

The success of such strategies depends on the efficiency with which the transgene is introduced and expressed into the target cell, the duration of transgene expression, and the ability of the transgene product to ultimately fulfil its role. Transfer vectors facilitate cellular penetration and intracellular trafficking of the transgene, and local delivery systems deliver the vector to the vicinity of the target cells. Transfer vectors are required to increase the efficiency of the process and may be viruses, non-viruses or mixed systems. There are two major categories of gene transfer systems, viral and non-viral. The most commonly used viral vectors for gene transfer are adenovirus, adeno-associated virus, and retrovirus. Non-viral methods include introduction of naked DNA (plasmid DNA with no additional vector) into the target area, and use of liposomes.

VEGF possesses several features that facilitate gene transfer. First, as previously mentioned, VEGF possesses a secretory signal sequence that permits the protein to be secreted naturally from intact cells, thus enabling a sequence of additional paracrine effects to be activated. Second, VEGF possesses an autocrine loop shared by most angiogenic cytokines, and facilitates modulation of EC behavior. When activated under hypoxic conditions, the autocrine loop serves to amplify and thereby protract the response in ECs stimulated by exogenously administered VEGF. Third, factors secreted by hypoxic myocytes upregulate VEGF receptor expression on ECs within the hypoxic milieu.[37] Such localised receptor expression may explain the finding that angiogenesis does not occur indiscriminately, but rather at sites of tissue ischaemia.

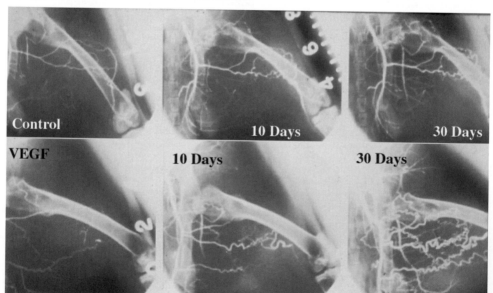

Figure 28.2. Angiogenesis in a rabbit model of hind-limb ischaemia. Rabbits treated with either a single intra-arterial bolus of VEGF or control. Angiograms taken at baseline, 10 days and 30 days after transfection. Note the rapid development of vessels in the VEGF-treated group compared to the control group. (From Takeshita S, Zheng LP, Brogi E et al. Therapeutic angiogenesis: A single intra-arterial bolus of vascular endothelial growth factor augments revascularization in a rabbit ischaemic hindlimb model. J Clin Invest 1994; 93:662-670, with permission).

Gene transfer of VEGF for cardiovascular disease

Coronary and peripheral atherosclerotic diseases remain leading causes of morbidity and mortality. Despite significant progress using medical, surgical and percutaneous therapies over the last three decades, there remains a significant population of patients who are not optimal candidates for surgical or percutaneous revascularisation. These patients continue to suffer from debilitating symptoms and remain at risk of myocardial events, limb loss or death. It is this clinical need, coupled with advances in the understanding of angiogenesis, which has led to efforts to develop angiogenic therapies for patients with peripheral and myocardial ischaemia.

Therapeutic angiogenesis is a novel strategy for the treatment of ischaemia

Evidence that VEGF stimulates angiogenesis *in vivo* had been developed in experiments performed on rat and rabbit cornea, the chorioallantoic membrane, and the rabbit bone graft model.[18,33] Preclinical studies have established proof of principle for the concept that the angiogenic activity of VEGF is sufficiently potent to achieve therapeutic benefit.[24] Doses of 500–1000 µg of phVEGF$_{165}$ produced statistically significant augmentation of angiographically visible collateral vessels (Fig. 28.2) and histologically identifiable capillaries in rabbits with severe, unilateral hind-limb ischaemia. Similar results were achieved in a separate series of experiments in which VEGF was administered by an intramuscular route daily for 10 days.[34]

Gene transfer of cDNA encoding for secreted protein may result in meaningful biological outcomes despite low transfection efficiency

It has been previously observed that site-specific transfection of genes encoding for a secreted protein may overcome the handicap of inefficient transfection by a paracrine effect, even when the number of transduced cells remains low, by secreting adequate protein to achieve local levels with physiologically meaningful biological effects. *In vitro*[35] and *in vivo*[36] models demonstrated that low-efficiency transfection (successful transfection in <1% of cells in the transfected arterial segment) with a gene encoding for a **secreted** protein may achieve therapeutic effects not realized by transfection with genes encoding for proteins that remain intracellular (e.g. bFGF).

Arterial gene transfer may also accomplish therapeutic angiogenesis. In rabbits with hind-limb ischaemia, 400 µg of phVEGF$_{165}$, delivered percutaneously via the hydrogel layer coating the outside of an angioplasty balloon catheter[37] augmented the development of collateral vessels as documented by serial angiograms *in vivo*, and increased capillary density at necropsy. Angiographic and histologic evidence of angiogenesis were subsequently demonstrated following intra-arterial gene transfer of phVEGF$_{165}$ in a human patient[25] (Fig. 28.3). These findings thus established that site-specific gene **transfer** can be used to achieve physiologically meaningful **therapeutic** modulation of vascular disorders.

Pre-clinical and clinical studies have established that intramuscular gene transfer may be utilised to successfully accomplish therapeutic angiogenesis

Ischaemic skeletal muscle itself serves to augment transfection efficiency five-fold. Meaningful biological outcomes have been observed following gene transfer of naked DNA by

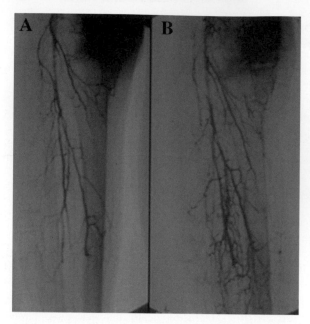

Figure 28.3. Selective digital subtraction angiograms performed in a patient with critical limb ischaemia due to occlusion of all three infrapopliteal vessels at mid-calf level. (A) immediately prior to and (B) 1 month after intra-arterial gene therapy with 2000µg naked plasmid DNA encoding VEGF. The post-gene transfer angiogram disclosed a plethora of new collateral vessels in the ischaemic limb. (From Isner JM, Pieczek A, Schainfeld et al. Clinical evidence of angiogenesis following arterial gene transfer of phVEGF$_{165}$, Lancet 1996; 348:370-374, with permission).

direct injection into skeletal muscle. Ten days after ischaemia was induced in one hind-limb of New Zealand White rabbits, 500 µg of phVEGF$_{165}$, or the reporter gene LacZ, were injected IM into the ischaemic hind-limb muscles. Site-specific transgene expression was documented by mRNA and immunohistochemistry. At 30-day follow-up, angiographically recognisable collateral vessels and histologically identifiable capillaries were increased in VEGF-transfectants compared to controls.[38]

It was subsequently shown that intramuscular gene transfer can be used to successfully accomplish therapeutic angiogenesis in critical limb ischaemia.[28] Gene transfer was performed in 10 limbs of nine patients with non-healing ischaemic ulcers (n=7) and/or rest pain (n=10) due to peripheral arterial disease. A total amount of 4000 µg naked plasmid DNA encoding the secreted 165-amino acid isoform of human VEGF (phVEGF$_{165}$) was injected into ischaemic muscles of the affected limbs. Gene expression was documented by a transient increase in serum levels of VEGF monitored by ELISA.

Therapeutic benefit was demonstrated by regression of rest pain and/or improved limb integrity. Based on criteria proposed by Rutherford, limb status improved in nine of 10 extremities treated. In one patient an ischaemic ulcer resolved sufficiently to permit placement of a split-thickness skin grafting, leading to absolute limb salvage (Fig. 28.4). In two patients in whom a major amputation would have been inevitable, retention of a functional foot by a minor (toe) amputation was reached.

The ankle systolic pressure index (ASPI) and/or the toe brachial index increased from 0.33±0.05 at baseline to 0.48±0.03 at 12 weeks. All patients experienced a significant increase in pain-free walking time and absolute, claudication-limited walking time. Digital subtraction angiography showed newly visible collateral vessels at the knee, calf and ankle levels in seven limbs. Magnetic resonance angiography showed qualitative evidence of improved distal flow with enhancement of signal intensity as well as an increase in the number of newly visible collaterals in eight limbs.

A similar form of therapy was used in 11 patients with Buerger's disease presenting with critical limb ischaemia, nine of whom were successfully treated.[39] These patients had resolution of nocturnal rest pain and healing of ulcers. The ankle-brachial index increased

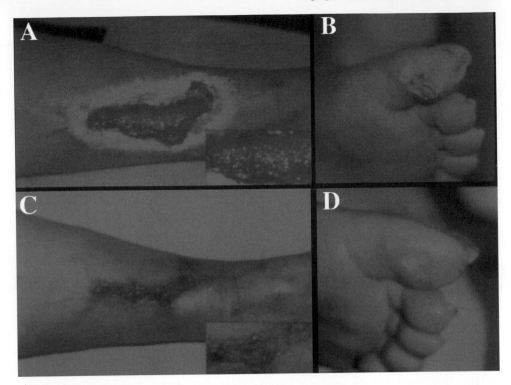

Figure 28.4. A patient with critical limb ischaemia-rest pain and non-healing ulcerations of the medial aspect of the left leg and the left great toe. (A, B) Prior to and (C, D) 12 months following two intramuscular (IM) injections of naked DNA encoding VEGF$_{165}$ (phVEGF$_{165}$). The patient's ABI increased from 0.28 to 0.55, angiography disclosed new collateral vessels in the ischaemic limb and successful split-thickness skin grafting to a 9x3 cm wound was achieved after the ulcerations had healed sufficiently. (From Baumgartner I et al. Constitutive expression of phVEGF$_{165}$ following intramuscular gene transfer promotes collateral vessel development in patients with critical limb ischemia. Circulation 1998; 97:1114-1123, with permission).

by greater than 0.1 (10%) and newly formed collateral vessels were seen on MRA and serial contrast angiography. Two of these patients needed below-knee amputation because of advanced gangrene at the time of treatment initiation, although the level of amputation was lowered in both patients.

Administration of human recombinant VEGF protein in myocardial ischaemia

Animal experiments utilising recombinant human VEGF (rhVEGF$_{165}$) protein administered directly into the left coronary ostium demonstrated significant augmentation of flow to collateral-dependent ischaemic myocardium. However, this was complicated by hypotension, apparently mediated by VEGF-induced release of NO.

The recently reported VIVA trial[40] (a double-blind, placebo-controlled, dose-escalating trial of patients with viable myocardium who were not optimal candidates for percutaneous or surgical revascularisation) which investigated the effect of intra-coronary followed by intravenous rhVEGF in more than 140 patients, failed to show any clinical benefit. Doses were limited by hypotension, which developed at higher doses in an earlier dose-ranging study. Exercise treadmill time and SPECT-sestambi scan did not show any significant change. An interesting finding was that two patients in the placebo group were diagnosed to have tumors after enrolment in this study.

Intramyocardial gene transfer can be safely and successfully achieved via a minimally invasive chest wall incision

Given that VEGF could augment myocardial angiogenesis in a porcine model of chronic myocardial ischaemia and previous experiments had demonstrated that direct intramuscular injection could be accomplished in smaller animal models,[41] experiments were extrapolated to establish the safety of performing intramyocardial gene transfer by direct intramuscular injection of plasmid DNA encoding VEGF$_{165}$ (phVEGF$_{165}$) to achieve therapeutic angiogenesis. Pilot experiments to determine appropriate dosing volumes using four intramyocardial injections indicated that a total volume of 8 ml was better than 2 ml; no further improvement was seen with 20 ml.

Intramyocardial injections caused no haemodynamic or arrhythmic complications. Online ultrasound monitoring documented that the administered plasmid DNA was distributed several cm beyond the site of needle entry. The electrocardiogram did not show evidence of myocardial infarction in any pig. Creatine phosphokinase (CPK) levels increased transiently, but the myocardial specific MB isoenzyme did not increase higher than the normal limits. The left ventricular ejection fraction (LVEF) remained unchanged irrespective of the volume injected. After 8 weeks, LVEF was 39±8%. Diagnostic coronary angiography typically showed enhanced filling (Rentrop score 3–4) of the left obtuse marginal branch of the left circumflex coronary artery, reconstituted by one or more collateral vessels from the left anterior descending (LAD) or diagonal branches of the LAD coronary artery.

Histologic examination of 276 sections retrieved at necropsy from 12 pigs disclosed only occasional foci of mononuclear inflammatory cells. Foci of necrosis or fibrosis were limited to myocardium subserved by the occluded artery in the porcine model of myocardial ischaemia. Histologic examination of sections retrieved from all non-cardiac sites showed no evidence of pathologic findings. Furthermore, Western Blotting demonstrated presence of VEGF protein in myocardial tissue, with the strongest band closest to the injection site.

Gene therapy for myocardial angiogenesis: initial clinical results with direct myocardial injection of phVEGF$_{165}$ as sole therapy for patients with chronic myocardial ischaemia

As a result of the animal experiments outlined above, a phase 1, dose-escalating, open label clinical study was initiated to determine the safety and bioactivity of direct myocardial gene transfer of phVEGF$_{165}$ as sole therapy (i.e. without angioplasty, stenting or by-pass graft surgery) for patients with stable exertional angina refractory to medical therapy, areas of viable but under-perfused myocardium on perfusion scanning, and multi-vessel occlusive coronary artery disease. Preliminary results of this trial suggest that safe and successful transfection can be achieved by this method with a favourable clinical effect.[42]

Patients received phVEGF$_{165}$ administered by direct myocardial injection in 4 aliquots of 2.0 ml via a 'mini-thoracotomy'; total dose 125 µg (n=10), 250 µg (n=10), 500 µg (n=10). An immobile field for intramyocardial injection was ensured by using a stabilising device that facilitates vascular anastomosis during beating heart bypass (Fig. 28.5). Continuous transoesophageal echocardiographic monitoring was performed throughout the procedure to monitor development of wall motion abnormalities associated with injections and to ensure that plasmid DNA was not injected into the LV cavity.

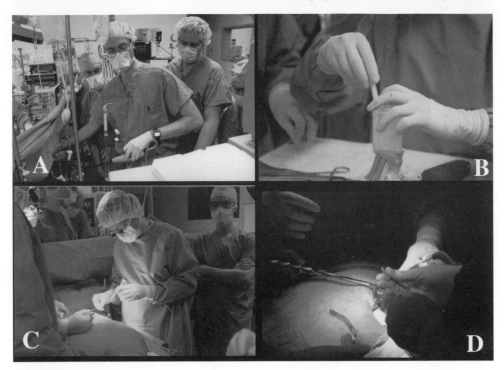

Figure 28.5. Direct myocardial injection of naked plasmid DNA encoding for VEGF via anterior thoracotomy. (A) Transoesophageal monitoring is performed throughout to monitor development of wall motion abnormalities associated with injections and ensure that plasmid DNA was not injected into the LV cavity. (B) Plasmid DNA is reconstituted with sterile saline and injected in 4 aliquots of 2.0ml. (C) Standard anterior thoracotomy is used similar to the incision made for beating heart bypass surgery. (D) The DNA is injected with a 27 guage needle that is protected by a rubber sleeve to prevent penetration through the ventricular wall into the LV cavity.

VEGF gene transfer was performed in 30 patients (23 males), aged 48–74 years. No perioperative complications were experienced. VEGF injections caused no significant changes in heart rate or blood pressure and were only associated with single ventricular premature contractions. There was no evidence of myocardial damage by cardiac enzyme analysis and patients maintained left ventricular function. Gene expression was documented by a transient but significant increase in plasma levels of VEGF monitored by ELISA assay.

All patients experienced marked symptomatic improvement and/or objective evidence of improved myocardial perfusion. At latest follow-up, 8 of 16 patients at 360 days, and 15 of 30 patients at 180 days were free of angina. Specifically, sublingual nitrate use fell from 60/week to 2.5/week at day 180, accompanied by a significant reduction in episodes of angina from 55/week to 3/week at day 180. Evidence of reduced ischaemia (SPECT-sestamibi myocardial perfusion scanning) was documented in 22/29 patients. The mean perfusion/ischaemia score decreased significantly in both stress (18.5 ± 3.7 vs 14.5 ± 3.4, p=0.010) and rest (14.2 ± 3.5 vs 11.0 ± 2.7, p=0.002) images at day 60 follow-up. It is intriguing that not only defects observed in the perfusion scans with pharmacologic stress, but also those observed at rest, improved post-gene transfer. This observation suggests that these pre-test defects may constitute foci of hibernating myocardium rather than myocardial scar and may have been successfully resuscitated as the result of therapeutic neovascularisation. Coronary angiography showed evidence of new collateral vessel development with improved collateral filling in at least 1 territory in 50% of patients.

This study provides the first evidence for a favourable clinical effect of direct myocardial injection of naked plasmid DNA encoding for VEGF as the sole therapeutic intervention. These subjective findings are supported by the results of objective testing, including the results of treadmill exercise tests and radionuclide pharmacological perfusion scans. This early experience, while encouraging from the standpoint of therapeutic angiogenesis and gene therapy, leaves multiple issues unresolved. Optimising the anatomic site, number, and dose of intramyocardial injections requires further investigation. The strategy of gene therapy alone administered via a mini-thoracotomy does not permit randomisation against placebo (untreated controls) or clinical testing of alternative dosing regimens including multiple treatments.

Catheter-based myocardial gene transfer using non-fluoro-scopic electromechanical LV mapping

While successful intravascular,[25] pericardial[43] and intramuscular[26] gene transfer have all been performed using minimally invasive delivery techniques, all of the clinical work involving myocardial gene transfer has to date required an operative mini-thoracotomy. While this approach has clearly reduced the length of hospital stay and morbidity associated with conventional bypass surgery, it nevertheless implies additional morbidity and limits the feasibility of repeat administrations. Percutaneously administered myocardial gene transfer could further reduce morbidity, allow incorporation of a control group, and facilitate repeat use of myocardial gene transfer.[90]

To determine if the delivery catheter could be employed in a site-specific manner, myocardial gene transfer was integrated with a previously described navigation system and catheter mapping technology[44] The injection catheter (NOGA™ Biosense-Webster, Warren, NJ) is a modified mapping catheter, the distal tip of which incorporates a 27G needle that can be protruded 3–5 mm, and was used to deliver six injections (1.0 ml per injection) to the myocardium of normal and ischaemic swine.[44] Injections caused no haemodynamic or arrhythmic complications including pericardial effusion and/or cardiac tamponade. Injections of methylene blue were identified at necropsy as discrete sites corresponding to injection sites indicated prospectively *in vivo* on the endocardial map (Fig. 28.6), suggesting reliable and reproducible targeting of endocardial sites. In addition, myocardial staining was limited to the myocardial wall and no epicardial staining was demonstrated. Reporter gene (pCMV-nls*LacZ*) delivery to a single (normal or ischaemic) LV myocardial region resulted in peak ß-galactosidase (ß-gal) activity in the target area. Low-level to negligible activity was seen in areas remote from the injection sites, suggesting relatively localised gene transfer to those sites indicated by pre-injection electroanatomical mapping (Fig. 28.7). In addition, ß-gal activity was greater in ischaemic versus non-ischaemic injected myocardium, indicating enhanced gene transfer in ischaemic myocardium.

The results of this preliminary study establish that percutaneous myocardial gene transfer can be successfully achieved in normal and ischaemic myocardium in a relatively site-specific fashion without significant morbidity or mortality. The mapping capabilities of the NOGA™ system utilised in this study were useful for demonstrating that gene expression could be directed to predetermined LV sites. This indicated that this technique may be advantageous for avoiding gene transfer to sites of myocardial scar, as well as accurately relocating the tip of an injection catheter to areas of myocardial ischaemia (or hibernating myocardium) where gene transfer may be potentially optimised. These findings thus establish the potential to replace currently employed operative approaches with a minimally invasive

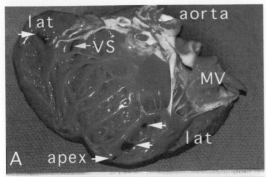

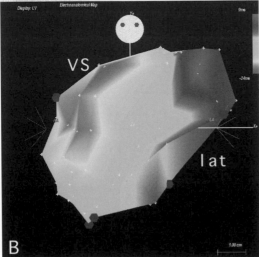

Figure 28.6 (top). A) The endocardial surface following dissection through the left lateral free wall following injections with methylene blue. Left ventricle with papillary muscles, left atrium and mitral valve apparatus are displayed. Lateral wall and septum are labelled. Methylene blue injection sites (arrows) are demonstrated at the apex, septum and posterolateral wall. B) Corresponding NOGA™ map (LAO projection) with injection sites indicated by red hexagons. LA = left arm; RA = right arm. (From Vale PR, Losordo DW et al. Catheter-based myocardial gene transfer utilizing non-fluoroscopic electromechanical left ventricular mapping. J Am Coll Cardiol 1999; 34:246-254 with permission).

technique for applications of cardiovascular gene therapy designed to target myocardial function.

Catheter-based gene transfer of VEGF may accomplish therapeutic angiogenesis

Subsequent investigations established the feasibility and safety of using LV mapping, coupled to a locatable injection catheter, to percutaneously deliver naked plasmid DNA encoding for vascular endothelial growth factor (phVEGF$_{165}$) to the myocardium of swine with myocardial ischaemia.[45] Consequently, this suggests that catheter-based myocardial gene transfer may ultimately achieve what operative delivery has so far achieved in terms of therapeutic angiogenesis. This catheter-based technique has already been used to deliver naked DNA encoding VEGF-2 to the myocardium of patients (Fig. 28.8). Such an approach, if efficacious, is attractive because it potentially replaces the morbidity and 2–4 day hospital stay of surgery with an outpatient procedure, and permits repeat therapy. Moreover, eliminating the need for thoracotomy has permitted the catheter trial to be performed in a randomised, placebo-controlled fashion.

Conclusions

The current clinical therapeutic strategy employed constitutes an extrapolation from initial applications of gene transfer to animal models and patients with limb ischaemia utilising

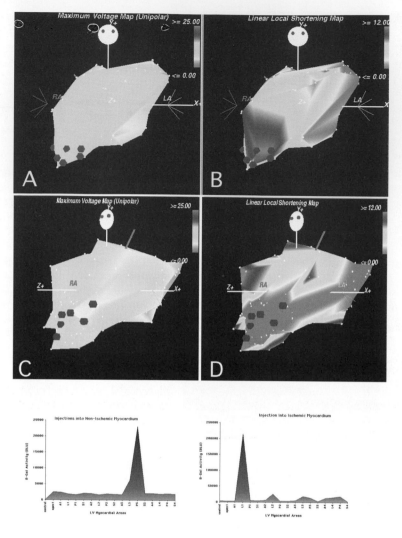

E

Figure 28.7. Catheter-based myocardial injections into swine left ventricle (LV). NOGA™ electrical (maximum unipolar voltage) and mechanical (linear log shortening) maps of the swine LV are shown. Note area of ischaemia in the lateral wall - normal electrical activity (blue/green) coupled with poor mechanical function (red). Images A and B represent anteroposterior projections demonstrating 6 injection sites (red hexagons) in an area of normal myocardial (apex) remote from the ischaemic zone. Images C and D depict LAO projections of indicated injection sites in the ischaemic lateral LV free wall. LA = left arm; RA = right arm. (E) Quantitative β-Galactosidase assays of catheter-based single site LV injections in swine models of chronic myocardial ischaemia (pigs 9-10). Injections into myocardium remote from the ischaemic zone are distinguished from injections made into the ischaemic lateral wall. A = anterior wall, L = lateral wall, P = posterior wall, S = septum. Numbers refer to the harvested tissue specimens; 1 being closest to the apex, and 4 being adjacent to the LV outflow tract and mitral valve ring. (From Vale PR, Losordo DW et al. Catheter-based myocardial gene transfer utilising non-fluoroscopic electromechanical left ventricular mapping. J Am Coll Cardiol 1999; 34:246-254 with permission).

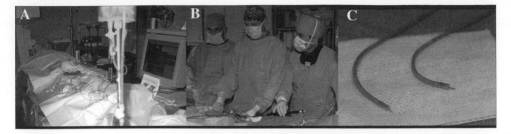

Figure 28.8. Catheter based gene therapy. (A) Cardiac Catheterisation Laboratory, St Elizabeth's Medical Center Boston, MA, USA. (B) Performing catheter-based myocardial gene transfer with VEGF-2, using NOGA™ LV electromechanical mapping. (C) Modified mapping-injection catheter (Biosense, Johnson & Johnson, Warren, NJ). Electrode at distal catheter tip enables annotation of electromechanical map to document sites of injection (gene transfer). In catheter shown on right, 27-guage needle has been advanced out of the distal catheter tip to simulate myocardial engagement in preparation for injection.

the 165-amino acid isoform of the VEGF-1 gene. These results, however, are likely to have generic implications for strategies of therapeutic neovascularisation using alternative candidate genes, vectors, and delivery strategies. Preclinical data supporting use of other VEGF-1 isoforms[46] as well as other VEGF genes,[31] have been previously reported, as have preclinical studies using fibroblast growth factor (FGF).[47, 48] All of these are being actively studied in ongoing clinical trials. Furthermore, the relative merits of gene transfer versus recombinant protein administration remain to be clarified. Additional investigations comparing doses of recombinant protein and routes of delivery are required to resolve this issue. Until all these studies are complete, the ideal method of achieving therapeutic angiogenesis remains unknown.

At this early stage of clinical trials into myocardial gene therapy, however, it has been shown conclusively that direct myocardial gene transfer utilising different doses of naked plasmid DNA encoding for $VEGF_{165}$ can be performed safely and that this approach achieves a sustained clinical benefit. In terms of safety, no operative complications, or deterioration in eyesight due to diabetic retinopathy,[49] or growth of latent neoplasms have been observed in any patient treated with $phVEGF_{165}$ gene transfer. Ongoing clinical studies will also determine the potential for neovascularisation gene therapy to be performed by non-surgical, catheter-based delivery.

References

1.   Folkman J: Tumor angiogenesis. Therapeutic implications. *N Engl J Med* 1971; **285**:1182–86.
2.   Isner JM, Asahara T. Angiogenesis and vasculogenesis as therapeutic strategies for postnatal neovascularisation (Perspective). *J Clin Invest* 1999; **103**:1231–36.
3.   D'Amore PA, Thompson RW. Mechanisms of angiogenesis. *Annu Rev Physiol* 1987; **49**:453–64.
4.   Ausprunk DH, Folkman J. Migration and proliferation of endothelial cells in preformed and newly formed blood vessels during tumor angiogenesis. *Microvasc Res* 1977; **14**:53–65.
5.   Schaper W, Brahander MD, Lewi P. DNA synthesis and mitoses in coronary collateral vessels of the dog. *Circ Res* 1971; **28**:671–79.
6.   Pasyk S, Schaper W, Schaper J *et al.* DNA synthesis in coronary collaterals after coronary artery occlusion in conscious dog. *Am J Physiol* 1982; **242**:H1031–H1037.
7.   White FC, Carroll SM, Magnet A, Bloor CM. Coronary collateral development in swine after coronary artery occlusion. *Circ Res* 1992; **71**:1490–1500.

8.   Takeshita S, Rossow ST, Kearney M *et al.* JM: Time course of increased cellular proliferation in collateral arteries following administration of vascular endothelial growth factor in a rabbit model of lower limb vascular insufficiency. *Am J Pathol* 1995; **147**:1649–60.

9.   Risau W, Flamme I. Vasculogenesis. *Ann Rev Cell Dev Biol* 1995; **11**:73–91.

10. Flamme I, Risau W. Induction of vasculogenesis and hematopoiesis *in vitro*. *Development* 1992; **116**:435–39.

11. Asahara T, Murohara T, Sullivan A *et al.* Isolation of putative progenitor endothelial cells for angiogenesis. *Science* 1997; **275**:965–67.

12. Shi Q, Rafii S, Wu MH-D *et al.* Evidence for circulating bone marrow-derived endothelial cells. *Blood* 1998; **92**:362–67.

13. Brogi E, Schatteman G, Wu T *et al.* Hypoxia-induced paracrine regulation of VEGF receptor expression. *J Clin Invest* 1996; **97**:469–76.

14. Joukov V, Pajusola K, Kaipainen A *et al.* A Novel vascular endothelial growth factor, VEGF-C, is a ligand for the Flt4 (VEGFR-3) and KDR (VEGFR-2) receptor tyrosine kinases. *EMBO J* 1996; **15**:290–98.

15. Olofsson B, Pajusola K, Kaipainen A *et al.* Vascular endothelial growth factor B, a novel growth factor for endothelial cells. *Proc Natl Acad Sci USA* 1996; **93**:2576–81.

16. Maglione D, Guerriero V, Viglietto G *et al.* Isolation of a human placenta cDNA coding for a protein related to the vascular permeability factor. *Proc Natl Acad Sci USA* 1991; **88**:9267–71.

17. Leung DW, Cachianes G, Kuang WJ *et al.* Vascular endothelial growth factor is a secreted angiogenic mitogen. *Science* 1989; **246**:1306–09.

18. Ferrara N, Henzel WJ. Pituitary follicular cells secrete a novel heparin-binding growth factor specific for vascular endothelial cells. *Biochem Biophys Res Commun* 1989; **161**:851–55.

19. Conn G, Soderman D, Schaeffer M-T *et al.* Purification of glycoprotein vascular endothelial cell mitogen from a rat glioma cell line. *Proc Natl Acad Sci USA* 1990; **87**:1323–27.

20. Breier G, Albrecht U, Sterrer S, Risau W. Expression of vascular endothelial growth factor during embryonic angiogenesis and endothelial cell differentiation. *Development* 1992; **114**:521–32.

21. Carmeliet P, Ferreira V, Breier G *et al.* Abnormal blood vessel development and lethality in embryos lacking a single VEGF allele. *Nature* 1996; **380**:435–39.

22. Peters KG, deVries C, Williams LT. Vascular endothelial growth factor receptor expression during embryogenesis and tissue repair suggests a role in endothelial differentiation and blood vessel growth. *Proc Natl Acad Sci USA* 1993; **90**:8915–19.

23. Tsurumi Y, Murohara T, Krasinski K *et al.* Reciprocal relationship between VEGF and NO in the regulation of endothelial integrity. *Nature Med* 1997; **3**:879–86.

24. Takeshita S, Zheng LP, Brogi E *et al.* Therapeutic angiogenesis: A single intra-arterial bolus of vascular endothelial growth factor augments revascularisation in a rabbit ischaemic hindlimb model. *J Clin Invest* 1994; **93**:662–70.

25. Isner JM, Pieczek A, Schainfeld R *et al.* Clinical evidence of angiogenesis following arterial gene transfer of phVEGF$_{165}$. *Lancet* 1996; **348**:370–74.

26. Baumgartner I, Pieczek A, Manor O *et al.* Constitutive expression of phVEGF$_{165}$ following intramuscular gene transfer promotes collateral vessel development in patients with critical limb ischaemia. *Circulation* 1998; **97**:1114–23.

27. Folkman J. Angiogenesis in cancer, vascular, rheumatoid and other disease. *Nature Med* 1995; **1**:27–30.

28. Couffinhal T, Kearney M, Witzenbichler B *et al.* Vascular endothelial growth factor/vascular permeability factor (VEGF/VPF) in normal and atherosclerotic human arteries. *Am J Pathol* 1997; **150**:1673–85.

29. Jeltsch M, Kaipainen A, Joukov V *et al.* Hyperplasia of lymphatic vessels in VEGF-C transgenic mice. *Science* 1997; **276**:1423–25.

30. Briddell R, Hartley C, Smith K, McNiece I. Recombinant rat stem cell factor synergizes with recombinant human granulocyte colony stimulating factor *in vivo* in mice to mobilize peripheral blood progenitor cells that have enhanced repopulating potential. *Proc Natl Acad Sci USA* 1990; **87**:5978–82.

31. Witzenbichler B, Asahara T, Murohara T *et al.* Vascular endothelial growth factor-C (VEGF-C/

VEGF-2) promotes angiogenesis in the setting of tissue ischaemia. *Am J Pathol* 1998; **153**:381–94.

32. Rivard A, Silver M, Chen D *et al.* Rescue of diabetes-related impairment of angiogenesis by intramuscular gene therapy with adeno-VEGF. *Am J Pathol* 1999; **154**:355–64.

33. Connolly DT, Hewelman DM, Nelson R *et al.* Tumor vascular permeability factor stimulates endothelial cell growth and angiogenesis. *J Clin Invest* 1989; **84**:1470–78.

34. Takeshita S, Pu L-Q, Zheng L *et al.* Vascular endothelial growth factor induces dose-dependent revascularisation in a rabbit model of persistent limb ischaemia. *Circulation* 1994; **90**:II-228–II-234.

35. Takeshita S, Losordo DW, Kearney M, Isner JM. Time course of recombinant protein secretion following liposome-mediated gene transfer in a rabbit arterial organ culture model. *Lab Invest* 1994; **71**:387–91.

36. Losordo DW, Pickering JG, Takeshita S *et al.* JM: Use of the rabbit ear artery to serially assess foreign protein secretion after site specific arterial gene transfer *in vivo*: Evidence that anatomic identification of successful gene transfer may underestimate the potential magnitude of transgene expression. *Circulation* 1994; **89**:785–92.

37. Riessen R, Rahimizadeh H, Blessing E *et al.* Arterial gene transfer using pure DNA applied directly to a hydrogel-coated angioplasty balloon. *Hum Gene Ther* 1993; **4**:749–58.

38. Tsurumi Y, Takeshita S, Chen D *et al.* Direct intramuscular gene transfer of naked DNA encoding vascular endothelial growth factor augments collateral development and tissue perfusion. *Circulation* 1996; **94**:3281–90.

39. Isner JM, Baumgartner I, Rauh G *et al.* Treatment of thromboangiitis obliterans (Buerger's disease) by intramuscular gene transfer of vascular endothelial growth factor: preliminary clinical results . *J Vasc Surg* 1998; **28**:964–75.

40. Henry TD, Rocha-Singh K, Isner JM *et al.* Results of intracoronary recombinant human vascular endothelial growth factor (rhVEGF) administration trial. *Circulation* 1998; **31**:65A(Abstract).

41. Gal D, Weir L, Leclerc G *et al.* Direct myocardial transfection in two animal models: Evaluation of parameters affecting gene expression and percutaneous gene delivery. *Lab Invest* 1993; **68**:18–25.

42. Losordo DW, Vale PR, Symes JF *et al.* JM Gene therapy for myocardial angiogenesis: initial clinical results with direct myocardial injection of phVEGF$_{165}$ as sole therapy for myocardial ischaemia. *Circulation* 1998; **98**:2800–04.

43. March KL. Methods of local gene delivery to vascular tissues. *Sem Interv Cardiol* 1996; **1**:215–23.

44. Vale PR, Losordo DW, Tkebuchava T *et al.* Catheter-based myocardial gene transfer utilising nonfluoroscopic electromechanical left ventricular mapping. *J Am Coll Cardiol* 1999; **34**:246–54.

45. Vale PR, Milliken CE, Tkebuchava T *et al.* Catheter-based gene transfer of VEGF utilising electromechanical LV mapping accomplishes therapeutic angiogenesis: pre-clinical studies in swine. *Circulation* 1999; **100**:I–512(Abstract).

46. Takeshita S, Tsurumi Y, Couffinhal T *et al.* Gene transfer of naked DNA encoding for three isoforms of vascular endothelial growth factor stimulates collateral development *in vivo*. *Lab Invest* 1996; **75**:487–502.

47. Giordano FJ, Ping P, McKirnan D *et al.* Hammond HK: Intracoronary gene transfer of fibroblast growth factor-5 increases blood flow and contractile function in an ischaemic region of the heart. *Nature Med* 1996; **2**:534–39.

48. Lopez JJ, Edelman ER, Stamler A *et al* Angiogenic potential of perivascularly delivered aFGF in a porcine model of chronic myocardial ischaemia. *Am J Physiol* 1998; **274**:H930–H936.

49. Vale PR, Rauh G, Wuensch DI *et al.* Influence of vascular endothelial growth factor on diabetic retinopathy. *Circulation* 1998; **17**:I-353(Abstract).

Chapter 29

Nursing Care of the Cardiac Catheterisation Patient

Kim L. Koo and S. Brouwer

Introduction

Nursing care of the patient in the cardiac catheterisation laboratory is an area that is neglected in most publications. Indeed, there is little literature available that supports the nursing perspective in the laboratory. Nursing responsibility in the catheter laboratory is an integral part of the clinical pathway and an area requiring further investigation and documentation. Up to the time of the IMPACT trial in 1996, standards of nursing care based on clinical trials following balloon angioplasty were not available.[1]

Patients may be admitted for cardiac catheterisation from various areas of the hospital, including the accident and emergency room, coronary care unit, a general or day-only ward, or by direct referral or transfer from another hospital.

Before transfer to the laboratory, use of appropriate materials such as information booklets, videos, teaching sessions and one-on-one explanation by the health care team all ensure that the patient has a reasonable understanding of what will occur. This allows the patient to ask questions about the procedure itself or specifics about what may happen in the laboratory. Additional information may be accessed from the Internet.[2] Reassurance and an explanation may help allay any anxiety patients may have and help them to relax both before and during the procedure. A premedication may also be ordered.

On arrival at the cardiac catheterisation laboratory

Patient identification is an essential part of the transfer/check-in process of the patient to the cardiac catheterisation laboratory.

This admission process is usually undertaken using a standard checklist to ensure that all vital information is examined, thus any discrepancies can be brought to the attention of the cardiologist. This checklist generally covers the following main areas of concern:

1. Patient identification is very important as it helps to ensure that the correct patient has arrived for the correct procedure. The patient's name and date of birth are confirmed verbally with the patient and checked with the wristband identification and the admission sheet. Similarly, patients should be asked which procedure is planned, and this should also be checked with the appropriate consent forms. This process may reveal any lack of understanding about the procedure and highlight any areas requiring further explanation or discussion.

2. Each hospital has its own policy for obtaining and witnessing a consent form. Staunton and Whyburn[3] contend that nursing staff should not be responsible for obtaining a

patient's signature on a consent form, that it is the responsibility of the treating doctor. It is the responsibility of the nurse checking the patient to inform the consultant if the patient expresses a lack of understanding regarding the proposed procedure, if the written consent does not correlate with the patient's understanding of the procedure, or if no consent is available. Consent is obtained prior to the administration of any premedication, to ensure that the patient has a full understanding of the procedure.

3. Allergies are noted to ensure that no antiseptics, sticking plaster, medication or contrast are administered that could place the patient at risk of allergic reaction. The cardiologist should be informed of any relevant allergies.

4. Fasting time is checked to ensure that the patient has been fasted for at least six hours prior to the procedure. This means that the patient has an empty stomach and reduces the chance of vomiting and/or aspiration should resuscitation or transfer to the operating room be required.

5. An intravenous cannula allows immediate venous access for delivery of medication and intravenous fluids, particularly in an emergency situation. This can be inserted prior to arrival in the cardiac catheter laboratory or as part of the check-in process.

6. A recent electrocardiogram (ECG) is essential to use as a baseline for comparison, particularly in the post-procedural phase.

7. Other useful information to collect at this time is whether the patient is on any anticoagulant or antiplatelet drugs. This may affect anticoagulant dosage during the procedure and also the method of post-procedural sheath removal.

8. Diabetic patients should have their blood sugar level checked, and those with impaired renal function should be considered for pre-hydration. Patients on metformin have the potential risk of drug accumulation and lactic acidosis from contrast-related renal impairment and should have their creatinine levels checked. If creatine level exceeds 0.15, metformin is withheld for 48 hours prior to the procedure and is not recommenced until the level returns to normal (0.15 or less). An alternative hypoglycaemic agent may be necessary during this period.

9. It is helpful to give an explanation of what happens in the procedure room, as it provides an opportunity for any last-minute questions to be answered.

10. The following explanation is an example of what the patient could be told:

'Most angiograms take about 20 to 30 minutes from the time you enter the procedure room to the end of the procedure. If you have had bypass surgery it may take a little longer. You will be lying flat on a very narrow bed. The groin area will be washed with an antiseptic and you will be covered with a sterile drape. The doctor will come in and give some local anaesthetic, which may sting a bit but the area will soon go numb, after which you should feel very little. During the procedure the doctor may ask you to take a deep breath. This allows clearer pictures to be taken. When the x-ray contrast is injected into the pumping chamber of the heart you will experience a brief hot sensation that spreads rapidly throughout your body. You may feel that you are passing water, but it is only the sensation of the heat. Occasionally some people feel nauseated for a few seconds. If you experience any pain or discomfort please let the doctor know straight away. The doctor may also ask you to cough during the procedure, as sometimes the injection of the contrast medium or dye may slow down your heart rate or your blood pressure may be affected.'

Angioplasty patients

If patients are to undergo a percutaneous transluminal coronary angioplasty (PTCA) or stent implantation, they will often have fluids running to maintain hydration as ordered by the consultant. A consent form must be signed for PTCA/stent and coronary artery bypass grafting (CABG) should this be required in an emergency.

Contrast allergy

If a patient claims to be allergic to contrast, iodine or seafood the cardiologist must be notified. Prophylactic intravenous hydrocortisone and intramuscular phenergan may be ordered by the consultant and should be administered prior to the procedure.

The procedure room

The registered nurse (RN) is responsible for checking emergency equipment in the procedure room. This equipment generally consists of a fully equipped emergency trolley with a defibrillator and temporary pacing box. Oxygen outlets and suction equipment should also be available if required. All RNs working in the procedure room should be trained in cardiopulmonary resuscitation and be able to defibrillate and administer first-line emergency drugs. Reasonable skills in ECG interpretation and cardiac rhythm are also useful. Major areas of concern for the RN in the procedure room are:

1. Infection control issues, utilising universal precautions and maintenance of aseptic technique of all staff within the laboratory.

2. Occupational health and safety issues incorporating radiation safety and manual handling are also of major concern in the laboratory to ensure safety of patients and staff.

Recovery room

The recovery process ensures early identification of complications and facilitates transfer of the patient to the patient care areas (wards) in a stable condition. The RN is responsible for safe delivery of quality care to all patients. It is the responsibility of the recovery room nurse to ensure that the emergency trolley has been checked and is fully stocked with required equipment and drugs. The emergency trolley should also have a defibrillator, oxygen, and suction readily accessible.

All patients undergoing a procedure in the cardiac catheterisation laboratory should be monitored in a recovery area prior to transfer to the ward. This involves close monitoring by trained personnel and in most cases involves removal of the arterial sheath.

One set of observations must be recorded on arrival at the recovery area as a baseline for further comparison during the recovery and sheath removal process. These observations should include blood pressure (BP), pulse, circulation check with peripheral pulse status. This information should be recorded accurately in the patient's medical record.

If the arterial sheath is to be removed, time of sheath removal and manner of haemostasis applied needs to be recorded, whether using manual compression or a mechanical device.[4]

The puncture site must be checked for signs of bleeding and bruising or haematoma[5] and should also be documented in the patient's medical record.

The sheath may have been removed in the procedure room by the consultant and a closure device such as AngioSeal™ or PerClose™ may be in place. The RN should follow the manufacturer's directions for correct or suggested care.

Sheath removal by RN

Only RNs trained to remove arterial sheaths should do so, preferably following established protocols.[6] It is helpful to have all the necessary equipment ready for use at the bedside. This will generally consist of the following:

Appropriate haemostasis device (unless using digital pressure)
Dry sterile gauze
Kidney tray
Gloves
Splash glasses
Preferred dressing
Scissors

It is also useful to have atropine ready for intravenous injection and normal saline 500 ml with giving set ready to connect, should intravenous fluids be required in the event of a vasovagal reaction.

Following is a suggested procedure for safe removal of a femoral arterial sheath. Other appropriate methods such as digital pressure should be employed for other puncture sites.

1. Assess vital signs (ECG, BP and pulse). If systolic blood pressure >160 mmHg, nitrates may be required; check with consultant.
2. Explain procedure to patient. A simple explanation can help to reassure the patient and decrease any anxiety likely to be experienced.
3. Appropriate aseptic technique is required for removing the sheath. The RN should wash hands using an appropriate antibacterial solution. Disposable gloves and splash glasses should be worn to protect against exposure to blood.
4. Palpate the pedal pulse distal to the puncture site and the femoral pulse above the puncture site. The surrounding skin is cleaned with appropriate solution. The preferred device is placed above the incision site and pressure is applied until a pedal pulse is absent, and the sheath is simultaneously removed in a downward motion toward the feet.
5. Pressure on the site is reduced until a pedal pulse is just palpable, ensuring that haemostasis is maintained.
6. Note the time of removal, and observe for 5 minutes.
7. If using C clamp, gradually reduce pressure over the next 20 minutes until haemostasis is achieved.
8. If using Femostop™, reduce pressure gradually and send back to patient care level with device *in situ*. Ensure that time/pressure schedule accompanies patient and is documented in the patient's record.

Complications

Cardiac catheterisation is a potentially dangerous procedure that requires constant supervision for some hours after the procedure. Evaluation of post-procedural complications rests almost entirely with nursing staff. Proper training in specifics of patient management is essential to recognise and manage any complications, by far the most serious of which are bleeding from the puncture site, vasovagal reactions and chest pain. Attention to the following guidelines is essential in securing patient safety and a successful release from the catheter laboratory.

Bleeding

1. Check the insertion site regularly for bleeding and/or haematoma.
2. If bleeding or haematoma is present, apply pressure to femoral artery. Note that pressure should be applied above puncture site. Remember that access was gained using a needle at an angle of 45°, so the actual puncture to the artery is slightly higher than the skin puncture site.

3. Ideally apply only enough pressure to stop the bleeding, although it is preferable to have some blood flow distally. The cardiologist should be notified that bleeding has occurred and the RN should anticipate the possibility of a vasovagal reaction to the bleeding and to the pressure being placed on the artery.

Vasovagal reaction

1. The signs and symptoms of a vasovagal reaction are nausea, sweating, bradycardia, and hypotension. The patient may complain of feeling dizzy or unwell. Immediate intervention is required.
2. Do not leave the patient, obtain help from other staff, and notify the cardiologist. The immediate nursing action is to elevate the foot of bed to increase blood to the head, and to ask the patient to cough, as this increases vagal tone.
3. Anticipate commencing or increasing intravenous fluids and preparing atropine for rapid infusion.

Chest pain

1. Assess whether the pain is cardiac in nature. Offer reassurance and ask the patient to relax.
2. Note clinical appearance, e.g. dyspnoea, cold and clamminess, anxiety and diaphoresis. Give oxygen at 6 L/min via a Hudson face mask. Assess blood pressure, pulse and respiration.
3. If systolic BP is greater than 100 mmHg, give nitrates sublingually (e.g. Anginine, Isordil) and inform doctor.
4. If there is no pain relief within 5 minutes, contact cardiologist and recheck blood pressure, pulse and respirations. If blood pressure is adequate, repeat nitrates.
5. Record 12-lead ECG and compare to the previous base line ECG. Note any changes and inform the consultant.
6. Anticipate morphine and/or GTN infusion.
7. Chest pain post PTCA is managed in a similar manner. The RN should anticipate a rapid return to the procedure room if re-catheterisation is necessary.

On return to ward

Patients are normally returned to their respective wards soon after cardiac catheterisation, where they are restricted to bed for 4–6 hours.[7] Nursing management in the wards usually follows a set of protocols depending on each procedure, but may vary due to unforeseen complications such as unexpected prolonged bleeding from the puncture site, haematoma requiring further investigations, stroke, or subsequent chest pain. In some instances patients may be returned to acute care units such as the coronary care ward or critical care unit depending on the type of procedure performed, the relative condition of the patient and whether or not the patient is intubated. This may also be required if complications are encountered, particularly in interventional procedures.

Day-only admissions are becoming increasingly common in today's health care environment.[8] Such patients may be returned to a coronary care or intensive care unit instead of a short-stay ward.

Limb observations

Patients with transfemoral sheaths *in situ* should have limb observations continued until sheaths are removed, following which limb observations are the same as for those undergoing diagnostic procedures. Patients usually have to stay in bed for 4–6 hours after transfemoral sheath removal. Limb observations are routinely performed half-hourly for two hours, then hourly for four hours for patients having diagnostic procedures. Some cases may vary if a patients's condition warrants further close observations, not only for limbs but also for haemodynamic status.

Patients having AngioSeal™ or PerClose™ application after transfemoral sheath removal in the cardiac catheterisation laboratory may be allowed out of bed earlier, depending on the doctor's instructions.

Vital signs

Vital signs are taken hourly for 4 hours and then four-hourly. Any change in the patient's haemodynamic status is reported to the doctor.

On discharge

Management of patient care following cardiac catherisation or interventional procedures depends on the cardiologist's instructions. These may vary slightly from one cardiologist to another and from one hospital to another. In many hospitals, patients may be discharged on the same day, usually six hours after the procedure. However, these patients must be reviewed by a doctor prior to discharge. Patients having interventional procedures such as PTCA with or without stenting, or mitral valvuloplasty, may be discharged the next day if there are no complications or changes in haemodynamic status. Some patients may have to remain for further observations or investigations if required.

Upon discharge, patients are informed of the cardiac health program undertaken by the cardiac rehabilitation team. Patients may consider joining the program after discharge.

Summary

Nursing care and management are basically similar in all units, and involve continual monitoring of all patients for 24 hours, particularly following interventional procedures. Vital signs and haemodynamic status are assessed and limb observations are routinely taken. Limb observation is very important for patients, as any changes in status may be a warning of complications. As post-procedural care is largely the responsibility of nursing staff, the nurse's role as part of the cardiology team is vital.

References

1. Juran NB, Smith DB, Rouse CL *et al.* Survey of patient practice patterns for percutaneous transluminal coronary angioplasty. *Am J Crit Care* 1996; **5**:442–448.
2. The Heart Centre, Akron General internet site: www.agmc.org/hrtcath.htm and Advocate Health Care internet site: www.advocatehealth.com/healthinfo/articles/heartcare/invasive/cardcath.html
3. Staunton P, Whyburn B. *Nursing and the law.* Sydney: WB Saunders 1989.
4. Lazzara D, Pfersdorf P, Sedlacek M. Femoral compression. *Nursing* 1997 (Dec):54–58.
5. Spokojny AM, Sanborn TA. Management of the arterial puncture site. *J Intervent Cardiol* 1994; **2**:187–93.
6. O'Brien C, Recker D. How to remove a femoral sheath. *AJN* 1992 (Oct):34–37.
7. University of Virginia Health Sciences Centre and School of Nursing. Reducing time in bed after cardiac catheterisation. *Am J Crit Care* 1996; **5**:277–81.
8. Montes P. Managing outpatient cardiac catheterization. *AJN* 1997; **97**:34–37.

Chapter 30

Vascular Access Site Management and Arterial Closure

Peter Hadjipetrou

Percutaneous catheterisation via the transfemoral route is a widely used technique for diagnostic and interventional cardiovascular procedures. When the procedure is completed, the femoral sheaths are removed and pressure must be applied to the artery until haemostasis is achieved. Meticulous management of the vascular access site is an integral part of patient care in order to avoid puncture-related complications. The number and complexity of catheterisations performed worldwide continues to increase, with vascular complications estimated to occur in 0.2–1.9% of patients undergoing elective diagnostic angiography, depending on the access site used, and up to 10% in patients undergoing certain interventional procedures.[1-5]

There has been considerable expansion in the indications for diagnostic and percutaneous coronary intervention. More high-risk patients are being included, necessitating a variety of new devices to improve success rates. The incidence of complications varies widely because of the diversity of procedures in an increasingly ageing population. Predictors associated with an increased incidence of vascular hazards include older age, presence of peripheral vascular disease, puncture of the superficial femoral artery, smaller body surface area, use of larger-calibre introducing sheaths, the brachial approach, duration and intensity of periprocedural anticoagulants and use of glycoprotein IIb/IIIa receptor inhibitors.[6,7]

Puncture technique and complications

A careful puncture technique is important to avoid risks associated with superficial femoral artery puncture and simultaneous artery and vein puncture. As a general guide, it is safer to puncture the artery directly above the inferior border of the femoral head. This may be facilitated by fluoroscopic guidance if necessary. The inguinal skin crease should be avoided as an anatomical landmark because of its variable location in relation to the common femoral artery. Puncture of the femoral artery above the inguinal ligament should also be avoided because of the increased risk of retroperitoneal haematoma. Other complications range from simple haematomas to more serious injuries that may require surgical repair, false aneurysms, arterio-venous fistulae, infection, arterial thrombosis leading to critical limb ischaemia, femoral neurological deficits and significant bleeding requiring transfusion, with its attendant risks of disease transmission. This can lead to potentially avoidable prolonged hospital stays, increased patient discomfort, inconvenience, periprocedural morbidity and added cost, regardless of how successful or elegant the procedure may otherwise have been.

It is important to recognise peripheral vascular complications early, and this can often be done at the bedside. External haemorrhage is easily recognised and should be managed by immediate compression. Retroperitoneal bleeding is often more difficult to diagnose. It should be suspected in any patient with unexplained hypotension or falling haemoglobin levels following femoral instrumentation. Common presenting symptoms include significant back or flank pain and suprainguinal tenderness and fullness.[8] It is more commonly seen following intensive anticoagulation in conjunction with glycoprotein IIb/IIIa receptor antagonists and prolonged sheath dwelling times. The diagnosis is often made clinically but can be confirmed if necessary by computed tomographic scanning. Femoral artery thrombosis is associated with loss of peripheral pulses and clinical signs of limb ischaemia. The diagnosis is usually confirmed by duplex sonography or angiography. Vascular duplex scanning is useful to distinguish a large haematoma from an expanding pseudoaneurysm or arterio-venous fistula. Duplex scanning is also an effective tool for non-surgical repair of pseudoaneurysms. This is achieved by Doppler guided compression until flow into the pseudoaneurysm is obliterated.

Access site

The femoral approach is used for access in the majority of patients, although the transradial artery puncture is becoming increasingly common. With current techniques it has become routine to use 6-French and 7-French procedural sheaths as a result of the steady improvement in accessibility to the lesion site in standard angioplasty. The radial approach has the advantage of minimising access site complications and is relatively easy to use, allowing immediate sheath removal even in anticoagulated patients. It is very comfortable for patients, and operator time is shorter, with earlier ambulation a distinct advantage.

With the femoral route, vascular complications may occur more frequently because of the larger sheaths and guiding catheters used for new techniques (e.g. directional and rotational atherectomy, thrombectomy, intra-aortic balloon pump).

Closure of puncture site

Vascular access complications, as well as the discomfort associated with manual compression and prolonged bed rest, have led to several new haemostatic devices for closure of the arterial puncture. These have been studied in several trials evaluating their safety, effectiveness and ease of handling compared with the conventional method of manual compression. There is also potential for improved cost-effectiveness from earlier ambulation and shortened hospital stays.

Direct closure by open suturing of the brachial artery was the first technique described by Sones for achieving haemostasis at the access site. Alternatively, with the introduction of Judkin's percutaneous femoral method for cardiac catheterisation, haemostasis is achieved with direct compression either manually or with a C-clamp device for 10 to 40 minutes. A pneumatic vascular compression device (Femostop,™ C.R. Bard, Billerica, MA) has also been developed to apply external femoral artery compression after sheath removal, with comparable success and complication rates.

Manual compression

The main issues with regard to management of the vascular access site are the safe removal of the catheter or sheath and accomplishing haemostasis without bleeding or arterial injury. This is most commonly achieved by digital or mechanical compression of the artery to control bleeding and to allow coagulation to occur. In manual compression, arterial sheath removal is usually delayed 4–6 h after interventional procedures or heparin discontinuation. Application of pressure is necessary for periods up to 20 minutes or longer and both hands are usually required for digital compression.

Mechanical devices

Mechanical devices such as the C-Clamp consist of a disk-shaped pressure pad attached to an inverted U-shaped structure that is in turn attached to a vertical shaft so that it can slide up and down. The device is supported by a broad base, which is slipped beneath the patient's hip. When the sheath is removed, downward pressure is applied on the arm, which lowers the disk-pad over the puncture site to compress the artery. The arm automatically locks in this position and is released when coagulation is estimated to have occurred. The height of the arm and the pressure applied can be easily adjusted. The main advantage of this device is that of convenience, allowing the operator to perform other duties while coagulation is taking place. In a randomised trial comparing the effectiveness of manual or C-clamp mechanical compression it was found that patients receiving mechanical compression had a lower incidence of haematoma formation and shorter time to haemostasis.[9,10]

The Femostop pneumatic compression device consists of an inflatable transparent bubble attached to an arch made of hard plastic. The plastic guard is secured with an adjustable belt around the patient's hips. Pressure is applied by gradually inflating the bubble as the sheath is removed, to temporarily occlude the vessel until haemostasis occurs. Advantages include the ability to accurately control compression pressure using the manometer, and the low risk of device malposition with patient movement. This device is safe and effective and seems to cause less discomfort than the C-clamp. It also allows application of gentle compression for prolonged periods, which may lead to a lower incidence of false aneurysm formation. This should be able to be performed with minimum patient discomfort, allowing early recovery, ambulation and discharge.

In general, several hours of bed rest with the patient immobilised are necessary following the haemostasis procedure.

Direct arterial closure devices

The major disadvantages of compression techniques are that they are time-consuming and anticoagulation has to be reduced before they can be performed safely. This prolongs bed rest, causes patient discomfort and delays convalescence. This has led to the development of several devices to facilitate direct closure of the femoral arteriotomy site, including collagen plug devices (VasoSeal™, AngioSeal™), and percutaneous suture closure (PerClose™). These devices can achieve satisfactory haemostasis with success rates equivalent to manual and mechanical compression. If used successfully they provide the advantage of allowing immediate sheath removal and early patient ambulation, shortening the convalescence period.

Collagen plugs

Several commercially available devices have been developed to allow delivery of collagen at the exterior of the vessel to achieve haemostasis after arterial puncture. These include the Vascular Haemostatic Device (VHD VasoSeal, Datascope Corp., Montvale, NJ) and Angioseal (Sherwood Davis & Geck, St Louis Missouri), which is a collagen plug with an anchor mechanism.

VasoSeal

The VasoSeal haemostatic device is the prototype bovine collagen device. It consists of purified collagen plugs that induce formation of a haemostatic cap directly over the arterial puncture site. The biodegradable collagen plug induces local platelet activation and aggregation, releasing coagulation factors and resulting in the formation of fibrin and thrombus. Collagen is ultimately degraded by granulocytes and macrophages. The delivery system uses two 90 mg collagen cartridges advanced through an 11.5 F sheath directly over the arterial surface, guided by pre-procedure needle depth measurements and use of a blunt-tipped dilator. After the application of the collagen plug, light pressure is sustained for 3–5 minutes to obtain haemostasis.

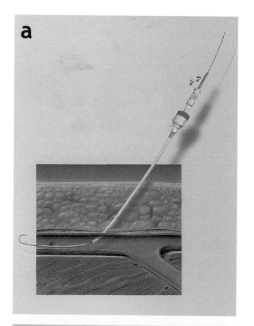

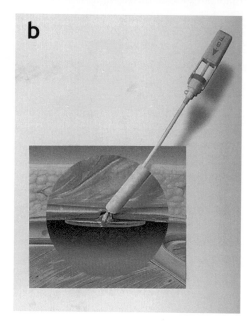

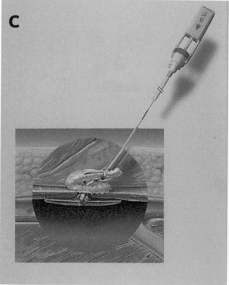

Figure 30.1. The AngioSeal device has 3 absorbable components: An anchor deployed intra-arterially, a collagen sponge positioned on the outer wall of the artery, and a suture. The procedure involves locating the artery (a), setting the anchor (b), and sealing the puncture (c) by applying tension on the suture to draw the collagen sponge and anchor together, 'sandwiching' the arteriotomy.

Collagen plugs are relatively safe and effective, allowing for earlier patient mobilisation compared with manual compression after diagnostic angiography, and are particularly helpful when haemostasis has to be achieved and uninterrupted anticoagulation is desirable. Compared with conventional manual compression the time needed to attain haemostasis using the collagen plug is decreased by about 14 minutes after diagnostic catheterisation (using 6F to 8F) and by about 25–30 minutes after angioplasty.[2,8] Shorter time to haemostasis is achieved if sealing is performed at a comparable prothrombin time with similar sheath dwell times as for manual compression.[11]

While VasoSeal does not influence the rate of minor local events, there appears to be an increase in the incidence of major complications. In a retrospective review of the VasoSeal haemostasis device in predominantly anticoagulated patients, complications included vascular surgery in 5%, failure to achieve haemostasis (2%), late external bleeding (2%), purulent discharge (1.5%) and large (>6 cm) haematomas (6%). Smaller (<6 cm) haematomas occurred in 7% and minor blood oozing in 7%. One or more complications were noted in 30.5% of cases.[12] These complication rates are similar to other reports and appear to be higher than with manual compression.[13] There is no difference regarding local complications between VasoSeal and manual compression when sheath dwell times are identical at similar levels of anticoagulation.

There are some other disadvantages to using this device. Delayed application carries a potential risk of infection and is not recommended. Repuncture of the same artery within 1 month should be avoided because of the risk of intraluminal dislocation of the collagen, which can cause local thrombosis or distal embolisation. Also, the late proliferative reaction induced by the collagen can lead to subcutaneous scar formation and make future arterial access more difficult.

Because of the relatively higher incidence of access site complications associated with this device its use has been mainly limited to those situations where immediate haemostasis is desirable in patients with high levels of anticoagulation. It has not been recommended for routine use after angioplasty.

Implantable collagen devices

The Haemostatic Puncture Closure Device (AngioSeal) produces direct femoral arterial haemostasis by deploying a bioabsorbable anchor through a carrier sheath to the anterior vascular wall. The anchor is drawn up tightly against the arteriotomy by means of an absorbable suture, while drawing down a small collagen plug. This combination of the anchor with the collagen plug retained by the suture forms a mechanical 'sandwich' around the arteriotomy (Fig. 30.1).

The success rate of device deployment is high and the time to haemostasis is considerably shorter, even in patients with higher levels of anticoagulation. In most patients this is almost immediate (within 1 minute). Compared with manual compression, complication rates appear to be lower for bleeding and haematoma but there is no difference in the incidence of pseudo-aneurysm, arterio-venous fistulae, limb ischaemia, or infection.[14–16]

AngioSeal allows earlier haemostasis and ambulation, without associated decrease in safety, compared with traditional methods such as manual compression. It is therefore particularly useful in patients who receive heparin and in those undergoing interventional procedures, allowing shorter sheath dwell times and earlier ambulation and discharge. Its major disadvantage is that re-puncture of the artery is not recommended for at least 3 months after use of the device.

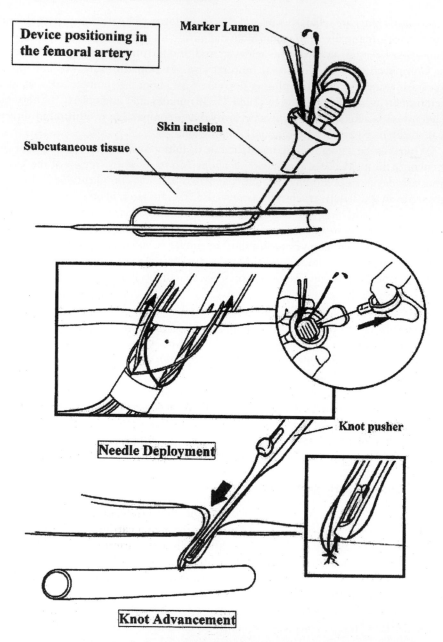

Figure 30.2. *Illustration of the percutaneous suture closure device (Perclose) in its correct position, indicated by pulsatile blood return from the dedicated marker lumen. The needles are unlocked and pulled through the arterial wall during deployment. The knot pusher is used to appose the knot to the arterial wall.*

Percutaneous suturing devices

Devices have been designed for percutaneous deployment of surgical sutures to the common femoral arterial puncture site during diagnostic or interventional procedures (Perclose,™ Techstar™/Prostar™). The needles, with attached sutures, are housed in a sheath delivery system, which is advanced through the arteriotomy over a wire. A dedicated marker lumen is incorporated to indicate that the needles and sutures are within the vessel lumen by pulsatile blood return. The needles carrying the sutures are then deployed through the edges of the arteriotomy and tied with a sliding knot and knot pusher to ensure apposition of the knot to the vessel wall (Fig. 30.2). These devices provide a safe and effective method of achieving haemostasis to allow early or immediate ambulation. They significantly shorten time to haemostasis, even when used in fully anticoagulated patients, without significant increase in the incidence of major access-site-related complications.[17,18] There is a relatively prolonged learning curve, with high volume users of the device generally achieving a higher success rate.

Conclusions

Use of mechanical devices to achieve arterial puncture site haemostasis can result in prolonged hospital stay, patient discomfort, and vascular complications. Various strategies to achieve more complete haemostasis and earlier patient ambulation have included use of smaller sheath sizes, C-clamps or pneumatic compression devices, plus a variety of arterial closure devices. Their effectiveness has been enhanced by the current practice in percutaneous interventions of reducing post-procedural anticoagulation. However, these various methods of securing haemostasis must be compared with the 'gold standard' of manual compression, which is safe and effective. Recently there has been a shift towards the use of ancillary devices to achieve haemostasis, as these permit immediate sheath removal and haemostasis.

Various factors influence the choice of haemostasis technique. Patient factors include the risk of complications and patient tolerance for the technique, taking into consideration body size, discomfort, and the expected duration of compression. Operator factors include individual preference for a device based on previous experience and the learning curve associated with the technique, ease of use and patient safety. Institutional factors include cost, availability of equipment and length of hospital stay. Regardless of the haemostatic device used, it is important for the groin access management scheme to be performed safely and with minimal discomfort to the patient.

References

1. Johnson LW, Lozner E, Johnson S *et al.* Coronary arteriography 1984–1987: A report of the registry of the society for cardiac angiography and interventions. I. Results and complications. *Cathet Cardiovasc Diagn* 1989; **17**:5–10.
2. Messina LM, Brothers TE, Wakefield TW *et al.* Clinical characteristics and surgical management of vascular complications in patients undergoing cardiac catheterization: Interventional versus diagnostic procedures. *J Vasc Surg* 1991; **13**:593–600.
3. Spokojny AM, Sanborn TA. Management of arterial puncture site. *J Interven Cardiol* 1994; **7**:187–93.
4. Johnson LW, Esente P, Giambartolomei A *et al.* Peripheral vascular complications of coronary angioplasty by the femoral and brachial techniques. *Cathet Cardiovasc Diagn* 1994; **31**:165–72.
5. Kaufman J, Moglia R, Lacy C *et al.* Peripheral vascular complications from percutaneous transluminal coronary angioplasty. A comparison with transfemoral cardiac catheterisation. *Am J Med Sci* 1989; **297**(1):22–5.
6. EPIC investigators. Use of a monoclonal antibody directed against the platelet glycoprotein IIb/IIIa receptor in high-risk coronary angioplasty. *N Engl J Med* 1994; **330**:956–61.
7. EPILOG investigators. Platelet glycoprotein IIb/IIIa blockade with abciximab with low-dose heparin during percutaneous coronary revascularization. *N Engl J Med* 1997; **336**:1689–96.

8.   Kent KC, Moscucci M, Mansour KA *et al*. Retroperitoneal haematoma after cardiac catheterisation: Prevalence, risk factors, and optimal management. *J Vasc Surg* 1994; **20**:905–13.

9.   Semler HJ. Transfemoral Catheterization: Mechanical versus Manual control of bleeding. *Radiology* 1985; **154**:234–5.

10. Semler HJ, Experience with an external clamp to control bleeding following transfemoral catheterization. *Radiology* 1974; **110**:225–6.

11. Silber S, Bjorvik A, Rosch A. Usefulness of collagen plugging with VasoSeal after PTCA as compared to manual compression with identical sheath dwell times. *Cathet Cardiovasc Diagn* 1998; **43**:421–7.

12. Carere RG, Webb JG, Miyagishima R *et al*. Groin Complications associated with Collagen Plug closure of femoral arterial puncture sites in anticoagulated patients. *Cathet Cardiovasc Diagn* 1998; **43**:124–9.

13. Camenzind E, Grossholz M, Urban P *et al*. Collagen application versus manual compression: A prospective randomized trial for arterial puncture site closure after coronary angioplasty. *J Am Coll Cardiol* 1994; **24**:655–62.

14. Cremonesi A, Castriota F, Tarantino F *et al*. Femoral arterial haemostasis using the Angio-Seal system after coronary and vascular percutaneous angioplasty and stenting. *J Invas Cardiol* 1998; **10**:464–9.

15. Fry SM. Review of the Angio-Seal hemostatic puncture closure device. *J Invas Cardiol* 1998; **10**(2):111–120.

16. Kussmaul III WG, Buchbinder M, Whitlow PL *et al*. Rapid arterial haemostasis and decreased access site complications after cardiac catheterization and angioplasty: Results of a randomized trial of a novel haemostatic device. *J Am Coll Cardiol* 1995; **25**:1685–92.

17. Chamberlin JR, Lardy AB, McKeveer LS *et al*. Use of vascular sealing device (VasoSeal and Perclose) versus assisted manual compression (Femostop) in transcatheter coronary interventions requiring Abciximab (Reopro). *Cathet Cardiovasc Interv* 1999; **47**:143–7.

18. Gerckens U, Cattelaens N, Lampe EG, *et al*. Management of arterial puncture site after catheterization procedures: evaluating a suture mediated closure device. *Am J Cardiol* 1999; **83**(12):1658–63.

Chapter 31

Medical Management of the Cardiac Patient Undergoing Coronary Angiography

Jerry Greenfield, Drew Mumford and Gerard Carroll

A ccess to cardiac catheterisation units and the advent of interventional cardiology have revolutionised the treatment of acute coronary syndromes in the last few decades. Emergency angioplasty and coronary artery stenting, together with the ongoing development of new anti-platelet agents, have dramatically altered the management of acute myocardial infarction (AMI) and unstable angina pectoris (UAP). This chapter examines the indications for cardiac catheterisation, preparation of the coronary care patient prior to angiography, potential complications of catheter procedures and the management of patients on return to the coronary care unit after angiography.

Indications for cardiac catheterisation

A prominent role of the coronary care unit is to determine which presentations of chest pain are due to acute coronary syndromes (i.e. UAP or AMI). Other frequent indications for admission and cardiac catheterisation include acute dyspnoea of cardiac origin or acute haemodynamic compromise due to arrythmias, pump failure or valvular disease. These may be classified under the following five major categories:

1. Diagnostic clarification of acute ischaemic syndrome

The decision and timing of cardiac catheterisation in individuals with acute ischaemic syndromes is variable. 'High-risk' patients (i.e. those with fluctuating S–T segments, prolonged rest pain and elevated troponins in the first 8 hours after onset of pain) should be considered for urgent catheterisation. In terms of completed myocardial infarction, the development of in-hospital complications, the most common of which is ongoing is-chaemia, is a common indication for coronary angiography before discharge. Ongoing ischaemia may be evident as rest angina or a positive sub-maximal exercise stress test prior to discharge. Other in-hospital complications requiring angiography following a myocardial infarction include cardiogenic shock, reinfarction, ventricular tachyarrythmias with accompanying haemodynamic instability and development of an infarct-related ventricular septal defect or papillary muscle infarction leading to severe mitral regurgitation.

There is some debate over the role and timing of angiography and angioplasty for acute coronary syndromes. Studies of patients with myocardial infarction and S–T segment elevation who achieve successful coronary artery opening following thrombolysis have shown that immediate angioplasty (without stenting or intensive platelet inhibition) offers no significant benefit in terms of mortality (4% immediate vs 1% elective; p=0.37), rates of reocclusion (11% immediate vs 13% elective; p=0.67) or improvement in ejection fraction when compared with patients who undergo angioplasty 7 days after the acute event.[1]

The TIMI IIIB trial[2] compared the effects of tissue plasminogen activator (t-PA) with placebo as well as an early invasive, conservative strategy in 1473 patients with non Q-wave infarction or UAP. The 12-month follow-up results for death and/or non-fatal infarction showed that early invasive procedures had no significant benefit over conservative management (10.8% vs. 12.2%, p=0.42), but did result in significantly shorter hospital stays and fewer subsequent readmissions. The study also revealed that administration of t-PA resulted in no survival benefit or reduction in reinfarction rates over placebo at one year for both the UAP and non Q-wave infarct groups, and was associated with significantly increased rates of haemorrhagic stroke. The group of patients with UAP treated with t-PA had an increased incidence of death and infarction compared to the placebo group. This difference was found not to be significant by one year (12.5% vs. 9.7% p=0.13).

More recently, results of the VANQWISH Trial[3] were published for 920 patients presenting with non Q-wave infarction. This study compared an early 'invasive' strategy (angiography followed by myocardial revascularistion, if appropriate) versus an early 'conservative' management plan (non-invasive, pre-discharge thallium stress-testing). In the latter group, myocardial revascularisation was indicated if patients developed ischaemia or had positive stress tests. The primary endpoint (death or non-fatal myocardial infarction) was found to be significantly lower in patients who were randomised to the 'conservative' group: at hospital discharge (15 vs 36 patients, p=0.004), at 30 days (26 vs 48 patients, p=0.012) and at 12 months (85 vs 111, p=0.025). Similarly, overall mortality was significantly lower in the non-invasive group at these times. It should be noted, however, that the primary reason for the higher incidence of adverse outcomes in the invasive group was an unusually high mortality rate in patients who required bypass graft surgery. The mortality curves tended to converge by the end of the follow-up period (approximately 1000 days).

2. Primary management in acute coronary occlusion

There is an increasing tendency in some major metropolitan centres to offer primary angioplasty, usually with stenting, for the unequivocal acute coronary occlusion. The argument for this aggressive approach is strongest in the case of significant coexistent contraindications to thrombolysis and when the patient is haemodynamically compromised, particularly with cardiogenic shock, which has a very poor prognosis when treated conservatively. The initial trials exploring whether primary angioplasty was superior to thrombolysis for the treatment of infarction yielded conflicting results. With the advent of improved antiplatelet therapy and more widespread use of stents, immediate intervention for acute coronary occlusion has now become a feasible and efficacious first-line treatment in selected cases.[4]

The Primary Angioplasty in Myocardial Infarction trial (PAMI)[5] was the first major study in its class. The purpose of this prospective, randomised multicentre trial, in which 395 patients were enrolled, was to compare use of intravenous t-PA with primary angioplasty in the treatment of myocardial infarction. Immediate angioplasty was successful in 97.1% of cases, with no patients requiring coronary artery bypass grafting as an emergency procedure. The in-hospital mortality rate was 2.6% in the angioplasty group and 6.5% in the t-PA group (p=0.06). The combined endpoint of reinfarction and in-hospital death was lower in the angioplasty group (5.1% for angioplasty group compared to 12% in the t-PA group; p=0.02) and this benefit continued to 6 months (8.5% angioplasty group vs 16.8% t-PA group; p=0.02). No haemorrhagic strokes occurred in the angioplasty group compared with 2% in the t-PA group (p=0.05). The left ventricular ejection fraction at 6 weeks was the same in both groups. The negatives of immediate angioplasty in this non-stent trial included a greater need for vascular surgical repair (2.1% angioplasty group vs 0% in t-PA group) and a significantly increased risk of ventricular fibrillation compared with treatment with t-PA (6.7% angioplasty group vs 2.0% in t-PA group, p=0.02).

Some of the trials that followed PAMI, which have incorporated longer follow-up periods, failed to show a significant advantage of angioplasty over thrombolysis. The GUSTO IIb Trial,[6] which involved 1138 patients with AMI, randomly assigned patients to angioplasty or an accelerated dose of t-PA. There was no statistically significant difference between the two groups in the mortality at 30 days (5.7% in the angioplasty group vs 7.0% in the t-PA group; p=0.37). There was, however, a statistically significant difference in the composite endpoint of death, non-fatal reinfarction and non-fatal disabling stroke at 30 days (9.6% in the angioplasty group vs 13.7% in the t-PA group; p=0.033). At 6 months there was no significant difference in the composite outcome (14.1% vs 16.1%).

A similar finding was reported by Every *et al.*,[7] who enrolled more than 3000 patients at the time of myocardial infarction. Over 1000 were assigned to the primary angioplasty arm and over 2000 to the thrombolytic arm. There was no statistically significant difference in the in-hospital mortality (5.6% in the thrombolytic group and 5.5% in the primary angioplasty group, p=0.93) or mortality at 3 years. There was no difference between the two groups in the proportion of patients requiring admission to hospital or bypass grafting at 1- or 3- year follow-up. In addition, there was a 13% lower cumulative cost at 3 years in the thrombolytic group.

In recent years, with the advent of abciximab and greater experience in primary angioplasty, there have been more favourable outcomes with early intervention. Two meta-analyses that include trials comparing primary angioplasty with thrombolytic regimens support this conclusion. Weaver *et al.*[8] identified 10 randomised trials from 1985-1996 and found that 30-day mortality was significantly lower in the primary angioplasty group (4.4% vs 6.5%, p=0.02). Rates of death or non-fatal infarction were also significantly reduced in the angioplasty group (7.2% vs 11.9%, p<0.001). There were also significantly fewer total strokes (0.7% vs 2.0%, p=0.007) and haemorrhagic strokes (0.1% vs 1.1%, p<0.001) in those who underwent angioplasty. Similarly, Michels and Yusuf[9] reported a meta-analysis of seven trials in which patients presenting with acute myocardial infarction were treated with either primary angioplasty or thrombolysis. They reported an odds ratio of 0.53 (95% CI 0.33–0.94) in favour of angioplasty for the combined endpoint of death or non-fatal reinfarction at 6 weeks but mortality rates were not significantly different at 1 year (odds ratio 0.91, 95% CI 0.42–2.00).

Outcomes can be further improved by judicious use of coronary stents and glycoprotein IIb/IIIa inhibition in the setting of AMI. In the Stent–PAMI trial,[10] although there was no difference in in-hospital outcomes, there was a statistically significant difference in event-free survival at 6 months in the stented patients, due principally to a reduction in need for repeat revascularisation procedures. Similarly, there appeared to be a small incremental benefit in both angioplasty and stent patients who were assigned to receive adjunctive abciximab in the CADILLAC trial,[11] a four-way comparison of angioplasty vs angioplasty and abciximab vs stent vs stent and abciximab. It should be noted that the outcomes were remarkably good in all four arms of this trial.

Therefore, in terms of the choice of primary therapy for acute coronary syndromes, there are data to support different approaches. The time from onset of symptoms to opening of the artery is critical, as final size of the infarct and the prognosis are directly related to the duration of coronary occlusion. Currently, only a minority of coronary care facilities are in a position to provide a 24-hour angioplasty service for AMI. The intuitive benefit of opening an artery by primary angioplasty compared to administration of a thrombolytic agent has not necessarily translated into a clear-cut improvement in outcome, but there does appear to be a reduction in the incidence of recurrent ischaemia in patients treated invasively.

3. Rescue angioplasty for failed thrombolysis, especially in the setting of ongoing ST segment and haemodynamic compromise

Rescue angioplasty involves angioplasty for persistent occlusion of the infarct-related artery in the case of failed thrombolytic therapy, especially when there are signs of haemodynamic compromise. In a recent meta-analysis,[1] there was a trend towards a reduction in both the 6-week and 1-year mortality in patients treated with rescue angioplasty compared with those treated with thrombolysis alone.

4. Management of valvular and congenital heart disease

Long-term success rates of percutaneous mitral balloon valvotomy for mitral stenosis in selected patients are comparable to surgical commissurotomy.[12] Echocardiography is a useful investigative tool in identifying patients who will have favourable outcomes (i.e. those with little or no valve calcification, good valve mobility, minimal valve thickening, minimal mitral regurgitation, no involvement of subvalvular structures and no intercurrent left atrial thrombus).[13] Complications of mitral valvuloplasty include death (0.5%), atrial septal defect (10%) (most are small and close spontaneously), severe mitral regurgitation (2%), ventricular perforation (1%), stroke (1%) and restenosis (10%).[14]

Balloon valvuloplasty for degenerative calcific aortic stenosis in adults has no long-term haemodynamic or symptomatic benefit.[15,16] There is a high restenosis rate (50% by 6 months) as well as a risk of aortic regurgitation, aortic rupture, leaflet avulsion, ventricular perforation, systemic embolisation or stroke and local vascular injury. Balloon valvuloplasty is therefore reserved for patients with critical aortic stenosis who are extremely unwell and are awaiting aortic valve replacement, or who require urgent non-cardiac surgery.[17]

Percutaneous balloon valvuloplasty for congenital pulmonary stenosis has been highly successful and is now the procedure of choice provided the valve is not heavily calcified. Long-term 'curative' outcomes have been achieved with very low procedural mortality (0.2%).[18] Balloon valvuloplasty for congenital non-calcific aortic stenosis has been performed successfully, but the procedural mortality is higher (2.4%)[19] and long-term follow-up studies have not yet been completed.

The first congenital heart lesion to be treated with non-surgical transcatheter devices in the 1970s was a patent ductus arteriosus (PDA). Since then, a number of other innovative devices have been developed for closure of atrial septal defects (ASD) and patent foramen ovale (PFO). The two ASD/PFO closure devices currently used are the Amplatzer™ Septal Occluder Device and the CardioSeal™.

There is growing experience with the use of the Amplatzer™ Septal Occluder, which consists of a self-expanding double-disc Nitinol™ wire mesh with polyester layers. The Amplatzer™ device may be deployed via a 6F to 12F sheath under guidance of simultaneous transoesophageal echocardiography. More than 4000 of these devices have been deployed worldwide, many in children. Complete shunt obliteration is achieved in approximately 94% of patients by 3 months.[20] Complication rates are low and include:[21]

Right ventricular embolism	0.9%
Transient ischaemic attack	0.4%
Endocarditis	0.4%

Patients undergoing transcatheter closure of an ASD, PFO or PDA are admitted on the same day of the procedure and are usually discharged the following morning. In addition to aspirin for 48 hours prior to the procedure, perioperative heparin (5000–15000 units) and antibiotic prophylaxis are given in the cardiac catheter suite. Post-procedure, a regimen of aspirin 300 mg daily for 6 months and clopidrogel 75 mg daily for one month is commenced. In addition, antibiotic prophylaxis is advised prior to invasive procedures for 6 months, by which time endothelialisation of the device is expected to have been completed. To determine whether successful closure has occurred, transthoracic echocardiograms are performed at 1, 3 and then 12 months post deployment. Despite shorter 'lengths-of-stay', high efficacy rates and comparable costs with surgery, non-surgical techniques for ASD and PDA closures remain largely experimental and await further large multicentre trial outcomes.

5. Other indications for cardiac catheterisation

Acute breathlessness is a common indication for admission to the coronary care unit. Cardiac catheterisation plays an important diagnostic role in determining the aetiology, e.g. left ventricular dysfunction secondary to either coronary artery disease or cardiomyopathy; valvular heart disease; pulmonary hypertension, or an intra-aortic shunt.

Primary arrhythmias such as ventricular tachycardia, and sometimes atrial fibrillation, may be a manifestation of significant coronary disease, even without clear-cut ST segment changes or chest pain. Patients with severe chest pain and left bundle branch block may benefit from early definition of their coronary anatomy.

Preparation for cardiac catheterisation

An important function of the coronary care unit is the preparation of the patient prior to coronary angiography. This includes patient education and obtaining informed consent. Most patients receive a premedication comprising of an oral benzodiazepine and/or a sedating antihistamine before transfer to the catheterisation laboratory. Patients with pre-existing renal disease are at increased risk of contrast nephropathy from the iodinated contrast used at cardiac catheterisation. This risk can be minimised by intravenous hydration before, during and after the procedure and strict limitation of contrast volume (i.e. omission of ventriculography or aortography).

Patients with diabetes make up a large proportion of patients undergoing coronary angiography, as a result of the markedly increased risk of coronary artery disease associated with diabetes. Patients with diabetes in the PROCAM study[22] had at least twice the risk of myocardial infarction compared with those without diabetes. The presence of other cardiovascular risk factors was found to increase this risk even further. Patients in the PROCAM population with both diabetes and hyperlipidaemia had a 15-fold increased risk of infarction. As reported by Haffner in 1998,[23] patients with diabetes without a history of ischaemic heart disease have as high a risk of infarction as non-diabetic patients with previous myocardial infarction.

Patients with diabetes require several special precautions prior to cardiac catheterisation, including prehydration to minimise the risk of contrast nephropathy and also in regard to the appropriate modification of oral hypoglycaemic agents and insulin therapy before and after angiography. As should occur perioperatively, patients with diabetes should omit their sulphonylurea whilst fasting. If the patient is taking metformin, this should be ceased 48 hours prior to angiography if possible, to minimise the potential risk of drug accumulation and lactic acidosis in the setting of contrast-related renal impairment.

Patients with a history of contrast allergy should be considered for pre-treatment with corticosteroid therapy. Those with a history of anaphylaxis to contrast media should receive at least 25 mg prednisone orally or 100 mg hydrocortisone intravenously at least 6 hours prior to the procedure.

Complications of cardiac catheterisation

Historically, two approaches to coronary arteriography have been used, one via the femoral and the other via the brachial artery. The CASS Registry[24] of more than 7500 procedures showed that the femoral approach has fewer complications, including death (0.14% vs 0.51%), stroke (0.08% vs 0.17%) and local vascular trauma (0.24% vs 1.85%), when compared with brachial techniques. The Judkins percutaneous puncture technique via the femoral artery has superseded the more traditional Sones cut-down technique via the arm.

The Registry of the Society for Cardiac Angiography and Interventions reported on 222 553 patients[25] who underwent cardiac catheterisation between 1984 and 1987. They found the following complication rates:

Death   0.10%
Myocardial infarction   0.06%
Stroke   0.07%
Local vascular complications (sheath haematomas, false aneurysms, arteriovenous fistulae and infection)   0.46%
Contrast reactions   0.23%

Other well-recognised complications include:[26]

Nephropathy   <0.5%
Serious arrhythmia   0.3–0.5%
Vasovagal reactions   1.5–2.5%

Patients identified at highest risk of death were those with left main coronary artery disease (0.55%), left ventricular ejection fractions < 30% (0.3%), NYHA functional class IV (0.29%)[25] and severe co-morbidities (eg. diabetes mellitus, renal impairment, chronic lung disease and peripheral vascular disease).[26]

Post-angiographic management in the coronary care unit

Following a routine cardiac catheterisation, the femoral sheath is removed and femoral haemostasis is achieved with digital pressure. In certain cases, a mechanical device such as a Femostop™ can be applied to maintain haemostasis, or to be used as surrogate for digital pressure (see Chapters 29,30). The aim of effective haemostasis following sheath removal is to prevent major blood loss, groin haematomas and false aneurysm formation. If this latter complication develops, Doppler ultrasound can be both diagnostic and therapeutic by compressing and closing the neck of the false aneurysm using the ultrasound probe. Several ingenious femoral artery closure devices that achieve haemostasis via a suture system or a patch on the wall of the affected femoral artery (e.g. Perclose™ and AngioSeal™ respectively) have been developed to minimise the risk of access site complications. There are theoretical risks with each of these devices, but they have the advantage of early mobilisation after successful deployment.

Post-procedurally, several anti-platelet regimens have been proposed. Providing there are no contraindications, patients who have had placement of an intra-arterial stent in our laboratory are given aspirin 600 mg and clopidogrel 300 mg immediately after the procedure. The following day they are commenced on aspirin 300 mg daily, which can be reduced to 150 mg after 3 months. In addition, clopidogrel 75 mg daily is continued for 1-month post-stenting. This corresponds to the time at which the risk of thrombosis of the coronary artery stent is increased.

Clopidogrel is a new anti-platelet agent similar to ticlopidine, with the added benefit of an almost negligible incidence of neutropaenia. Clopidogrel is a rapidly absorbed thienopyridine which irreversibly inhibits platelet aggregation by blocking the ADP receptor, thereby preventing the subsequent binding of fibrinogen to the glycoprotein IIb /IIIa complex.[27] Clopidogrel has an excellent overall safety profile, which in the CAPRIE study was found to be comparable to medium-dose aspirin. In particular, the incidence of neutropaenia (neutrophil count $< 1.2 \times 10^9/L$) in the group treated with clopidogrel was less than those prescribed aspirin (0.10 % vs 0.17%). Due to its relatively low side-effect profile, clopidogrel has largely superseded ticlopidine (an older thienopyridine derivative) for post-stent treatment. Ticlopidine therapy is associated with significant risk of neutropaenia (2.4%).[28]

The advent of abciximab (ReoPro™) has reduced the complication rate following angioplasty and stent insertion. It may also reduce the incidence of restenosis in both acute and elective patients.[29] Abciximab is the Fab fragment of the chimeric monoclonal antibody 7E3 which is directed against the glycoprotein IIb/IIIa receptor located on the surface of the human platelet. Abciximab is said to inhibit platelet aggregation by preventing the binding of von-Willebrand's factor, fibrinogen and other adhesive molecules to the above-mentioned receptor sites on activated platelets. The EPIC trial[30] was designed to assess whether abciximab could reduce the incidence of restenosis post-angioplasty in 2099 patients. These patients were considered to have high-risk angiographic lesions, unstable angina and recent or evolving myocardial infarctions. They were randomly assigned to receive either an abciximab bolus and 12-hour infusion, an abciximab bolus and placebo infusion or placebo bolus and infusion. The patients were followed for at least 6 months to determine the incidence of repeat angioplasty or surgical intervention and the recurrence of unstable angina or myocardial infarction. At 30-day follow-up there was a significant reduction in combined endpoints of 35% in the group who received the abciximab bolus and infusion compared with the placebo group (8.3% vs 12.8%, p=0.008). The abciximab bolus only group showed a 10% reduction in combined endpoints, but this was not statistically significant (11.4%, compared to the 12.8% described above; p= 0.43). This benefit was also apparent at 6 months, at which time the bolus and infusion group experienced a 23% reduction in the combined endpoint. At the expense of reduced coronary reocclusion rates in the EPIC trial, there was an excess of major bleeding and transfusions at 1 month compared with placebo (14%) in the abciximab bolus and infusion group vs 7% in placebo group; p=0.001). No difference was found in the incidence of intracranial haemorrhage in the three groups.

The other major trial involving use of abciximab in the setting of high- and low-risk angioplasty or atherectomy, the EPILOG trial,[31] found similar findings to those of the above study in terms of benefits, but there was no statistically significant increase in the incidence of haemorrhagic complications in the 30-day follow-up.

The use of abciximab is limited by its cost and is generally tailored to patients who develop complications during angioplasty and stenting. Broad guidelines[32] include the following:

Acute MI
Early post-infarction angina
UAP with fluctuating ST-T segments
Visible thrombus at the site of intervention

Degenerated saphenous vein grafts
Interventions in the sole patent coronary artery

All such patients are at risk of bleeding from their femoral puncture sites and therefore are usually maintained on bed rest for the period before the femoral sheath is removed (i.e. 4-6 hours) and for a further 4 hours post sheath removal.

Use of abciximab may be obviated by precatheterisation infusions of tirofiban (Aggrastat™), a short-acting non-peptide inhibitor of the platelet glycoprotein IIb/IIIa receptor. In the PRISM-PLUS trial,[33] tirofiban was reported to reduce ischaemic endpoints at 7 days in patients with unstable angina pectoris and non-Q wave infarcts when combined with heparin and aspirin. Published concurrently was the PRISM Trial,[34] which demonstrated a significant reduction in 30-day mortality in patients with UAP who received tirofiban in addition to aspirin, when compared with the group of patients who were treated with heparin and aspirin alone. The reduction in the composite end-point (death, myocardial infarction or refractory ischaemia) in the tirofiban/aspirin group (risk ratio 0.67, 95% CI 0.48–0.92, p=0.01) at 48 hours was not found to be significant at 30 days (risk ratio 0.92, 95% CI 0.78–1.09, p=0.34). Tirofiban treatment was not associated with a significant increase in major bleeding complications in either trial. Whether tirofiban will have a role in the management of patients post-angioplasty has not yet been established.

Conclusion

The coronary care unit is complementary to the successful functioning of any cardiac catheterisation laboratory. Recent advances in the treatment of congenital heart disease and acute coronary events have paved the way to a very exciting and promising future for cardiac medicine in the new millenium.

References

1.   Topol EJ, Califf RM, George BS *et al.* A randomised trial of immediate versus delayed elective angioplasty after intravenous tissue plasminogen activator in acute myocardial infarction. *N Engl J Med* 1987; **317**:581–8.
2.   Anderson HV, Cannon CP, Stone PH *et al.* One-year results of the thrombolysis in myocardial infarction (TIMI) IIIB clinical trial. A randomised comparison of tissue-type plasminogen activator vs placebo and early invasive vs conservative strategies in unstable angina and non-Q wave myocardial infarction. *J Am Coll Cardiol* 1995; **26**: 1643–50.
3.   Ferry DR, O'Rourke RA, Blaustein AS *et al.* Design and baseline characteristics of the Veterans Affairs non Q-wave infarction strategies in-hospital (VANQWISH) trial. *J Am Coll Cardiol* 1998; **31**:312–20.
4.   Stone GW, Brodie BR, Griffin JJ *et al.* Prospective, multicentre study of the safety and feasibility of primary stenting in acute myocardial infarction: In-hospital and 30-day results of the PAMI stent pilot trial. *J Am Coll Cardiol* 1998; **31**:23–30.
5.   Grines CL, Brown KF, Marco J *et al.* A comparison of immediate angioplasty with thrombolytic therapy for acute myocardial infarction. *N Engl J Med* 1993; **328**:673–9.
6.   GUSTO Angiographic Investigators. A clinical trial comparing coronary angioplasty and tissue plasminogen activator for acute myocardial infarction. The global use of strategies to open occluded coronary arteries in acute coronary syndrome (Gusto IIb). *N Engl J Med* 1997; **336**:1621–8.
7.   Every NR, Parsons LS, Hlatky M *et al.* A comparison of thrombolytic therapy with primary coronary angioplasty for acute myocardial infarction. *N Engl J Med* 1996; 335:1253–60.

8.   Weaver WD, Simes RJ, Betriu A *et al.* Comparison of primary coronary angioplasty and intravenous thrombolytic therapy for acute myocardial infarction. A quantitative review. *JAMA* 1997; **278**:2093–98.

9.   Michels KB and Yusuf S. Does PTCA in acute myocardial infarction affect mortality and reinfarction rates? A quantitative overview (meta-analysis) of randomised clinical trials. *Circulation* 1995; **91**:476 85.

10. Grines CL, Cox DA, Stone GW *et al.* Coronary angioplasty with or without stent implantation for acute myocardial infarction. Stent primary angioplasty in myocardial infarction study group. *N Engl J Med* 1999; **341**; (26)1949–56.

11. Stone G. Interim CADILLAC. Results underscore success rates of PTCA and stenting. American Heart Association Meeting, November 1999.

12. Reyes VP, Raju BS, Wynne J *et al.* Percutaneous balloon valvuloplasty compared with open surgical commissurotomy for mitral stenosis. *N Engl J Med* 1994; **331**:961–67.

13. Wilkins GT, Weyman AE, Abascal VM *et al.* Percutaneous mitral valvotomy: An analysis of echocardiographic variables related to outcome and the mechanism of dilatation. *Br Heart J* 1988; **60**:299–308.

14. Braunwald E. *Heart disease. A textbook of cardiovascular medicine*, 5th ed. Philadelphia: W.B.Saunders 1997, pp1016–17.

15. Lieberman EB, Bashore TM, Hermiller JB, *et al.* Balloon aortic valvuloplasty in adults: failure of procedure to improve long-term survival. *J Am Coll Cardiol* 1995; **26**:1522–28

16. Otto CM, Mickel MC, Kennedy JW *et al.* Three year outcome after balloon aortic valvuloplasty: Insights into prognosis of valvular aortic stenosis. *Circulation* 1994; **89**:642–50.

17. Braunwald E. *Heart disease. A textbook of cardiovascular medicine*, 5th ed. Philadelphia: W.B.Saunders 1997, p1044.

18. Stranger P, Cassidy SC, Girod DA *et al.* Balloon pulmonary valvuloplasty: Results of the valvuloplasty and angioplasty of congenital anomalies registry. *Am. J. Cardiol.* 199; **65**:775–783.

19. O'Conner BK, Beckman RH, Rocchini AP, Rosenthal A. Intermediate-term effectiveness of balloon valvuloplasty for congenital aortic stenosis: a prospective follow-up study. *Circulation* 1991; **84**:732–738.

20. Thanopoulos BV, Laskari CV, Tsaosis GS *et al.* Closure of atrial septal defects with the Amplatzer Occlusion device: Preliminary results. *J Am Coll Cardiol* 1998; **31**(5)1110–16.

21. Masura J, Lange PE, Hijazi ZM *et al.* US/International multicenter trial of atrial septal catheter closure using the Amplatzer septal occluder: Inital results (Abstract 804-1). *J Am Coll Cardiol* 1998; **31**(2)57A

22. Assmann G, Schulte H. Diabetes and hypertension in the elderly: concomitant hyperlipidaemia and coronary heart disease risk. *Am J Cardiol* 1989; **63**:33H–37H.

23   Haffner SM, Seppo L, Ronema *et al.* Mortality from coronary heart disease in subjects with type 2 diabetes and in non diabetic subjects with and without prior Myocardial infarction. *N Engl J Med* 1998; **339**:229–34.

24. Davis K, Kennedy JW, Kemp HG Jr *et al.* Complications of coronary arteriography for the collaborative study of coronary artery surgery (CASS). *Circulation* 1979; **59**:1105–12.

25. Johnson LW, Lozner EC, Johnson S *et al.* Coronary arteriography 1984–1987: A report of the Registry of the Society for Cardiac Angiography and Interventions: I Results and complications. *Cathet Cardiovasc Diagn* 1989; **17**:5.

26. Adair OV, Havranek EP. *Cardiology secrets*. Philadelphia: Hanley & Belfus 1995 p50.

27. Coukell AJ, Markham A. Clopidogrel: Adis New. Drug profile *Drugs* 1997; **54**; (5)745–50.

28. CAPRIE Steering Committee. A randomised, blinded, trial of clopidogrel versus aspirin in patients at risk of ischaemic events (CAPRIE). *Lancet* 1996; **348**:1329–39.

29. The EPISTENT investigators. Randomised placebo-controlled and balloon-angioplasty-controlled trial to assess safety of coronary stenting with use of platelet glycoprotein-IIb/IIIa blockade. *Lancet* 1998; **32**:87–92.

30. The Epic Investigators. Use of a monoclonal antibody directed against the platelet glycoprotein IIb/IIIa receptor in high-risk coronary angioplasty. *N Engl J Med* 1994; **330**:956–61.

31. The EPILOG Investigators. Platelet glycoprotein IIb/IIIa receptor blockade and low-dose heparin during percutaneous coronary revascularisation. *N Engl J Med* 1997; **336**:1689–96.
32. St Vincent's Hospital Drug Committee. *Formulary and guide to prescribing*, 2nd ed. St Vincent's Hospital, Sydney, 1998, p76.
33. The PRISM-PLUS Study Invesigators. Inhibition of the platelet glycoprotein IIb/IIIa receptor with Tirofiban in unstable angina and non-Q-wave myocardial infarction. *N Engl J Med* 1998; **338**:1488–97
34. The PRISM Study Investigators. A comparison of aspirin plus tirofiban with aspirin plus heparin for unstable angina. *N Engl J Med* 1998; **338**:1498–1505.

Chapter 32

The Intra-aortic Balloon Pump

Principles and use

Anthony Nicholson

Introduction

The intra-aortic balloon pump (IABP) is a device used to provide temporary support for the circulation during times of actual and potential cardiac dysfunction and is the most frequently used ventricular-assist device available today.[1] The intra-aortic balloon (IAB) is inserted into the aorta, usually via the femoral artery. Circulatory support is provided by counterpulsation, whereby the intra-aortic balloon is systematically inflated during early diastole and deflated just prior to systole. This increases coronary perfusion during the diastolic phase. By this means counterpulsation provides diastolic augmentation of intrinsic myocardial activity to supply blood to the heart and peripheral organs.

History

In 1968 Kantrowitz described the first clinically successful use of an IAB.[2] Since then many developments have occurred, to the extent that IABPs are now in their fourth generation.[3] Newer models are smaller, lighter and able to support patients during transport. Improvements in electronics have resulted in ease of use, increased automation and sophisticated alarm systems. Improvements have also been made in balloon design, particularly in regard to insertion and removal, which can both be performed without surgical assistance. This has resulted in increased portability and availability, as surgical expertise and operating conditions are no longer necessary. Current estimates suggest that IABPs are used in 70 000 patients annually.[4]

Indications

The IABP is primarily used in patients with heart failure that is severe but potentially reversible.[5] Other common reasons for using an IABP are situations of potential heart failure, where the IABP may be used to rest the myocardium, or where the myocardium may undergo a temporary insult due to an intervention or procedure such as surgery or percutaneous transluminal coronary angioplasty (PTCA).

Specific indications for use of IABP:

i)   left ventricular failure or cardiogenic shock
ii)   myocardial infarction
iii) refractory unstable angina

iv) failure to wean from heart-lung machine
v)   post cardiac transplant
vi) as a bridge to cardiac transplantation
vii) high-risk patients undergoing PTCA
viii) those in whom angioplasty has failed and their condition is subsequently unstable
ix) high-risk patients undergoing non-cardiac surgery requiring general anaesthesia
x)   papillary muscle rupture.[6]

There is increased prophylactic use of the IABP prior to cardiac surgery especially in patients with particularly compromised ventricular function (i.e. those in whom left ventricular ejection fraction [LVEF] <30%) who are considered to be at high risk.[7,8] Associated with this is a trend towards presurgical insertion of the IAB in patients where perioperative use is indicated. However, published studies have not demonstrated any significant improvement in outcomes.[4,8] Overall, the majority of IABs (30–50%) are inserted intraoperatively, most commonly due to failure to wean from cardiopulmonary bypass.[4,9] Perioperative use of IABP support occurs in 2–12% of all adult cardiac operations in the United States, and reported outcomes for these patients is relatively poor.[9]

Contraindications

Contraindications to IABP use can be either absolute or relative, in part depending on patient circumstances or status, and clinical judgement.
      Absolute contraindications include:

i)   irreversible brain damage
ii) end-stage heart disease, unless as support until transplantation
iii) dissecting aortic or thoracic aneurysms, as there is risk of further dissection.

Relative contraindications include:

i)   aortic incompetence, as counterpulsation may worsen the patient's condition by increasing myocardial workload
ii) severe peripheral vascular disease, which may hinder balloon insertion.[10,11]

Physiology of intra-aortic balloon pumping

The use of an IABP is aimed at:

i)   improving coronary artery perfusion
ii) increasing myocardial oxygen delivery as a result of increased aortic root and coronary perfusion pressures
iii) decreasing myocardial oxygen consumption by reduction of left ventricular afterload.

Other effects of IAB pumping include a decrease in left ventricular (LV) systolic wall tension, decreased LV end-systolic and end-diastolic volumes, reduced preload, and increased cardiac output.[4,12] Certain aspects of cardiovascular physiology have been presented in Chapter 9. However, to better appreciate the benefits of IABP specific physiological concepts need to be reviewed.

Cardiac cycle

Normal heart contractions are initiated by electrical signals generated within the sino-atrial node of the right atrium. In response to this electrical activity the myocardium of the ventricles contracts. The first phase is the period of **isovolumetric contraction**. At the

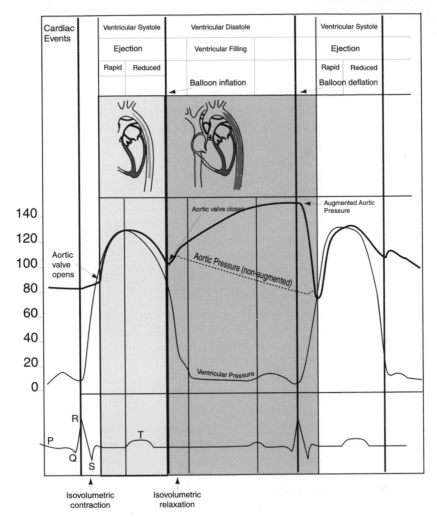

Figure 32.1. *Graphic representation of temporal changes in left ventricular and aortic pressures during two cardiac cycles and the associated electrocardiographic signals. Also displayed are the periods of IAB inflation and deflation relative to intrinsic pressure changes.*

beginning of this phase the mitral valve shuts and, with the aortic valve still closed, the ventricle starts to contract. This increases pressure within the left ventricle. When ventricular pressure exceeds that within the aortic root, the aortic valve opens. This marks the end of isovolumetric contraction, at which point the phase of **rapid ejection** begins, during which the ventricle continues to contract. This continued contraction increases ventricular and aortic pressures to their maximum values, the peak systolic pressures. The period of **reduced ejection** follows on immediately from that of rapid ejection. Ventricular pressure falls during this phase until pressure within the aorta is greater than that in the ventricle, which causes the aortic valve to shut. This marks the end of **ventricular systole**.

 Ventricular diastole starts with a period of **isovolumetric relaxation,** during which pressure within the left ventricle falls to a level below that of the atrium so that the mitral valve opens and the phase of **rapid filling** begins. This is followed by a period of **reduced ventricular filling** that continues until atrial systole, at which time the atrial muscle contracts and completes ventricular filling. Atrial contraction contributes 25–30% of ventricular filling volume in the normal heart.[13] The temporal relationships between the electrocardiogram (ECG) and the pressure changes in the left ventricle and aorta are demonstrated in Fig. 32.1.

Haemodynamics and contractility

The efficiency with which the heart pumps blood is dependent on many factors, some of which can be influenced by the IABP. Clinically, the effectiveness of the heart as a pump is assessed by measuring the **cardiac output** (CO). The CO is dependent on heart rate (HR) and stroke volume (SV), which can be represented by the formula:

$$CO = HR \times SV$$

Stroke volume is the volume of blood ejected by the heart during each systole and is influenced by preload, afterload and myocardial contractility. It can be calculated from the difference between left ventricular end-diastolic volume (LVEDV) and left ventricular end-systolic volume (LVESV):

$$SV = LVEDV{-}LVESV$$

Preload refers to the degree of stretch of the myocardium at the point of ventricular contraction; the best representation is the amount of ventricular filling during diastole, referred to as the **left ventricular end-diastolic volume** which depends on the amount of blood returning to the heart. Clinically, the left ventricular preload is assessed by measurement of the **left ventricular end-diastolic pressure** (LVEDP), the filling pressure of the left side of the heart. In many instances LVEDP is estimated by measurement of **pulmonary capillary wedge pressure** (PCWP).

    Afterload is the wall stress of the myocardium during left ventricular ejection and is generally referred to as the load against which the myocardium exerts its contractile force, i.e. the impedance to left ventricular ejection. It is a major determinant of myocardial oxygen consumption.[5] An approximation of afterload, useful for clinical assessment, is made by measuring **mean arterial pressure** (MAP), or preferably, if CO is measured, by calculation of the **systemic vascular resistance** (SVR), where:

$$SVR = (MAP{-}CVP) / CO$$

and CVP is the **central venous pressure**—a measure of the filling pressure of the right side of the heart (vascular resistance is expressed either in Wood units or as dynes-sec-cm^{-5}).

    The other contributor to stroke volume, and hence cardiac output, is **contractility**, an intrinsic property of myocardium, which reflects the mechanical work performed by the heart. Contractility is dependent on many factors, including preload, afterload, heart rate, sympathetic and parasympathetic stimulation and, clinically, administration of drugs that can directly alter myocardial contractility. Clinically, the most frequently used indicator of myocardial contractility is the **ejection fraction** (EF). This can be estimated either by echocardiography or ventriculography. The ejection fraction is normally about 65–75% of ventricular blood volume.[13]

Coronary blood supply

During the normal cardiac cycle, oxygenated blood is delivered to the myocardium and peripheral tissues and organs. In contrast to other tissues and organs, the majority of myocardial blood supply is delivered during diastole when the muscular tissue is relaxed.

Coronary blood flow is dependent on the diastolic gradient between pressure in the aortic root and that within the LV. Due to high metabolic demands placed upon it, the heart normally extracts 65–70% of delivered oxygen.[13] The balance between oxygen delivered to the heart and oxygen utilisation needs to be closely regulated, and is referred to as oxygen supply and demand. Any decrease in supply or increase in demand without compensatory mechanisms being invoked can be detrimental to the myocardium.

Oxygen demand will increase with increases in HR, preload, afterload, and contractility; oxygen supply can decrease due to decreases in coronary blood flow arising from tachycardia, diastolic hypotension, increased preload, hypocapnia or coronary spasm. Decreased oxygen delivery may also occur due to anaemia, or increased 2,3 DPG.[13]

The intra-aortic balloon pump

The IABP is a ventricular assist device used when the myocardium is unable to provide sufficient cardiac output to maintain oxygen delivery adequate for basal metabolic demands. The pump provides augmentation to the body's intrinsic cardiac output, so by definition can only work properly if some effective myocardial activity is present.

The IABP consists of three parts: a catheter-mounted balloon, a gas delivery module, and a control console. The long balloon catheter has two lumens and is usually inserted via the femoral artery. The central lumen, which runs the full length, is attached to a standard pressure transducer mounted on or near the pump console. This permits measurement of aortic blood pressure. The second, larger, lumen carries the driving gas for the balloon, which is usually helium.[14] This lumen ends distally by emptying into an elongated balloon that surrounds the catheter; it is this balloon that inflates to assist the left ventricle. The balloon is made of either polyurethane or cardiothane-51,[1] which have low thrombogenic surface properties and reliable durability.

Originally carbon dioxide was used as the shuttle gas but helium is now used exclusively. Helium has a lower molecular weight and density which, together with a much higher viscosity to density ratio, result in faster balloon inflation and deflation.[3,14,15] The significantly lower density of helium contributes greatly to its ability to maintain a laminar flow at higher flow rates than carbon dioxide, which more readily becomes turbulent.[15] However, helium has a very low solubility in blood, which creates greater problems when balloons rupture because it tends to form large bubbles that are poorly absorbed and act as large emboli.[12] Because of helium's very poor blood solubility, any bubbles that do form tend to remain stable and cause prolonged vessel obstruction.[15] The low molecular weight of helium also results in diffusion of very small amounts of gas through the balloon membrane. This slow gas leakage is not of clinical significance but does mean that the balloon needs to be refilled; most balloon pumps automatically refill the balloon to compensate for this, in some cases as frequently as every two hours. Just as helium leaks out of the balloon, water vapour tends to leak into the balloon and accumulate in the delivery tubing. Significant accumulation of condensate can impair gas shuttling, and for this reason most pumps have a collection and purging system to deal with this problem.[3,15]

Mechanism of augmentation

When implementing IAB pumping there are two major considerations to achieve maximum benefit:

1. Triggering The signal used to trigger balloon inflation and deflation.
2. Timing The points in the cardiac cycle when the balloon is inflated and deflated.

Ventricular assistance using an IABP is often referred to as **counterpulsation** because, with proper timing, the balloon is deflated while the ventricle is contracting, and inflated while the ventricle is in diastole, i.e. it cycles counter to the cardiac cycle. Counterpulsation relies on phasic displacement of blood, equal in volume to that of the inflated balloon, within a fixed intravascular space.[1,5] Hence, balloon inflation improves myocardial oxygen delivery by an increase in coronary artery blood flow from augmentation of diastolic blood pressure, which increases **coronary perfusion pressure**. Balloon deflation decreases myocardial oxygen demand by lowering the aortic end-diastolic pressure (AEDP). This decreases afterload, which enables the left ventricle to deliver blood into the aorta at a lower pressure so that less work is performed to achieve ejection, as well as allowing an increase in stroke volume.

The mechanism for balloon assistance is related to the timing of balloon inflation and deflation and associated changes in aortic volume and pressure. An understanding of balloon events and effects is made easier by starting with the beginning of diastole. Appearance of the dicrotic notch on the arterial waveform (Fig. 32.1) indicates the beginning of diastole. The **dicrotic notch** (DN) represents closure of the aortic valve. Ideally, balloon inflation is timed to occur at the dicrotic notch. Balloon inflation increases the total volume contained within the aorta. As a result of this sudden increase in aortic volume and the relative rigidity of the aorta, there is a sudden increase in aortic pressure. As a result, blood already contained within the aorta is displaced superiorly and inferiorly and there is a consequent increase in coronary perfusion pressure and systemic perfusion pressure. With proper balloon functioning and timing, this peak diastolic aortic pressure is higher than the patient derived systolic pressure, hence the term **augmentation**.[14,16]

The balloon remains inflated until the beginning of the next systole. At this point the balloon is rapidly deflated to create a relative vacuum. With correct timing, this causes a fall in aortic pressure just as the left ventricle is generating sufficient pressure to open the aortic valve and begin ventricular ejection. This means the required ventricular-generated pressure is reduced, which subsequently reduces oxygen demand. The reduction in afterload allows the ventricle to empty more effectively, which increases SV, which in turn may lead to a decrease in preload. These effects combine to improve cardiac output.[14,17]

In summary, the major benefits of IAB counterpulsation are:
i)   increased myocardial oxygen delivery
ii)   decreased myocardial oxygen demand
iii)   decreased afterload
iv)   decreased preload
v)   increased cardiac output.

Changes to the arterial waveform

Figure 32.2 outlines the normal radial arterial waveform together with that recorded from the proximal aorta as seen with an IAB. There are several notable differences between these two curves. The systolic peak of the radial trace is greater and narrower than that of the aorta, and the diastolic hump following the dicrotic notch is generally more marked in the radial trace. Features that are common to both, and relevant to IAB pumping, include: the **peak systolic pressure** (PSP), the dicrotic notch and the **aortic-end diastolic pressure** (AEDP),[13,18,19] as indicated in Fig. 32.3.

Figure 32.3 displays the arterial pressure (radial artery) trace during IABP augmentation, at an assist ratio of 1:2, where the balloon inflates at every second cardiac cycle. This ratio is chosen initially to assist with selection of the most effective timing of inflation and deflation. Features of this trace include the marked and sudden increase in diastolic

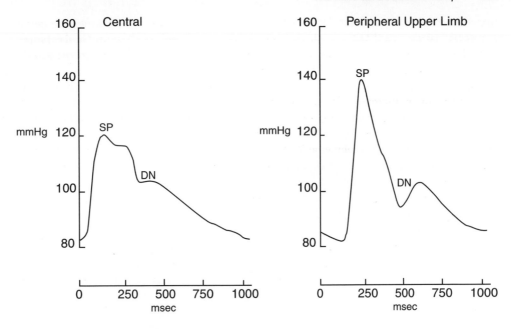

Figure 32.2. *Diagram displaying shape characteristics of pressure waveforms recorded from near the aortic root and from a peripheral artery. Note the increase in systolic peak (SP) and the more pronounced dicrotic notch (DN) in the peripheral trace.*

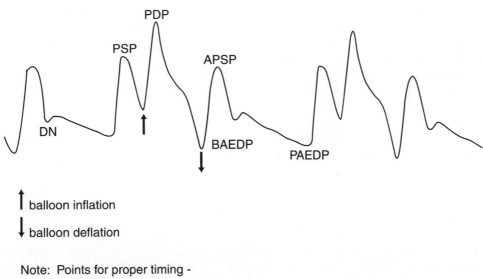

Figure 32.3. *Example of radial pressure trace during IAB pumping of every second beat, i.e. 1:2 counterpulsation. Features to note include: peak systolic pressure (PSP), which should be greater than the assisted peak systolic pressure (APSP); the peak diastolic pressure (PDP); the balloon aortic end-diastolic pressure (BAEDP), which should be less than the patient aortic end-diastolic pressure (PAEDP), and the dicrotic notch (DN).*

pressure with balloon inflation at the expected point of the DN; this becomes the **peak diastolic pressure** (PDP). Also highlighted are the **assisted peak systolic pressure** (APSP), the **balloon aortic end diastolic pressure** (BAEDP), and the **patient aortic end diastolic pressure** (PAEDP).[18,20,21]

Peak diastolic pressure is the increase in diastolic pressure due to balloon inflation (augmentation), which should be greater than the peak systolic pressure. Assisted peak systolic pressure is the systolic pressure generated by the myocardium immediately following balloon deflation. With correct timing this pressure should be less than PSP, as there is reduction in afterload associated with balloon deflation.

The balloon aortic end-diastolic pressure is the lowest pressure in the cardiac cycle that results from balloon deflation, whilst the patient aortic end-diastolic pressure is the lowest pressure in the cardiac cycle due to intrinsic myocardial activity. Correct timing will cause the BAEDP to be less than the PAEDP, suggested to be 10–15 mmHg lower.[1,3,14,22]

There are three goals to aim for with IAB pumping that indicate good timing of inflation and deflation. These are:

1. PDP >PSP
2. PSP > APSP
3. BAEDP < PAEDP.

Timing

Optimal timing is determined by assessment of the haemodynamic response to counter-pulsation.[5] Where possible, it is better to use the IAB central lumen aortic pressure trace to fine tune the timing, rather than the radial artery trace. There is less distortion of the aortic trace, which makes timing more accurate, and there is less delay in the pressure signal.[14] Quaal[18] stated that the time delay to the dicrotic notch due to differences in pulse wave velocity and blood flow velocity is the same, 40–50 msec, for the IAB central lumen, the

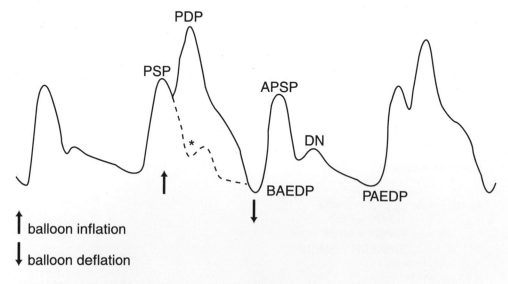

Figure 32.4. *Example of early balloon inflation, with absence of dicrotic notch. Representative traces of timing errors are all displayed at a ratio of 1:2.*

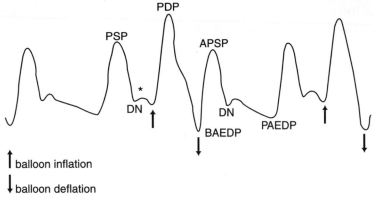

balloon inflation

balloon deflation

Note: Appearance of dicrotic notch (*) prior to balloon inflation

Figure 32.5. *With late deflation the balloon is inflated well after the dicrotic notch, which is clearly visible between PSP and the augmented PDP.*

subclavian and radial arteries. Despite this, the aortic trace is preferred for adjusting the timing of the IABP as it is a more accurate reflection of cardiac and pressure events. The differences can be observed when both a radial arterial trace and the balloon aortic trace are available.

Timing errors

Early inflation

With early inflation the balloon is inflated well before the dicrotic notch (Fig. 32.4). This results in premature closure of the aortic valve, which reduces SV and CO, with an increase in LVEDV. If this situation persists, myocardial work and oxygen consumption will increase, which is likely to worsen the patient's condition.

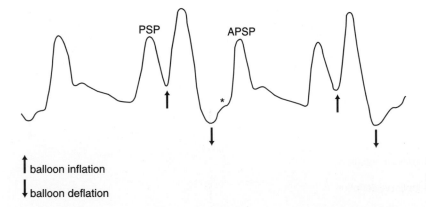

balloon inflation

balloon deflation

Note: Increase in end diastolic pressure before (*) next systole. May get APSP ≥ PSP (unassisted operation APSP < PSP)

Figure 32.6. *If the IAB is deflated too early, prior to the next systolic ejection, there is often an increase in the end-diastolic pressure (*) with an associated increase in the assisted peak systolic pressure (APSP).*

Late inflation

In this situation the balloon is inflated well after the dicrotic notch which is clearly visible between PSP and the augmented PDP (Fig. 32.5). In this instance the balloon inflates after the aorta is maximally filled with blood, so that the increase in volume and subsequent pressure is less than it could be; this results in a diminution in augmented coronary and peripheral perfusion.

Early deflation

Early deflation will result in the BAEDP reaching its nadir well before the beginning of the next systole. This will let the pressure within the aorta rise again as the left ventricle is about to begin emptying (Fig. 32.6). The APSP will rise due to an increase in afterload because of retrograde flow of blood which fills the 'space' left by the deflated balloon.[22]

Late deflation

With late deflation of the balloon, the left ventricle has to open the aortic valve at a higher pressure, resulting in increased left ventricular work (Fig. 32.7). As the LV work increases so does oxygen consumption, increasing the delivery demand. This is compounded by an associated decrease in CO due to increased afterload.[3,18]

Triggering modes

ECG triggering

There are two patient-derived physiological signals used for balloon triggering, and one console-generated signal. Most commonly, pumping will be triggered using the patient's ECG, which is the default trigger mode on most IABPs. This signal may be established through direct skin leads from the patient to the console, or via a slave cable from the anaesthetic or other monitor to the appropriate input jack on the console. Choice between these two triggers is often dependent on circumstances at the time of balloon insertion.

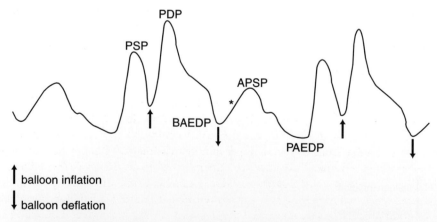

↑ balloon inflation

↓ balloon deflation

Note : Rate of rise of assisted peak systolic pressure (*) may be prolonged, and BAEDP ≥ PAEDP (unassisted operation BAEDP < PAEDP)

Figure 32.7. With late deflation of the balloon the left ventricle has to open the aortic valve at a higher pressure, which may result in an increase in the balloon-assisted end-diastolic pressure (BAEDP) and a decrease in the slope of the following systole (*).

The ability to apply IABP-specific patient ECG electrodes during surgery is limited, so that a slave signal is most commonly used. In most situations this signal is adequate for reliable pumping; however, the signal may be degraded at times, requiring an alternative trigger. This is particularly the case with intrinsically reduced signal strength from the patient. Apart from this situation, there is little difference with regard to triggering and pumping reliability between these two ECG sources.

When the heart is paced, either temporarily following surgery or with a permanent pacemaker, the appropriate trigger mode will need to be selected on the console. The exact type will depend on the individual IABP being used. All consoles have at least one pacing mode, designed to ignore/reject the pacing spike(s) and trigger from the ECG (T and R waves). Some consoles distinguish between atrial, ventricular or A-V sequential pacing. When slaving from another monitor whilst the heart is being paced, it is important to determine whether the pacing spike is suppressed or transmitted from the monitor to the IABP console. If the pacing spike is suppressed and the trigger mode is ECG with pacing, then the console will be aiming to detect a pacing spike. In this situation the pump may trigger irregularly and erratically due to inappropriate trigger selection. With a regular rhythm, newer balloon pumps are capable of reliable triggering at heart rates up to 180 bpm.[3] It has been recommended that during periods of tachycardia (HR >110–120 bpm) the IABP be set to inflate on every second beat;[4] this allows for complete balloon filling on alternate beats rather than only partial filling for every beat.

Pressure triggering

Pressure triggering is most frequently achieved from the aortic pressure signal obtained via the IAB catheter. In this instance the pressure transducer is connected directly to the balloon console. Alternatively, the pressure signal may be slaved from the anaesthetic monitor, which most often is derived from the radial artery. In either case the size of the pulse pressure must be above a certain threshold to enable reliable triggering. In many newer machines the pressure trigger mode detects both magnitude of the pressure increase with systole and the rate of rise, which helps to eliminate artefactual interference. The sensitivity with respect to pulse pressure size can generally be adjusted for very low output states. This triggering mode is less reliable than ECG triggering when the heart rate is very high, i.e. >150, or when the rhythm is irregular.[3]

Internal triggering

The internal asynchronous triggering mode is only used when there is no intrinsic myocardial activity, which means this mode is generally reserved for intraoperative use during cardiopulmonary bypass (CPB). The standard default rate for this mode is 80 inflations per minute but is variable from as low as 10 per minute to as high as 120 per minute, depending on the particular model. It must be remembered that when using this mode there is **no** synchronisation between the balloon inflation/deflation cycle and activity of the heart. Consequently, internal triggering may worsen ventricular failure if used inappropriately.

Internal triggering is used during CPB to avoid thrombus formation on the balloon. This precaution is taken even though the patient is fully heparinised for bypass. Although the default internal trigger rate is 80 per minute, this is generally reduced to as little as possible during bypass to minimally interfere with the surgery. The lowest rate available varies with the make of pump, from a low of 10 per minute up to about 32. If this frequency still results in surgical interference, then the balloon inflation volume may also be reduced.

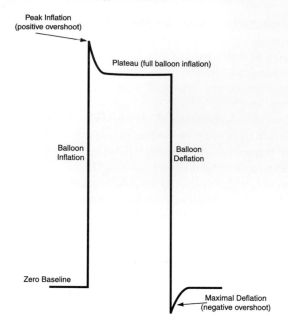

Peak Inflation
(positive overshoot)

Plateau (full balloon inflation)

Balloon
Inflation

Balloon
Deflation

Zero Baseline

Maximal Deflation
(negative overshoot)

Figure 32.8. Example trace of a normal balloon pressure waveform. Features to note include balloon pressure baseline; rapid balloon inflation; peak inflation artefact (pressure artefact); balloon pressure plateau; rapid balloon deflation; deflation undershoot (vacuum artefact), and the console zero baseline.

Balloon pressure waveform

All IABP models currently available enable display of the waveform, which represents pressure changes within the balloon associated with inflation and deflation; this is referred to as the **balloon pressure waveform** (BPW).

This pressure trace has characteristic features, deviations from which can be used for troubleshooting. A normal balloon pressure waveform is presented in Fig. 32.8, features of which include: balloon pressure **baseline**; **rapid balloon inflation**; **peak inflation artefact** (pressure artefact); balloon pressure **plateau**; **rapid balloon deflation**; **deflation undershoot** (vacuum artefact); and the **console zero baseline**.[14,23]

The width of the balloon pressure waveform represents duration of balloon inflation and consequently will change with changes in heart rate.

The level of the balloon pressure plateau reflects the pressure within the aorta during balloon inflation. The balloon wall material is highly compliant so there is rapid pressure equalisation across the wall. This means that the plateau pressure should be within 10–15 mmHg of the peak diastolic pressure on the arterial trace. The level of the plateau pressure will change in response to changes in aortic pressure. During periods of relative hypertension the plateau level will rise, reflecting the higher pressure needed to achieve full balloon inflation. Similarly, during periods of decreased aortic pressure the plateau level will fall accordingly.

Low balloon pressure baseline: Normally the baseline pressure is 5–10 mmHg. If the baseline value falls below this, likely causes include insufficient filling initially or loss of helium either through a leak in the circuit or normal diffusion of helium through the balloon wall.

High balloon pressure baseline: The baseline may rise in response to over-pressurisation of the gas system due to a kink in the tubing or the balloon. Otherwise a baseline increase signifies overfilling, implying an internal fault.

High plateau pressure: with an increase in the plateau pressure there is also generally a change in shape of the BPW, where the plateau rises and becomes rounded. Causes for this include: a kink in the catheter; balloon occlusion; balloon not fully unwrapped or unsheathed if percutaneously inserted; balloon too large for the aorta; or the patient may be hypertensive.

Balloon insertion

The preferred method of insertion is percutaneously into the femoral artery using the Seldinger technique. If difficulty is encountered in locating the artery a surgical cutdown may be required. In either case, once localised a sheath is inserted into the artery through which the fully deflated balloon is passed. To ensure complete deflation prior to insertion, the balloon should be fully evacuated using a 50 cc syringe and the one-way valve supplied with the balloon. It is crucial that the balloon not be inflated or unfurled prior to insertion, as this will make insertion impossible. Advancement of the balloon is over a guidewire, until the balloon catheter tip is just distal to (below) the origin of the subclavian artery. When in this position the proximal end of the balloon should be situated close to, but above, the renal arteries. It has been recommended that, where possible, the balloon be restricted to the descending thoracic aorta as this usually has less atheromatous plaques than the abdominal aorta.[3] Complications associated with percutaneous insertion are most commonly related to puncture of an inappropriate site or use of excessive force to advance the guidewire or balloon catheter.[14]

A recent development in balloon insertion and design is the sheathless balloon. This is also inserted percutaneously, but no guiding sheath is placed into the femoral artery. This results in less obstruction to blood flow in the affected femoral artery and a 30% reduction in cross-sectional area of the arterial puncture site. Reports to date are equivocal about advantages of the sheathless balloon catheters.[3,22,24]

Less frequently, IABs are inserted surgically. This technique involves suturing a Dacron graft side-arm onto the vessel wall, through which the balloon is passed.[1] Most commonly the femoral artery is used, although there are reports of antegrade insertion into the thoracic aorta at the time of cardiac surgery.[14]

Balloon sizes

The most commonly inserted balloon has a volume of 40 cc. This size is suitable for most adults, whilst a 30 or 34 cc balloon can be used in smaller patients. Paediatric balloons, with volumes as low as 2.5 cc, are also available. Rarely, very large patients require a 50 cc balloon.[14] It is recommended that, when inflated, the balloon occupy 75–95% of the aortic lumen.[3,11,12,14] This reduces the amount of direct contact between the balloon and the intimal surface of the aorta and results in less damage to both surfaces and to red blood cells.[14] Tate[24] has outlined two general principles regarding balloon size: (i) that the balloon lie between the subclavian artery and the renal arteries, and (ii) that the diameter be such that there is maximal volume displacement of blood on inflation without distension of the aorta. Studies have demonstrated that 90% of patients have aortic diameters in excess of 19 mm and subsequently most balloon catheters have diameters between 14 and 16.5 mm.[24]

Weaning

Weaning is considered likely to be successful if the patient can maintain a cardiac index greater than 2 L/min/m², PCWP <18 mmHg, and left ventricular stroke work index (LVSWI) >20 g/m/m².[5] Pharmacological support is reduced prior to weaning, so that it may then be increased if necessary during the weaning process. The weaning process itself involves a reduction in the frequency of augmentation, by changing the pumping ratio from 1:1 to 1:2 in the first instance, and if this is well tolerated then reducing the ratio further. The degree to which the ratio may be reduced varies with different models, but in some instances it may not be sufficiently low to enable gradual weaning from counterpulsation. In these situations the volume to which the balloon is inflated may also be reduced gradually. The time frame for this will depend on how well the patient copes with each change in pump settings. Several hours should be allocated for each change.

Complications

Use of the IABP is fraught with a degree of morbidity and mortality. Death resulting directly as a consequence of balloon insertion and counterpulsation is reported to be less than 1%. Reported rates for complications vary from 5–35%, with significant complication rates reported to be between 10 and 20%, and permanent morbidity less than 5%.[1,3,14,25]

Mortality in those patients who receive IABP support is in the range of 26–50%, largely because of the nature of the cardiac problems that necessitate IABP use.[4] Risk factors for mortality in patients receiving counterpulsation identified by McCarthy and Golding[4] include advanced age, female sex, high New York Heart Association (NYHA) classification, preoperative glycerol trinitrate (GTN), operative or post-operative balloon insertion, and transthoracic insertion. Despite the high mortality and the well recognised risk factors, McCarthy and Golding[4] consider that since the IAB is inserted for compelling indications, identification of risk factors does not influence (patient) management, except to encourage removal of the device as soon as the cardiac status of the patient permits.

Kesselbrenner and colleagues[22] have identified several categories of complication associated with IABP therapy. These include:

i)   trauma to the arterial wall during insertion
ii)   limb ischaemia
iii) dislodged thrombus
iv)   haematologic (thrombocytopaenia, haemolysis, haemorrhage)
v)   balloon leak or rupture
vi)   infection.

Limb ischaemia is the most common complication, occurring in 9–25% of patients. In the great majority of cases ischaemia resolves with balloon removal; however, in 1–2% of cases ischaemia may persist and result in some degree of lower limb amputation.[1,4,26] Risk factors associated with limb ischaemia include severity of peripheral vascular disease, extent of myocardial failure, presence of significant longstanding hypertension, diabetes mellitus, female sex, smoking and duration of therapy.[4,22]

Infection associated with presence of the balloon catheter is the second most common complication (3–4% incidence).[1] Balloon rupture occurs in 1–4% of cases, although a study cited by Baldyga[26] reported a mean incidence for 2 years of 9% and 10.1%, with a range up to 17%. Balloon rupture and leakage is assumed to occur due to plaque abrasion. It is more likely to occur in patients with a history of hypertension, those who display a marked diastolic augmentation from the IABP, and in women.[4,26] Consequences of IAB rupture are gas embolism and vascular entrapment of the balloon. Gas embolism resulting in neurological sequelae is a very rare occurrence, even following balloon rupture.[26] Balloon entrapment may occur following slow leakage as well as sudden rupture. Rupture and leakage are often first detected by presence of blood in the shuttle gas tubing, although the gas leak alarm may sound, or an increased frequency in balloon refilling may be noted.[26]

Set up

The procedures involved in setting up for IAB pumping are similar for all models of IABP currently available. There will be slight differences depending on which particular unit is in use, but the following guidelines apply to all:

1. Ensure there is sufficient helium in the cylinder and turn on the cylinder.
2. Where possible, connect to mains power. Turn on power switch on the console.
3. Establish a reliable triggering mode. In many instances in the operating theatre this is best achieved initially by using a slave cable from the anaesthetic monitor to establish an ECG signal. Subsequent to balloon insertion, the aortic pressure signal may be used as the balloon trigger. This is particularly useful if significant electrical interference from electrocautery is present.
4. After the balloon has been inserted into the patient and the one-way valve removed, connect the helium delivery hose to the appropriate port on the console.
5. Connect the aortic pressure monitoring line to the nearby pressure transducer. This may be mounted onto the console, but for safety reasons this practice is not recommended. Ensure that the pressure transducer has been zeroed to the patient's approximate mid-chest height. Use of a pressurised continuous flush device is recommended to avoid blood clotting within the central lumen and to ensure a good, reliable aortic pressure trace. Heparin, at a concentration of 4 IU/ml may also be added to the bag of flush. It is extremely important that the flush device be carefully set up to avoid air bubbles, which will dampen the trace and potentially form emboli within the patient.
6. Confirm console settings for initiation of pumping. These are:
   a) Inflation and deflation triggering set to middle of their respective ranges.
   b) Augmentation ratio 1:2, which allows for comparison between augmented and non-augmented beats.
   c) Ensure there is a triggering signal (usually a flashing display) for each cardiac signal.
   d) Where appropriate, ensure balloon inflation volume is zero.
7. Fill the balloon; most consoles have an automated filling function.
8. Start pumping; in certain models it is necessary to increase the volume of helium delivered to the balloon until it is maximal, or until maximal augmentation is achieved.
9. Establish maximal augmentation by adjustment of both the time of inflation and time of deflation.
10. Increase augmentation ratio to 1:1 when satisfied with timing.

The latest models (e.g. Datascope® System 98 IABP, Datascope Corporation, Fairfield, NJ) are fully automated.

References

1. Craver JM, Connolly MW. The percutaneous intraaortic balloon pump and ventricular assist devices. In: Alexander RW, Shiant RC, Fuster A *et al.* eds. *Hurst's The heart, arteries and veins,* Vol. 1. 8th ed. New York: McGraw-Hill 1998, pp. 621–8.
2. Kantrowitz A. Origins of intraaortic balloon pumping. *Ann Thorac Surg* 1990; **50:**672–4.
3. Anonymous. Evaluation: Intra-aortic balloon pumps. *Health Devices* 1997; **26**(5):184–216.
4. McCarthy PM, Golding LAR. Temporary mechanical support. In: Edmunds LH (ed). *Cardiac surgery in the adult.* New York: McGraw-Hill 1997 pp. 319–38.
5. Underwood, M.J, Firmin RK, Graham TR. Current concepts in the use of intra-aortic balloon counterpulsation. *Br J Hosp Med* 1993; **50** (7):391–7.

6.   Quaal SJ. Indications. In: Quaal SJ (ed). *Comprehensive intraaortic balloon counterpulsation*, 2nd ed. St Louis: Mosby 1993, pp. 118–43.

7.   Christenson JT, Simonet F, Badel P, Schumuziger M. Evaluation of preoperative intra-aortic balloon pump support in high risk coronary patients. *Eur J Cardio-thorac Surg* 1997; **11**:1097–103.

8.   Torchiana DF, Hirsch G, Buckley MJ *et al.* Intraaortic balloon pumping for cardiac support: Trends in practice and outcome, 1968 to 1995. *J Thorac Cardiovasc Surg* 1997; **113**(4):758–69.

9.   Anstadt MP and Newman MF. Use of the intra-aortic balloon pump for post-cardiotomy support. In: Maccioli GA (ed). *Intra-aortic balloon pump therapy*. Baltimore: Willams & Wilkins 1997, pp. 107–125.

10.   Quaal SJ. Contraindications. In: Quaal SJ (ed). *Comprehensive intraaortic balloon counterpulsation*, 2nd ed. St Louis: Mosby 1993, pp. 144–5.

11.   Kahn JK. *Intra-aortic balloon pumping: Theory and clinical applications – A monograph for the clinician*. Princeton: Communications Media for Education Inc 1991.

12.   Weber KT, Janicki JS. Intraaortic balloon counterpulsation: A review of physiological principles, clinical results, and device safety. *Ann Thor Surg* 1974; **17**(6):602–36.

13.   Berne RM, Levy MN. *Cardiovascular physiology*, 3rd ed. St Louis: Mosby 1977.

14.   Aroesty JM , Shawl FA. Circulatory assist devices. In: Baim DS, Grossman W (eds). *Cardiac catheterization, angiography, and intervention*, 5th ed. Baltimore: Willams & Wilkins 1996, pp. 421–445.

15.   Shedlick RR, Maccioli GA. Physical and medical aspects of inflation gases: Helium vs carbon dioxide. In: Maccioli GA (ed). *Intra-aortic balloon pump therapy*. Baltimore: Willams & Wilkins 1997, pp. 43–50.

16.   Quaal SJ. Basic priciples of IABC. In: Quaal SJ (ed). *Comprehensive intraaortic balloon counterpulsation*, 2nd ed. St Louis: Mosby 1993, pp. 93–100.

17.   Quaal SJ. Interactive hemodynaics of IABC. In: Quaal SJ (ed). *Comprehensive intraaortic balloon counterpulsation*, 2nd ed. St Louis: Mosby 1993, pp. 101–17.

18.   Quaal SJ. Conventional timing using the arterial pressure waveform. In: Quaal SJ (ed). *Comprehensive intraaortic balloon counterpulsation*, 2nd ed. St Louis: Mosby 1993, pp. 246–59.

19.   Lucas WJ, Anstadt MP. Triggering and timing of the intra-aortic balloon pump. In: Maccioli GA (ed). *Intra-aortic balloon pump therapy*. Baltimore: Willams & Wilkins 1997, pp. 57–67.

20.   Datascope Clinical Suppport Services. *Technical seminar for intra-aortic balloon pumping*. Fairfield (NJ): Datascope Corp. 1993.

21.   Aries Medical Incorporated. *Model 700 control system operator's manual*. Woburn (MA): Aries Medical Incorporated 1986.

22.   Kesselbrenner MB, Weinberg HM, Reemstma K, Bregman D. Intra-aortic balloon counterpulsation. In: Ayres SM, Grenvik A, Holbrook PR, Shoemaker WC (eds). *Textbook of critical care*, 3rd ed. Philaldelphia: WB Saunders 1995, pp. 538–53.

23.   Kalina J. Use of the bloon pressure waveform in conjunction with the augmented arterial pressure waveform. In: Quaal SJ (ed). *Comprehensive intraaortic balloon counterpulsation*, 2nd ed. St Louis: Mosby 1993, pp. 295–308.

24.   Tate DA. Physical and clinical aspects of intra-aortic balloon pump catheters. In: Maccioli GA (ed). *Intra-aortic balloon pump therapy*. Baltimore: Willams & Wilkins 1997, pp. 51–56.

25.   Lange SS. Complications associated with IABC. In: Quaal SJ (ed). *Comprehensive intraaortic balloon counterpulsation*, 2nd ed. St Louis: Mosby; 1993, pp. 146–64.

26.   Baldyga AP. Complications of intra-aortic balloon pump therapy. In: Maccioli GA (ed). *Intra-aortic balloon pump therapy*. Baltimore: Willams & Wilkins 1997, pp. 127–161.

Chapter 33

An Evidence-based Guide to Cardiac Catheterisation

Steven Faddy

The concept of evidence-based medicine (EBM), which employs only the best sources of evidence to address a clinical question, has become increasingly accepted in recent years. It relies on a thorough literature search, appraisal of relevant papers, analysis of results obtained and application of these results to a population or clinical condition. The *JAMA* series titled 'Users' Guide to the Medical Literature'[1-19] provides complete guidelines for appraising all types of studies and clinical questions, and is strongly recommended for those wishing to further their expertise in this area. This chapter examines the practice of EBM in the cardiac catheterisation laboratory.

The literature search

The literature search is the first and possibly most important step in the process. The emphasis is on finding results of **all** studies performed in the area of interest. This includes searching several electronic databases (Medline, EMBASE, Cochrane Database of Systematic Reviews, etc.) and may involve hand searching through numerous volumes of non-electronic indexes (Medical Subject Heading index, Cumulated Index Medicus, etc.). Reference lists uncovered by the literature search should also be examined for references that have not previously been identified.

A complete literature search also involves contact with experts in the field in question to find results of unpublished trials that may be included in the analysis. This step, which may seem somewhat extreme, avoids publication bias: trials that show positive results are more likely to be submitted and accepted for publication than trials that fail to demonstrate a significant effect.

The best source of evidence

A literature search will commonly uncover many types of studies and publications. It is important to identify which studies may give satisfactory results and which have results that are subject to bias. A summary of the most common study designs and publication types is presented below.

Systematic review

Often called an 'overview' or 'meta-analysis', this type of publication incorporates all steps necessary for obtaining the best available answer to the clinical question. A well performed systematic review includes a thorough literature search, critical appraisal of the studies identified, analysis of pooled results and identification of the population to which these results apply. The reader need only assess the paper to evaluate the quality of the literature search, adequacy of the methods of appraisal and the generalisability of the results to their individual patient(s). If these criteria are satisfactorily met, the results of the systematic review can be easily applied to the patient or clinical condition in question.

Randomised controlled trial

The randomised controlled trial (RCT) is considered to be the study type that provides the best evidence of association between an exposure and an outcome. The strength of this

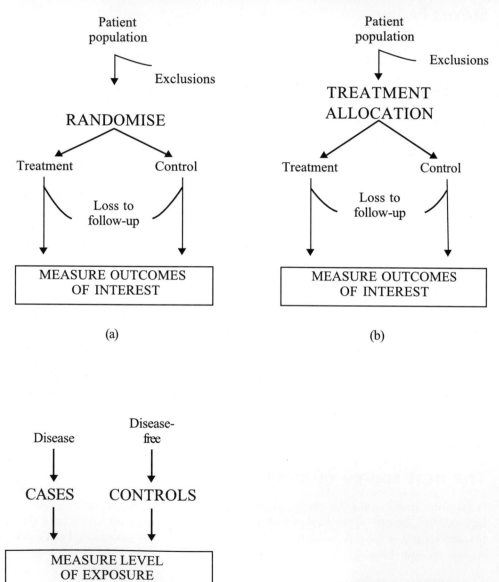

Figure 33.1. Common controlled trial designs. (a) Randomised controlled trial; (b) Cohort study; (c) Case-control study.

study type lies largely in the random assignment of patients to the exposure under examination (a drug, intervention or therapy) or to a control (current therapy or placebo). Completely random allocation of patients to the study groups should ensure that baseline characteristics of the groups are almost identical, provided enough patients are included in the study. Confounders are variables that alter the strength of association between an exposure and an outcome. Study results can be adjusted for confounders if they are known to occur. However, unidentified confounders have the potential to alter the observed strength of association. By randomly assigning patients to either study group, unidentified confounders should be evenly distributed between the groups and should not bias the strength of association. In this way, the only difference between study groups should be exposure to the study factor. The groups are then followed prospectively to the end of the trial and assessed for the outcome (Fig. 33.1).

Cohort study

Like an RCT, a cohort study follows patients prospectively from an exposure to an outcome. Unlike an RCT, the assignment of exposure is non-random and is based on patients' individual characteristics (such as cigarette smoking or cholesterol level). Non-random assignment introduces bias from confounding factors. For example, consider a study investigating the relationship between smoking and coronary artery disease. The exposure factor is cigarette smoking, and it is neither ethical nor sensible to randomise patients to be smokers or non-smokers. Instead, allocation to a study group is guided by the patients' own habits. Cigarette smoking may be associated with higher coffee consumption, higher stress levels, less exercise, or a tendency towards other negative lifestyle habits. These confounding factors may thus have an independent association with coronary artery disease. The absence of randomisation may result in these factors being unevenly distributed between the smoking and non-smoking groups and bias the observed strength of association between smoking and coronary artery disease.

Case-control study

A case-control study identifies positive outcomes first and works backwards to identify the levels of exposure. A control population can be chosen from a number of sources. A poorly defined control group (hospital-based controls) is chosen from a narrow section of the community and is often not representative of the whole population. A well-defined control group (population-based controls) is drawn from the same geographical areas at the same time as the cases being evaluated, and is often well representative of the section of the community from which it is drawn.

In an attempt to obtain some equality in baseline characteristics of the study groups, controls are often age- and sex-matched to cases. However, matching has been shown to have little effect on the estimate of association, and extreme care must be taken to ensure that results are not biased by other unidentified confounding variables.

The advantages of a case-control study are the ability to study exposures for which it is unethical to randomise patients, and the ability to study outcomes that are rare. For example, consider a study examining the relationship between a hypothetical industrial solvent (HIS) and atrial myxoma. Obviously it would be unwise to expose patients to this chemical simply to see if atrial myxoma develops. Further, atrial myxoma is a rare disease and it may be necessary to expose many thousand subjects to the chemical in order to detect two or three cases. In these situations it would be far better to identify as many cases as possible, obtain a suitable control group, and study both groups for their relative rates of exposure to HIS.

Case series

Case series and case reports are simply a description of the course of single or small groups of patients. The benefits of randomisation are lost, since only those patients treated are reported and there is generally no control group to compare with the group receiving the new treatment or medication. As such, it is not possible to draw any conclusions about cause and effect from these reports.

Critical appraisal

Having identified all trials addressing the clinical question, it is necessary to analyse the quality and content of the reports. The exact method of appraisal will vary with different study types, publication types and clinical questions. The 'Users' Guide to the Medical Literature' series[1-19] divides most appraisals into two basic units: 'Are the results of the study valid?' and 'What are the results and how will they help me in caring for my patients?'.

Critical appraisal of a systematic review starts with validation of the criteria used to select articles for inclusion, including the literature search. The review is assessed to ensure that the validity of each primary study has been appraised. The results are reviewed to ensure consistency and reproducibility between trials. When these criteria have been met it is possible to adopt the results, assuming there is adequate precision (results lie within a statistically suitable range). The study population is assessed for relevance to the physician's own patient population.[8]

Papers concerning therapies or interventions are checked for random allocation of patients to treatment groups, adequate retention of subjects, sufficient follow-up, similarity of baseline characteristics, adequate blinding and analysis by intention-to-treat. Assessment can then be made of the significance of the treatment effect, the precision of the results and the relevance of the patient population to the clinician's own patients.[2,3]

Trials assessing harms of an exposure require a clearly defined comparison group with similar baseline characteristics, outcomes measured the same way for both groups, sufficient follow-up and investigation for a dose-response gradient. Appraisal is made of the strength of association between exposure and outcome (and the precision of this estimate) along with the relevance to the clinician's practice.[6] The relative harms of a therapy can then be weighed against benefits for individual patients.[20]

Articles concerning diagnostic tests require an independent, blind comparison of all patients against a reference standard. All patients should have the reference test to be compared with the new test. The patient population should be representative of those patients on whom the test would normally be performed. Likelihood ratios, sensitivity, specificity, positive predictive value and negative predictive value can be assessed to determine whether the new test provides any additional benefit in diagnosis of the target disease.[4,5]

Aspects of study design

Randomisation

The benefits of randomisation have already been discussed. They primarily revolve around equality of baseline characteristics. If the study groups are similar for all measurable variables, it can be assumed that the distribution of any unidentified confounding variables will also be evenly distributed. In this way, study groups should be similar in every respect except for the treatment or intervention being applied. The results will reflect the true effect of the new treatment without bias from uneven distribution of covariates.

Power and sample size

In any analysis of cause and effect, chance plays a part in the results obtained. A trial may correctly detect an effect of treatment when such an effect truly exists, or detect no effect when none exists. In either case, no error has been made. However, a trial may detect a treatment effect when no effect exists. This is referred to as type I (or α) error and is equal to the P value.[21] If the significance level is set at P=0.05 then there is a 5% chance that the difference observed between the study groups has occurred entirely by chance. Type II (or β) error occurs when a trial fails to detect an effect where one actually exists. The power of a study is defined as the probability that the study will correctly detect an effect of treatment when such an effect exists. This is given by the term 1-β (i.e. the probability of detecting a treatment effect is equal to 1 minus the probability of failing to detect the effect). Hence, if type II error (β, the probability of not detecting the effect) is 20% then the power of the study (1-b, the probability of correctly detecting the effect) is 1-0.20=0.80. This means that there is an 80% chance of correctly detecting a treatment effect of specified size.

Sample size is calculated taking account of type I and II errors. If a large treatment effect is expected, a relatively small number of patients may be required to demonstrate this effect. Conversely, if a small treatment effect is expected, a larger number of subjects may be required before it can confidently be concluded that the small difference between the study groups is due to the treatment and not to chance.

When a trial does not have a sample size large enough to adequately detect the difference expected, it loses power. That is, the probability that the trial will demonstrate a statistically significant effect of the specified magnitude is reduced. Adequate sample size is calculated taking account of the expected magnitude of the treatment effect (from previous research, pilot studies etc.), the type I error and the required power.

In the planning stage of a clinical trial, sample size calculations should be performed to determine how many patients will be required to have a sufficient chance of demonstrating an effect. In the appraisal of a clinical trial that does not show a significant effect, sample size calculations will determine whether there are sufficient patients to adequately detect the observed effect. Conversely, the sample size calculation can be used to evaluate the power of the study according to the number of patients actually enrolled. Ideally, a study should have a power of at least 80% to detect the specified treatment effect.

Blinding

An important aspect of any clinical trial is the blinding of study participants and investigators to the patient's treatment group. Surveillance bias occurs when an investigator is aware of the patient's treatment group and preferentially investigates more thoroughly for an outcome or side effect. Any investigator involved in collecting data should not be aware of the patient's treatment group, particularly in the case of subjective measurements such as pain, which are open to interpretation. A patient may be treated differently if the physician is aware of the study group to which the patient has been randomly assigned. This is referred to as treatment bias. A patient's response to a disease is also affected by his or her perception of the adequacy of the treatment being applied. Patients who know they are receiving a placebo or the currently accepted treatment may not respond as well as patients who know they are receiving the new 'wonder drug', simply by virtue of the former group's perception of sub-optimal treatment. The 'placebo effect' is a response to a placebo treatment simply because patients think they are being treated, and has been reported to be higher than 30%.[22-24] Others have refuted that this phenomenon exists[25-26] and suggest other mechanisms for the apparent cure of untreated patients. The placebo effect will bias results towards 'no effect of treatment' and should always be considered when interpreting results.

Control group

Choice of an appropriate control group is vital to ensure applicability of the results of a study to the patient population. If a current treatment or practice exists, this should be the intervention applied to the control group in the study. Patients are often unaware of this and incorrectly assume that a control group receives no treatment, whereas a control group in fact receives the best known alternative treatment to that of the experimental group. A placebo control is only appropriate if no current treatment exists for the disease.

Analysis by intention-to-treat

Study participants in an RCT should be analysed in the group to which they were randomised, regardless of the treatment they received. This is referred to as analysis by intention-to-treat. There are many reasons why a patient may not comply with a medication regimen, including adverse effects of the drug, cost of the treatment, clerical errors or misinterpretation of the dosing instructions. All of these factors are likely to occur if the drug is made widely available. The overall efficacy of the drug will be altered by the level of compliance in the general community. Hence, analysis of the effect of a drug should include those patients who were intended to take the drug but for one reason or another failed to do so.

Loss to follow-up

A clinical trial should strive to account for most, if not all, patients enrolled. Loss of contact with some patients is inevitable, particularly in trials with a long follow-up period. With careful planning and data collection, however, it is often possible to collect data on almost all patients enrolled in the trial. Omission of data from missing patients can alter the observed strength of association between an exposure and outcome. In trials where loss to follow-up is excessive (more than about 20%) a best case/worst case analysis should be performed. The best case assumes that all missing patients from the active treatment group have survived (or been cured) and all missing controls have died (or still have the

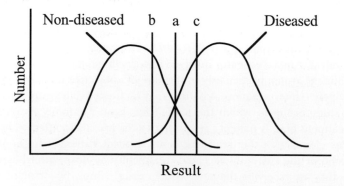

Figure 33-2. Distribution of continuous results of a test in diseased and non-diseased patients, with three possible threshold values for distinguishing positive from negative results.

disease). Conversely, the worst case assumes that all missing patients receiving the active treatment have died and all missing controls have survived. The true level of effect will lie somewhere between these two values.

Generalisability

Results of a clinical trial cannot always be applied to every patient or population. If a patient is different in some way from those involved in the trial, there may be a characteristic that alters the strength of effect in this patient. A classic example is the aborted CAST Trial[22] in which patients who had suffered myocardial infarction were given flecainide with the intention of suppressing ventricular ectopy and improving survival. It had been demonstrated previously that suppressing ventricular ectopic beats improved survival, and studies had shown that flecainide was effective in suppressing ventricular ectopics. The CAST Trial investigators found a death rate 3.5 times higher in the flecainide group than the control group. The previous studies with flecainide had been performed on patients with long QT syndromes and were not applicable to post-myocardial infarct (MI) patients with ischaemic myocardial disease.

Evaluating diagnostic tests

Diagnostic tests may lead to erroneous conclusions regarding the presence or absence of disease, particularly when nominal threshold values (or cut-points) are assigned to distinguish positive from negative results.

For a given disease there will be a range of results in which both diseased and non-diseased patients fall. This concept is illustrated in Fig. 33.2, which also shows three possible cut-points. The threshold marked 'a' will correctly distinguish between positive (diseased) and negative (non-diseased) patients, but some patients with disease will be incorrectly identified as not having disease; similarly, some disease-free patients will be incorrectly identified as having disease. If the threshold is set at 'b' nearly all of the patients with disease will be detected, but more of the non-diseased patients will be incorrectly labelled as having disease. Setting the threshold at 'c' will lead to very few non-diseased patients being identified as having the disease, and will result in failure to identify a greater number of patients with disease.

When deciding upon threshold values it is necessary to balance the need to detect all patients with a disease against the need to be sure that all patients who test negative are actually free of disease. The terms assigned to these conditions to describe the characteristics of the test are 'sensitivity' and 'specificity'.

Sensitivity describes the ability of a test to detect patients with the disease of interest. It is also called the 'True Positive Rate' and can be remembered as 'Positive in Disease'. Specificity describes the ability of a test to correctly exclude patients without disease. It is also called the 'True Negative Rate' and can be remembered as 'Negative in Health'.

Therefore, any test that gives a dichotomous result (positive/negative) has the potential to give one of four results. If the result is positive in a patient who has disease, this is a 'true positive'. If the test is positive and the patient does not have disease, this is a 'false positive'. Likewise, a 'true negative' is a negative result in a patient who is disease-free and a 'false negative' result is obtained when a patient tests negative but does have the disease. These tests are summarised in Table 33.1.

Sensitivity and specificity can be derived mathematically from Table 33.1. Sensitivity is the number of diseased patients who have a positive test (true positives) divided by the total number of patients with disease and is therefore represented by [a/(a+c)]. Speci-

Table 33.1. Possible outcomes for tests with dichotomous results

		Disease Present	Disease Absent	Total
Test	*Positive*	(a) True Positive	(b) False Positive	a + b
	Negative	(c) False Negative	(d) True Negative	c + d
	Total	a + c	b + d	

ficity is the number of true negatives divided by the total number of patients who are disease-free and is depicted as [d/(b+d)]. These values are normally expressed as percentages.

Discussion

The concepts of EBM provide the basis of critical appraisal of the literature to find the best source(s) of evidence addressing a clinical or research question. EBM encourages the reader to seek out high-quality studies and avoid those that may provide biased or misleading results.

These concepts can also be applied to the design stage of a clinical trial, to ensure that the best quality results are obtained. Knowledge of the techniques for producing high-quality results allows careful design and implementation of the study and it ensures that future researchers need not repeat poorly designed or poorly conducted trials, but can direct their funds and efforts towards improving further the advances already made.

References

1. Oxman AD, Sackett DL, Guyatt GH *et al.* for the Evidence-based Medicine Working Group. User's Guides to the Medical Literature: 1-How to get started. *JAMA* 1993; **270**(17):2093–5.
2. Guyatt GH, Sackett DL, Cook DJ *et al.* for the Evidence-based Medicine Working Group. User's Guides to the Medical Literature: II-How to use an article about therapy or prevention. A. Are the results of the study valid? *JAMA* 1993; **270**(21):2598–601.
3. Guyatt GH, Sackett DL, Cook DJ *et al.* for the Evidence-based Medicine Working Group. User's Guides to the Medical Literature: II-How to use an article about therapy or prevention. B. What were the results and will they help me in caring for my patients? *JAMA* 1994; **271**(1):59–63.
4. Jaeschke R, Guyatt GH, Sackett DL *et al.* for the Evidence-based Medicine Working Group. User's Guides to the Medical Literature: III-How to use an article about a diagnostic test. A. Are the results of the study valid? *JAMA* 1994; **271**(5):389–91.
5. Jaeschke R, Guyatt GH, Sackett DL *et al.* for the Evidence-based Medicine Working Group. User's Guides to the Medical Literature: III-How to use an article about a diagnostic test. B. What are the results and will they help me in caring for my patients? *JAMA* 1994; **271**(9):703–7.
6: Levine M, Walter S, Lee H *et al.* for the Evidence-based Medicine Working Group. User's Guides to the Medical Literature: IV-How to use an article about harm. *JAMA* 1994; **271**(20):1615–9.
7. Laupacis A, Wells G, Richardson S, Tugwell P for the Evidence-based Medicine Working Group. User's Guides to the Medical Literature: IV-How to use an article about prognosis.

JAMA 1994; **272**(3):234–7.

8. Oxman AD, Cook DJ, Guyatt GH *et al.* for the Evidence-based Medicine Working Group. User's Guides to the Medical Literature: VI-How to use an overview. *JAMA* 1994; **272**(17):1367–71.

9. Richardson WS, Detsky AS for the Evidence-based Medicine Working Group. User's Guides to the Medical Literature: VII-How to use a clinical decision analysis. A.Are the results of the study valid? *JAMA* 1995; **273**(16):1292–5.

10. Richardson WS, Detsky AS for the Evidence-based Medicine Working Group. User's Guides to the Medical Literature: VII-How to use a clinical decision analysis. B.What are the results and will they help me in caring for my patients? *JAMA* 1995; **273**(20):1610–3.

11. Hayward R, Wilson MC, Tunis SR *et al.* for the Evidence-based Medicine Working Group. User's Guides to the Medical Literature: VIII-How to use clinical practice guidelines. A. Are the recommendations valid? *JAMA* 1995; **274**(7):570–4.

12. Wilson MC, Hayward R, Tunis SR *et al* for the Evidence-based Medicine Working Group. User's Guides to the Medical Literature: VIII-How to use clinical practice guidelines. B. What are the recommendations and will they help you in caring for your patients? *JAMA* 1995; **274**(20):1630–2.

13. Guyatt GH, Sackett DL, Sinclair JC *et al.* for the Evidence-based Medicine Working Group. User's Guides to the Medical Literature: IX-A method for grading health care recommendations. *JAMA* 1995; **274**(22):1800–4.

14. Naylor CD, Guyatt GH for the Evidence-based Medicine Working Group. User's Guides to the Medical Literature: X-How to use an article reporting variations in the outcomes of health services. *JAMA* 1996; **275**:554–8.

15. Naylor CD, Guyatt GH for the Evidence-based Medicine Working Group. User's Guides to the Medical Literature: XI-How to use an article about a clinical utilization review. *JAMA* 1996; **275**(18):1435–9.

16. Guyatt GH, Juniper E, Heyland DK *et al.* User's Guides to the Medical Literature: XII-How to use an article about health-related quality of life. *JAMA* 1997; **277**:1232–7.

17. Drummond MF, Richardson WS, O'Brien BJ *et al.* User's Guides to the Medical Literature: XIII-How to use an article on economic analysis of clinical practice: A. Are the results of the study valid? *JAMA* 1997; **277**(19):1552–7.

18. O'Brien BJ, Heyland D, Richardson WS, Drummond MR. User's Guides to the Medical Literature: XIII-How to use an article on economic analysis of clinical practice: B. What are the results and will they help me in caring for my patients? *JAMA* 1997; **277**(22):1802–6.

19. Dans A, Dans LF, Guyatt GH, Richardson S, for the EBM Working Group. Users' Guides to the Medical Literature. XIV. How to decide on the applicability of clinical trial results to your patient. *JAMA* 1998; **279**(7):545–9.

20. Glasziou PP, Irwig LM. An evidence-based approach to individualising treatment. *BMJ* 1995; 311:1356–9.

21. Hennekens CH, Buring JE, Mayrent SL (eds). *Epidemiology in medicine.* Boston: Little Brown 1987, p259.

22. McQuay H, Carroll D, Moore A. Variation in the placebo effect in randomised controlled trials of analgesics: all is as blind as it seems. *Pain.* 1996; 64(2):331–5.

23. Bostrom H. Placebo – the forgotten drug. *Scand J Work, Envir & Health* 1997; **23**(Suppl 3):53–7.

24. Blair DT. The placebogenic phenomenon: art in psychiatric nursing. *J Psycosoc & Mental Health Services* 1996; **34**(8):11–5.

25. Kienle GS, Kiene H. The powerful placebo effect: fact or fiction? *J Clin Epidem* 1997; **50**(12):1311–8.

26. Kienle GS, Kiene H. Placebo effect and placebo concept: a critical methodological and conceptual analysis of reports on the magnitude of the placebo effect. *Alternative Therapies in Health and Medicine* 1996; **2**(6):39–54.

Appendix

Hemodynamic Calculations

The following is a list of formulae commonly used to calculate essential parameters during cardiac catheterisation. All computerised monitoring systems require manually entered data or electronically measured data to calculate automatically derived functions. (Modified courtesy of G.E./Marquette, as applied to the Maclab physiological monitoring system.

Manually Entered Data

WT	Weight	(Kg), (lbs)
HT	Height	(cm), (ins)
VO_2	Oxygen consumption	(L/min)
Hb	Haemoglobin	(g/dl)
ARTSAT	Arterial saturation	(%)
VENSAT	Venous saturation	(%)
PAO_2	Pa saturation	(%)
PVO_2	Pv saturation	(%)
CO	Cardiac output	(L/min)
VeSTPD	Minute vol @ ATPS	(L/min)
Pb	Barometric Pressure	(mmHg)
T	Room Temp	(°C)
FEO_2	O_2 expired air	(%)
FIO_2	O_2 inspired air	(%)
PO_2	Dissolved oxygen	(%)

Automatically Measured Data

ARTsdm	Arterial pressure	(mmHg)
PAsdm	Pulmonary artery pressure	(mmHg)
LAavm	Left atrium pressure	(mmHg)
CVP	Central venous press	(mmHg)
SPsdm	Special pressure	(mmHg)
LVsdme	Left ventricle pressure	(mmHg)
RVsdm	Right ventricle pressure	(mmHg)
RAavm	Right atrium pressure	(mmHg)
PCWavm	Wedge pressure	(mmHg)
VEN	Venous pressure	(mmHg)
FAsdm	Femoral artery pressure	(mmHg)
AOsmd	Aortic pressure	(mmHg)
HR	Heart rate	(BPM)
AVG	Aortic valve gradient	(mmHg)
MVG	Mitral valve gradient	(mmHg)
PVG	Pulmonary valve gradient	(mmHg)
TVG	Tricuspid valve gradient	(mmHg)

LVET	(SEP/b) left ventricular ejection time	(msec)
LVFT	(DFP/b) left ventricular filling time	(msec)
RVET	(SEP/b) right ventricular ejection time	(msec)
RVFT	(DFP/b) right ventricular filling time	(msec)
COtd	CO Thermal dilution	(L/min)

Automatically Derived Functions

BSA	Body surface area	$HT^{0.725} \times WT^{0.425} \times 0.007184$	(m²)
CI	Cardiac index	CO + BSA	
SVR	Systemic vascular resistance	((MAP − VP) x 79.92) + CO	(d/s/cm-5)
SVRI	SVR index	SVR x BSA	
PVR	Pulmonary vascular resistance	((PAm − WEDGE) x 79.92)+CO	(d/s/cm-5)
PVRI	PVR index	PVR x BSA	(d/s/cm-5)
TPR	Total pulmonary resistance	PAm + CO	(d/s/cm-5)
TPRI	TPR index	TPR + BSA	
LVSW	Left ventricular stroke work	CO + HR x 1000 x (Ao-WEDGE) x 0.0136 (gm)	
LVSWI	Left ventricular stroke work index	LVSW+BSA	
RVSW	Right ventricular stroke work	CO+HR x 1000 x (PAm − VP) x 0.0136 (gm)	
RVSWI	Right ventricular stroke work index	RVSW + BSA	
SEPa	Aortic Systolic ejection period	(LVET x HR) + 1000	(sec/min)
SEPp	Pulmonary Systolic ejection period	(RVET x HR) + 1000	(sec/min)
DFPm	Mitral Diastolic filling period	(LVET x HR) + 1000	(sec/min)
DFPt	Tricuspid Diastolic filling period	(RVET x HR) + 1000	(sec/min)
AVF	Aortic valve flow	CO + SEPa	(ml/sec)
MVF	Mitral valve flow	CO + DFPm	(ml/sec)
PVF	Pulmonary valve flow	CO + SEPp	(ml/sec)
TVF	Tricuspid valve flow	CO + DFPt	(ml/sec)
AVA	Aortic valve area	AVF + (44.5 x √AVG)	(cm²)
MVA	Mitral Valve Area	MVF + (38 x √MVG)	(cm²)
PVA	Pulmonary valve area	PVF + (44.5 x √PVG)	(cm²)
PVI	Pulmonary valve index	PVA + BSA	
TVI	Tricuspid valve index	TVA + BSA	

VO$_2$ VO$_2$ is calculated, estimated or manually entered. If the VO$_2$ field is blank, the MACLAB tries to calculate it using VeSTPD, Pb, T, FIO$_2$, FEO$_2$, as follows:

$$VO_2 = VeSTPD \times (273 + (273 + T)) \times ((Pb - ((1.18 \times T) - 6)) + 760) \times 10 \times (FIO_2 - FEO_2) \quad (ml/min)$$

The MACLAB tries to estimate VO$_2$ if any of the previous fields are blank but SEX, BSA, AGE and HR are available as follows:

MALE VO$_2$ = BSA x (138.1 − (log(AGE) x 11.49 + 0.378 x HR)   (ml/min)
FEMALE VO$_2$ = BSA x (138.1 − (log(AGE) x 17.04) + 0.378 x HR) (ml/min)

FCa   Arterial content is calculated as follows:
If FEO$_2$ and Pb are available
FCa=ARTSAT x Hb x 1.36 + (PO$_2$ x 0.003026)   (ml/dl)
otherwise FCa=ARTSAT x Hb x 1.36 + 0.3   (ml/dl)

| FCv | Mixed venous content | VENSAT x Hb x 1.36 + 0.2 | |
| FCpa | Pulmonary arterial content | PAO$_2$ x Hb x 1.36 + 0.2 | (ml/dl) |

FCpv   Pulmonary venous content is calculated as follows:
       If FE02 and PB are available
       $FCpv = PVO_2 \times Hb \times 1.36 + (PO_2 \times 0.003026)$ (ml/dl)
       otherwise $FCpv = PVO_2 \times Hb \times 1.36 + 0.3$ (ml/dl)
Qs   Systemic flow $(VO_2 + (FCa-FCv))+10$ (L/min)
Qp   Pulmonary flow $(VO_2+(FCpv-FCpa))+10$ (L/min)
QpQs   Shunt calculation is the ratio between Pulmonary flow and Systemic flow (%)
       If Pulmonary flow <Systemic flow then RIGHT TO LEFT SHUNT
       If Pulmonary flow >Systemic flow then LEFT TO RIGHT SHUNT
       If Pulmonary flow equals Systemic flow then NO SHUNT
COf   FICK cardiac output $(VO_2 + (FCa-FCv)) + 10$ (L/min)
FCl   FICK cardiac index   COf + BSA

Index

action of thrombin on, 121
as inglammatory marker, 108–9
assays, 15, 18–20
in coagulation, 93–9, 121
in fibrinolysis, 101
in platelet binding, 153
in thrombolysis, 148
with abciximab, 359
Fibrinolysis, 99
Fibroblast growth factor (FGF), 325
Fick, 12, 65–6, 80, 197–202, 299
Filament (cathode), 3, 5
Flecainide, 143
FloWire, 269
Fluvastatin, 108
Fractional flow reserve (FFR), 269
Fractional saturation, 25
Frank Starling, 55, 72, 75
Frusemide (furosemide), 139
Functional saturation, 25

Gamma radiation, 264–5
Gene transfer, 321, 325–8
Glycoproteins, 95
Gorlin formula, 64, 65–7, 78–9
GPIIb/IIIa (see abciximab)
Graft angiography, 190, 194
Grey level, 6
Guidelines for
abciximab use, 359
angiography, 184
clinical trials,, 379
IABP setup, 377
infection control, 47–9
INR and valve surgery, 318
safe fluoroscopy, 43–5
sheath removal, 342
waste disposal, 49
Guidewire use,
in atherectomy, 260
in brachial approach, 187, 194
in femoral approach, 193
in IABP insertion, 375
in IVUS, 267
in jugular cannulation, 299
in laser angioplasty, 262
in mammary grafts, 195
in peripheral interventions, 273
in radial approach, 188, 194
in Seldinger technique, 185–6

Haematoma, 186, 341, 342–9, 358
Haemoglobin
concentration, 27, 30–2, 198
structure, 29

Haemorrhage,
cerebral in PTCA, 89, 92, 359
complication of IABP, 376
subarachnoid, 37
with femoral puncture, 346
Haemostasis, 93
Haemoximetry (co-oximetry), 33
Heart sounds, 59
Hemi–block, 178
Heparin,
and ACT, 17–18
and angioplasty, 155
and cofactor II, 101–2, 105
and GISSI trial, 148
and GUSTO trial, 149
and thrombosis, 120–2
and warfarin, 96, 147
anticoagulation effect, 146
blood clotting tests, 15
monitoring, 122–4
neutralisation, 18
rebound, 18, 19
Response Test (HRT), 18
structure of, 120
unfractionated, 154
Hereditary effects, 40
Heterotopic transplantation, 301
Hexagonal system, 171
Hibernating myocardium, 227
High dose thrombin time (HiTT), 18
Hirudin, 121, 151, 155–6
HOCM, 73, 76–7, 90
Holter monitor, 292
Homocysteine, 108, 109
Hydrostatic pressure, 12, 24
Hyperobstructive cardiomyopathy, *see* HOCM
Hypertension, 107, 108, 310
Hypotension, 310

IABP,
contraindications for use, 364
complications, 97, 376
description, 363–7
for rescue angioplasty, 73,
history of, 363
in SHOCK trial, 34
indications for use, 363–4
physiology, 364–7
pressure waveforms, 369–74
Idioventricular tachycardia, 177
Image intensifier, 1–8, 12, 42–4, 189, 190
Indications for
cardiac catheterisation, 183–4, 353–7
IABP, 238
valve surgery, 315